Guidelines for Reporting Healt
A User's Manual

Guidelines for Reporting Health Research: A User's Manual

EDITED BY

David Moher

Ottawa Hospital Research Institute and University of Ottawa, Ottawa, Canada

Douglas G. Altman

Centre for Statistics in Medicine, University of Oxford and EQUATOR Network, Oxford, UK

Kenneth F. Schulz

FHI360, Durham, and UNC School of Medicine, Chapel Hill, North Carolina, USA

Iveta Simera

Centre for Statistics in Medicine, University of Oxford and EQUATOR Network Oxford, UK

Elizabeth Wager

Sideview, Princes Risborough, UK

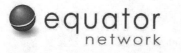

WILEY Blackwell   BMJ|Books

This edition first published 2014 © 2014 by John Wiley & Sons, Ltd.

Registered office: John Wiley & Sons, Ltd, The Atrium, Southern Gate, Chichester, West Sussex, PO19 8SQ, UK

Editorial offices: 9600 Garsington Road, Oxford, OX4 2DQ, UK
    The Atrium, Southern Gate, Chichester, West Sussex, PO19 8SQ, UK
    111 River Street, Hoboken, NJ 07030-5774, USA

For details of our global editorial offices, for customer services and for information about how to apply for permission to reuse the copyright material in this book please see our website at www.wiley.com/wiley-blackwell

Library of Congress Cataloging-in-Publication Data

Guidelines for reporting health research : a users manual / editors, David Moher, Douglas G. Altman, Kenneth F. Schulz, Iveta Simera, Elizabeth Wager.
  p. ; cm.
Includes bibliographical references and index.
ISBN 978-0-470-67044-6 (pbk.)
I. Moher, David, 1957- editor of compilation. II. Altman, Douglas G., editor of compilation.
III. Schulz, Kenneth F., editor of compilation. IV. Simera, Iveta, editor of compilation.
V. Wager, Elizabeth, editor of compilation.
[DNLM: 1. Biomedical Research–methods.
2. Research Report–standards. 3. Peer Review, Research–standards. W 20.5]
R850
610.72′4–dc23

                  2014000621

A catalogue record for this book is available from the British Library.

Wiley also publishes its books in a variety of electronic formats. Some content that appears in print may not be available in electronic books.

Cover design by Rob Sawkins a Opta Design Ltd.

Typeset in 9.5/13pt MeridienLTStd by Laserwords Private Limited, Chennai, India
Printed and bound in Malaysia by Vivar Printing Sdn Bhd

1 2014

Contents

Part III

Part IV

List of Contributors

Douglas G. Altman
Centre for Statistics in Medicine, University of Oxford, Oxford, UK

Andrew Booth
Cochrane Collaboration Qualitative Research Methods Group

Andrew H. Briggs
Health Economics and Health Technology Assessment, Institute of Health & Wellbeing, University of Glasgow, Glasgow, UK

Patrick M.M. Bossuyt
Department of Clinical Epidemiology & Biostatistics, Academic Medical Center, University of Amsterdam, Amsterdam, the Netherlands

Isabelle Boutron
Centre d'Epidémiologie Clinique, Assistance Publique-Hôpitaux de Paris, Paris, France

Centre Cochrane Français, INSERM U738, Université Paris Descartes, Paris, France

Marion K. Campbell
Health Services Research Unit, University of Aberdeen, Aberdeen, UK

Margaret M. Cavenagh
Cancer Diagnosis Program, Division of Cancer Treatment and Diagnosis, National Cancer Institute, Bethesda, MD, USA

Myriam Cevallos
CTU Bern and Insititute of Social and Preventative Medicine, University of Bern, Bern, Switzerland

An-Wen Chan
Women's College Research Institute, Toronto, ON, Canada

ICES@UofT, Toronto, ON, Canada

Department of Medicine, Women's College Hospital, University of Toronto, Toronto, ON, Canada

Mike Clarke
All-Ireland Hub for Trials Methodology Research, Centre for Public Health, Queens University Belfast, Belfast, Northern Ireland

Frank Davidoff
Annals of Internal Medicine, Philadelphia, PA, USA

Don C. Des Jarlais
Baron Edmond de Rothschild Chemical Dependency Institute, Beth Israel Medical Center, New York, NY, USA

Michael F. Drummond
University of York, York, UK

Matthias Egger
Institute of Social and Preventive Medicine (ISPM), University of Bern, Bern, Switzerland

Diana R. Elbourne
London School of Hygiene and Tropical Medicine, London, UK

Jeremy Grimshaw
Ottawa Hospital Research Institute and University of Ottawa, Ottawa, ON, Canada

Karin Hannes
Cochrane Collaboration Qualitative Research Methods Group

Angela Harden
Cochrane Collaboration Qualitative Research Methods Group

Janet Harris
Cochrane Collaboration Qualitative Research Methods Group

Allison Hirst
Nuffield Department of Surgical Sciences, University of Oxford, Oxford, UK

John Hoey
Queen's University, Kingston, ON, Canada

Sally Hopewell
Centre for Statistics in Medicine, University of Oxford, Oxford, UK

INSERM, U738, Paris, France

AP-HP (Assistance Publique des Hôpitaux de Paris), Hôpital Hôtel Dieu, Centre d'Epidémiologie Clinique, Paris, France

Univ. Paris Descartes, Sorbonne Paris Cité, Paris, France

Timothy T. Houle
Department of Anesthesiology, Wake Forest University School of Medicine, Winston-Salem, NC, USA

Samuel J. Huber
University of Rochester School of Medicine and Dentistry, Rochester, NY, USA

John P.A. Ioannidis
Stanford Prevention Research Center, Department of Medicine and Division of Epidemiology, Department of Health Research and Policy, Stanford University School of Medicine, and Department of Statistics, Stanford University School of Humanities and Sciences, Stanford, CA, USA

Thomas A. Lang
Tom Lang Communications and Training International, Kirkland, WA, USA

Julian Little
Department of Epidemiology and Community Medicine, Canada Research Chair in Human Genome Epidemiology, University of Ottawa, Ottawa, ON, Canada

Elizabeth W. Loder
British Medical Journal, London, UK

Division of Headache and Pain, Department of Neurology, Brigham and Women's Hospital, Boston, MA, USA

Harvard Medical School, Boston, MA, USA

Hugh MacPherson
Department of Health Studies, University of York, York, UK

Lisa M. McShane
Biometric Research Branch, National Cancer Institute, Bethesda, MD, USA

Donald Miller
Department of Anesthesia, The Ottawa Hospital, Ottawa Hospital Research Institute and University of Ottawa, Ottawa, ON, Canada

David Moher
Clinical Epidemiology Program, Ottawa Hospital Research Institute, Ottawa, ON, Canada

Jane Noyes
Centre for Health-Related Research, School for Healthcare Sciences, College of Health & Behavioural Sciences, Bangor University, Bangor, UK

Mary Ocampo
Ottawa Hospital Research Institute, Ottawa, ON, Canada

Greg Ogrinc
Dartmouth Medical School, Hanover, NH, USA

Donald B. Penzien
Department of Psychiatry, Wake Forest University School of Medicine, Winston-Salem, NC, USA

Gilda Piaggio
Statistika Consultoria Ltd, São Paulo, Brazil

Jason L. Roberts
Headache Editorial Office, Plymouth, MA, USA

Philippe Ravaud
Centre d'Epidémiologie Clinique, Assistance Publique-Hôpitaux de Paris, Paris, France

Centre Cochrane Français, INSERM U738, Université Paris Descartes, Paris, France

John F. Rothrock
Department of Neurology, University of Alabama at Birmingham, Birmingham, AL, USA

Margaret Sampson
Children's Hospital of Eastern Ontario, Ottawa, ON, Canada

Willi Sauerbrei
Department of Medical Biometry and Medical Informatics, University Medical Centre, Freiburg, Germany

David L. Schriger
UCLA Emergency Medicine Center, Los Angeles, CA, USA

Kenneth F. Schulz
FHI 360, Durham, and UNC School of Medicine, Chapel Hill, NC, USA

Dugald Seely
Ottawa Integrative Cancer Centre, Ottawa, ON, Canada

Iveta Simera
Centre for Statistics in Medicine, University of Oxford, Oxford, UK

George C. M. Siontis
Clinical Trials and Evidence-Based Medicine Unit, Department of Hygiene and Epidemiology, University of Ioannina School of Medicine, Ioannina, Greece

Cassandra Talerico
Neurological Institute Research and Development Office, Cleveland Clinic, Cleveland, OH, USA

Sheila E. Taube
ST Consulting, Bethesda, MD, USA

Jennifer Tetzlaff
Ottawa Methods Centre, Clinical Epidemiology Program, Ottawa Hospital Research Institute, Ottawa, ON, Canada

Allison Tong
Sydney School of Public Health, University of Sydney, Sydney, Australia

Dana P. Turner
Department of Anesthesiology, Wake Forest University School of Medicine, Winston-Salem, NC, USA

Elizabeth Wager
Sideview, Princes Risborough, UK

Laura Weeks
Ottawa Integrative Cancer Centre, Ottawa, ON, Canada

Merrick Zwarenstein
Schulich School of Medicine and Dentistry, Western University, London, ON, Canada

Foreword
Guides to guidelines

Drummond Rennie, MD

University of California, San Francisco, USA

Introduction

Good patient care must be based on treatments that have been shown by good research to be effective. An intrinsic part of good research is a published paper that closely reflects the work done and the conclusions drawn. This book is about preventing, even curing, a widespread endemic disease: biased and inadequate reporting. This bias and poor reporting threatens to overwhelm the credibility of research and to ensure that our treatments are based on fiction, not fact.

Over the past two decades, there has been a spate of published guidelines on reporting, ostensibly to help authors improve the quality of their manuscripts. Following the guidelines, manuscripts will include all the information necessary for an informed reader to be fully persuaded by the paper. At the same time, the articles will be well organized, easy to read, well argued, and self-critical. From the design phase of the research, when they may serve as an intervention to remind investigators, editors, and reviewers who find it easy to get the facts, and to note what facts are missing, all the way through to the reader of the published article who finds it easy to access the facts, all of them in context.

To which, given the ignorance, ineptitude, inattention, and bias of so many investigators, reviewers, and journal editors, I would add a decisive "Maybe!"

How did it start? How did we get here?

In 1966, 47 years ago, Dr Stanley Schor, a biostatistician in the Department of Biostatistics at the American Medical Association, in Chicago, and Irving Karten, then a medical student, published in *JAMA* the results of a careful examination of a random sample of published reports taken from the

10 most prominent medical journals. Schor and Karten focused their attention on half of the reports that they considered to be "analytical studies," 149 in number, as opposed to reports of cases. They identified 12 types of statistical errors, and they found that the conclusions were invalid in 73%. "None of the ten journals had more than 40% of its analytical studies considered acceptable; two of the ten had no acceptable reports." Schor and Karten speculated on the implications for medical practice, given that these defects occurred in the most widely read and respected journals, and they ended presciently: "since, with the introduction of computers, much work is being done to make the results of studies appearing in medical journals more accessible to physicians, a considerable amount of misinformation could be disseminated rapidly." Boy, did they get that one right!

Better yet, this extraordinary paper also included the results of an experiment: 514 manuscripts submitted to one journal were reviewed by a statistician. Only 26% were "acceptable" statistically. However, the intervention of a statistical review raised the "acceptable" rate to 74%. Schor and Karten's recommendation was that a statistician be made part of the investigator's team and of the editors' team as well [1]. Their findings were confirmed by many others, for example, Gardner and Bond [2].

I got my first taste of editing in 1977 at the *New England Journal of Medicine*, and first there and then at *JAMA* the *Journal of the American Medical Association*, my daily job has been to try to select the best reports of the most innovative, important, and relevant research submitted to a large-circulation general medical journal. Although the best papers were exciting and solid, they seemed like islands floating in a swamp of paper rubbish. So from the start, the Schor/Karten paper was a beacon. Not only did the authors identify a major problem in the literature, and did so using scientific methods, but they tested a solution and then made recommendations based on good evidence.

This became a major motivation for establishing the Peer Review Congresses. Exasperatedly, in 1986, I wrote:

> One trouble is that despite this system (of peer review), anyone who reads journals widely and critically is forced to realize that there are scarcely any bars to eventual publication [3].

Was the broad literature so bad despite peer review or because of it? What sort of product, clinical research reports, was the public funding and we journals disseminating? Only research could find out, and so from the start the Congresses were limited strictly to reports of research.

At the same time, Iain Chalmers and his group in Oxford were struggling to make sense of the entire literature on interventions in health care, using and refining the science of meta-analysis to apply it to clinical reports.

This meant that, with Chalmers' inspired creation of the Cochrane Collaboration, a great many bright individuals such as Altman, Moher, Dickersin, Chalmers, Schulz, Gøtzsche, and others were bringing intense skepticism and systematic scrutiny to assess the completeness and quality of reporting of clinical research and to identify those essential items, the inadequate reporting of which was associated with bias. The actual extent of biases, say, because of financial conflicts or failure to publish, could be measured, and from that came changes in the practices of journals, research institutions, and individual researchers. Eventually, there even came changes in the law (e.g., requirements to register clinical trials and then to post their results). Much of this research was presented at the Congresses [4–6]. The evidence was overwhelming that poor reporting biased conclusions – usually about recommended therapies [7]. The principles of randomized controlled trials, the bedrock of evidence about therapies, had been established 40 years before and none of it was rocket science. But time and again investigators had been shown to be making numerous simple but crucial mistakes in the reporting of such trials.

What to do about it?

In the early 1990s, two groups came up with recommendations for reporting randomized trials [8, 9]. These were published but produced no discernible effect. In discussions with David Moher, he suggested to me that *JAMA* should publish a clinical trial according to the SORT recommendation, which we did [10], calling for comments – which we got in large numbers. It was obvious that one of the reasons that the SORT recommendations never caught on was that while they were the product of a great deal of effort by distinguished experts, no one had actually tried them out in practice. When this was done, the resultant paper was unreadable, as the guidelines allowed no editorial flexibility and broke up the logic and flow of the article.

David and I realized that editors were crucial in this process. Put bluntly, if editors demanded it at a time when the authors were likely to be in a compliant frame of mind – when acceptance of their manuscript depended on their following orders, then editorial policy would become the standard for the profession.

Owing to the genius, persistence, and diplomacy of David Moher, the two groups got their representatives together, and from this CONSORT was born in 1996 [10–13]. Criticism was drowned in a flood of approval. This was because the evidence for inclusion of items on the checklist was presented, and the community was encouraged to comment. The backing of journal editors forced investigators to accept the standards, and the cooperation of editors was made easier when they were reassured, on Doug Altman's suggestion, that different journals were allowed flexibility in where they asked authors to include particular items. The guidelines were provisional, they were to be studied, and that there was a process for revision as new evidence accumulated.

The acceptance of CONSORT was soon followed by the creation and publication of reporting guidelines in many other clinical areas. The founding of the EQUATOR (Enhancing the QUAlity and Transparency Of health Research) [14] Network in 2008 was not only a recognition of the success of such guidelines but also the need to get authors to write articles fit for purpose and provide much needed resources for all those involved with medical journals. As such, it represents a huge step in improving the transparency and quality of reporting research.

Are we there yet?

Forty-seven years later, Lang and Altman, referring to the Schor/Karten article that I mentioned at the beginning, write about the changes that seem to have occurred.

> Articles with even major errors continue to pass editorial and peer review and to be published in leading journals. The truth is that the problem of poor statistical reporting is long-standing, widespread, potentially serious, concerns mostly basic statistics, and yet is largely unsuspected by most readers of the biomedical literature [15].

Lang and Altman refer to the statistical design and analysis of studies, but a study where these elements are faulty cannot be trusted. The report IS the research, and my bet is that other parts of a considerable proportion of clinical reports are likely to be just as faulty. That was my complaint in 1986, and it is depressing that it is still our beef after all these efforts. I suspect there is more bad research reported simply because every year there are more research reports, but whether things are improving or getting worse is unclear. What it does mean is that we have work to do. This book is an excellent place to start the prevention and cure of a vastly prevalent malady.

References

1 Schor, S. & Karten, I. (1966) Statistical evaluation of medical journal manuscripts. *JAMA*, **195**, 1123–1128.
2 Gardner, M.J. & Bond, J. (1990) An exploratory study of statistical assessment of papers published in the British Medical Journal. *BMJ*, **263**, 1355–1357.
3 Rennie, D. (1986) Guarding the guardians: a conference on editorial peer review. *JAMA*, **256**, 2391–2392.

4 Dickersin, K. (1990) The existence of publication bias and risk factors for its occurrence. *JAMA*, **263**, 1385–1389.

5 Chalmers, T.C., Frank, C.S. & Reitman, D. (1990) Minimizing the three stages of publication bias. *JAMA*, **263**, 1392–1395.

6 Chalmers, I., Adams, M., Dickersin, K. *et al.* (1990) A cohort study of summary reports of controlled trials. *JAMA*, **263**, 1401–1405.

7 Schulz, K.F., Chalmers, I., Hayes, R.J. & Altman, D.G. (1995) Empirical evidence of bias. Dimensions of methodological quality associated with estimates of treatment effects in controlled trials. *JAMA*, **273**, 408–412.

8 The Standards of Reporting Trials Group. (1994) A proposal for structured reporting of randomized controlled trials. *JAMA*, **272**, 1926–1931.

9 Working Group on Recommendations for Reporting of Clinical Trials in the Biomedical Literature (1994) Call for comments on a proposal to improve reporting of clinical trials in the biomedical literature. *Annals of Internal Medicine* **121**, 894–895.

10 Rennie, D. (1995) Reporting randomised controlled trials. An experiment and a call for responses from readers. *JAMA*, **273**, 1054–1055.

11 Rennie, D. (1996) How to report randomized controlled trials. The CONSORT Statement. *JAMA*, **276**, 649.

12 Begg, C., Cho, M., Eastwood, S. *et al.* (1996) Improving the quality of reporting of randomized controlled trials. The CONSORT Statement. *JAMA*, **276**, 637–639.

13 (1996) Checklist of information for inclusion in reports of clinical trials. The Asilomar Working Group on Recommendations for reporting of Clinical Trials in the Biomedical Literature. *Ann Intern Med.*, **124**, 741–743.

14 http://www.equator-network.org/resource-centre/library-of-health-research-reporting/reporting-guidelines/

15 Lang, T. & Altman, D. (2013) Basic statistical reporting for articles published in clinical medical journals: the SAMPL guidelines. In: Smart, P., Maisonneuve, H. & Polderman, A. (eds), *Science Editors' Handbook*. European Association of Science Editors, Redruth, Cornwall, UK.

Preface

Medical research is intended to lead to improvements in the knowledge underpinning the prevention and treatment of illnesses. The value of research publications is, however, nullified if the published reports of that research are inadequate. Recent decades have seen the accumulation of a vast amount of evidence that reports of research are often seriously deficient, across all specialties and all types of research. The good news is that many of these problems are correctable. Reporting guidelines offer one solution to the problem by helping to increase the completeness of reports of medical research. At their core the vast majority of reporting guidelines consist of a checklist which can be thought of as reminder list for authors as to what information should be included when reporting their research. When endorsed and implemented properly by journals, reporting guidelines can become powerful tools.

Since the original CONSORT Statement, published in 1996, the development of reporting guidelines has been quite prolific. By early 2014 there were more than 200 reporting guidelines listed in the EQUATOR Network's library with several more in development. This book brings together many of the most commonly used reporting guidelines along with chapters on the development of the field itself. We encourage authors and peer reviewers to use reporting guidelines, and editors to endorse and implement them. Together this will help reduce waste and increase value. Using reporting guidelines will help to produce research papers that are able to pass future scrutiny and contribute usefully to systematic reviews, clinical practice guidelines, policy decision making and generally advance our scientific knowledge to improve patients' care and life of every one of us.

The reporting guidelines field is evolving quickly, which makes it a challenge to keep an 'old' technology – a hard copy book – up-to-date. In this regard readers should consult the EQUATOR web site (www.equator-network.org) for the most recent reporting guideline developments.

David Moher
Douglas G. Altman
Kenneth F. Schulz
Iveta Simera
Elizabeth Wager
10th March 2014

PART I
General Issues

CHAPTER 1

Importance of Transparent Reporting of Health Research

Douglas G. Altman[1] *and David Moher*[2]

[1] *Centre for Statistics in Medicine, University of Oxford, Oxford, UK*
[2] *Clinical Epidemiology Program, Ottawa Hospital Research Institute, Ottawa, ON, Canada*

"Reporting research is as important a part of a study as its design or analysis." [1]

"Poorly conducted trials are a waste of time, effort, and money. The most dangerous risk associated with poor-quality reporting is an overestimate of the advantages of a given treatment … Whatever the outcome of a study, it is really hard for the average reader to interpret and verify the reliability of a poorly reported RCT. In turn, this problem could result in changes in clinical practice that are based on false evidence and that may harm patients. The only way to avoid this risk and to be sure that the final message of a RCT can be correctly interpreted is to fulfill the items listed in the CONSORT statement." [2]

Introduction

Research related to the health of humans should have the potential to advance scientific understanding or improve the treatment or prevention of disease. The expectation is that an account of the research will be published, communicating the results of the research to other interested parties. Publication is generally in the form of articles in scientific journals, which should describe what was done and what was found. Reports of clinical research are important to many groups, especially other researchers, clinicians, systematic reviewers, and patients.

What do readers need to know? While there are multiple aspects to that question, and the specifics vary according to the nature of both the research and the reader, certain broad principles should be unarguable. Obviously, research reports should be truthful and should not intentionally mislead.

Guidelines for Reporting Health Research: A User's Manual, First Edition. Edited by David Moher, Douglas G. Altman, Kenneth F. Schulz, Iveta Simera and Elizabeth Wager.
© 2014 John Wiley & Sons, Ltd. Published 2014 by John Wiley & Sons, Ltd.

As noted by the International Committee of Medical Journal Editors, "In return for the altruism and trust that make clinical research possible, the research enterprise has an obligation to conduct research ethically and to report it honestly" [3]. In addition, research reports must be useful to readers – articles should include all the information about methods and results that is essential to judge the validity and relevance of a study and, if desired, use its findings [4]. Journal articles that fail to provide a clear account of methods are not fit for their intended purpose [4].

A vast literature over several decades has documented persistent failings of the health research literature to adhere to those principles. Systematic reviews are a prime source of evidence of these failings (Box 1.1). In addition, hundreds of reviews of published articles, especially those relating to randomized controlled trials (RCTs), have consistently shown that key information is missing from trial reports [5, 6]. Similar evidence is accumulating for other types of research [7–11]. Without a clear understanding of how a study was done, readers are unable to judge whether the findings are reliable. Inadequate reporting means that readers have to either reject an article or take on trust that the study was done well in order to accept the findings.

Box 1.1: Examples of poor reporting highlighted in systematic reviews

"Risk of bias assessment was hampered by poor reporting of trial methods [64]."

"Poor reporting of interventions impeded replication [65]."

"15 trials met the inclusion criteria for this review but only 4 could be included as data were impossible to use in the other 11 [66]."

"Poor reporting of duration of follow-up was a problem, making it hard to calculate numbers needed to treat to benefit … one of the largest trials of the effects of cardiac rehabilitation, which found no beneficial effect, is yet to be published in a peer-reviewed journal over a decade after its completion [67]."

"Four studies compared two different methods of applying simultaneous compression and cryotherapy, but few conclusions could be reached. Poor reporting of data meant that individual effect size could not be calculated for any of these studies. Furthermore, two studies did not provide adequate information on the mode of cryotherapy, and all failed to specify the duration and frequency of the ice application [68]."

"With more complete reporting, the whole process of evaluating the quality of research should be easier. In my work as a systematic reviewer, it is such a joy to come across a clearly reported trial when abstracting data [69]."

This situation is unacceptable. It is also surprising, given the strong emphasis on the importance of peer review of research articles. Peer review is used by journals as a filter to help them decide, often after revision, which articles are good enough and important enough to be published. Peer review is widely believed to be essential and, in principle, it is valuable. However, as currently practised peer review clearly fails to prevent inadequate reporting of research, and it fails on a major scale. This is clear from the fact that the thousands of studies included in the literature reviews already mentioned had all passed peer review. And articles published in the most prestigious (and highest impact) journals are not immune from errors as many of those literature reviews focussed entirely on those journals [12–14]. Peer review (and other quality checks such as technical editing) clearly could be much more effective in preventing poor quality reporting of research [15].

The abundant evidence from reviews of publications shows that ensuring that reports are useful to others does not currently feature highly in the actions, and likely the thinking, of many of those who write research articles. Authors should know by now that it is not reasonable to expect readers to take on trust that their study was beyond reproach. In any case, the issue is not just to detect poor methods but, more fundamentally, simply to learn exactly what was done. It is staggering that reviews of published journal articles persistently show that a substantial proportion of them lack key information. How can it be that none of the authors, peer reviewers, or editors noticed that these articles were substandard and, indeed, often unfit for purpose?

In this chapter, we explore the notion of transparent reporting and consider how to achieve it.

What do we mean by inadequate reporting of research?

Reporting problems affect journal articles in two main ways. First, the study methods are frequently not described in adequate detail. Second, the study findings are presented ambiguously, incompletely, or selectively. The cumulative effect of these problems is to render many reports of research unusable or even harmful; at the very least, such papers certainly represent a waste of resources [16].

Systematic assessments of published articles highlight frequent, serious shortcomings. These include but are not limited to

- omissions of crucial aspects of study methods, such as inclusion and exclusion criteria, precise details of interventions [17], measurement of outcomes [18, 19], statistical methods [20, 21],
- statistical errors [22, 23],
- selective reporting of results for only some of the assessed outcomes [24–26],
- selective reporting of statistical analyses (e.g. subgroup analyses) [27],
- inadequate reporting of harms [28],
- confusing or misleading presentation of data and graphs [29],

- incomplete numerical presentation of data precluding inclusion in a later meta-analysis [30]
- selective presentation of results in abstracts or inconsistency with the main text [31, 32]
- selective or inappropriate citation of other studies [33, 34]
- misinterpretation of study findings in the main article and abstract ("spin") [35, 36].

A further concern is the clear evidence of frequent inconsistencies between details reported in a publication and those given in the study protocol or on a register [25, 37, 38]. Clear evidence of such discrepancies exists only for randomized trials, but the same concern applies to all research [39]. When researchers change details in the version written for a journal, we should suspect manipulation to enhance "publishability" [40].

All these deficiencies of the published research evidence are compounded by the fact that for many studies no results are ever published [41], a phenomenon often called publication bias although it results from selective *non*-publication, our preferred term. Failure to publish the results of completed research is surprisingly common [24, 42]. Furthermore, there is clear evidence that when results are published, studies with statistically significant results are published much more rapidly than those without [41].

Consequences of nonpublication and inadequate reporting

Nonpublication of the findings of some research studies, either through suppression of complete studies or selective reporting within publications, always diminishes the evidence base. Whether this diminution is due to carelessness, ignorance, or deliberately incomplete or ambiguous reporting, it creates avoidable imprecision and may mislead. The main concern is that the choices about whether and what to publish are driven by the results, specifically favoring the publication of statistically significant or otherwise favoured findings at the expense of so-called "negative" results [43]. Therefore, in the worst case, bad publication practices lead to both a biased and overly imprecise answer. This behavior has a harmful impact on patient care [44, 45].

Inadequate reporting of methodology can also seriously impede assessment of the reliability of published articles. For example, systematic reviewers and other readers should avoid making assumptions about the conduct of trials based on simple phrases about the trial methodology, such as "intention to treat" or "double blind," rather than a full description of the methods actually used [46] as there is evidence that such phrases may be misleading. Indeed, even experts are confused by so-called "standard terminology," and authors can facilitate the understanding of research reports by avoiding the use of jargon and being more explicit [47]. Knowing how a study was conducted really matters – there is clear evidence that poor conduct of research is associated with biased findings [48, 49]. Thus, poor reporting may have serious consequences for clinical practice, future research, policy making, and ultimately for patients, if readers cannot judge whether to use a treatment or data cannot be included in a systematic review.

Poor reporting practices seriously distort the available body of research evidence and compromise its usefulness and reliability [16]. Such practices are unacceptable whether deliberate or resulting from lack of knowledge of what to report. Failure to publish may be seen as a form of scientific misconduct [50, 51]. It is also a moral hazard. A similar view may apply to inadequate reporting that renders a study's findings unusable; the term "poor reporting" is thus rather kind. Overall, therefore, not only is there considerable waste of research that has been funded and performed [16], with both financial and scientific consequences, bad reporting of research breaches moral and ethical standards [52–54].

Principles of reporting research

From the preceding discussion on common deficiencies of research publications, several principles of good research reporting become evident. Box 1.2 shows one set of key principles of responsible research reporting. An

---

Box 1.2: Key principles of responsible research reporting

The research being reported should have been conducted in an ethical and responsible manner and should comply with all relevant legislation.

Researchers should present their results clearly, honestly, and without fabrication, falsification, or inappropriate data manipulation.

Researchers should strive to describe their methods clearly and unambiguously so that their findings can be confirmed by others.

Researchers should follow applicable reporting guidelines. Publications should provide sufficient detail to permit experiments to be repeated by other researchers.*

The decision to publish should not be based on whether the results were "positive" or "negative."*

Researchers should adhere to publication requirements that submitted work is original, is not plagiarized, and has not been published elsewhere.

Authors should take collective responsibility for submitted and published work.

The authorship of research publications should accurately reflect individuals' contributions to the work and its reporting.

Funding sources and relevant conflicts of interest should be disclosed.

*Reproduced from the International standards for authors of scholarly publications [70] augmented by two items marked.

important additional point is that the numerical results should be presented in a form suitable for inclusion in meta-analyses.

The over-arching principle behind these specific ideas is that research reports should maximize the value derived from the cost and effort of conducting a trial. Currently, however, there is a massive amount of waste because of nonpublication and inadequate reporting [16, 55].

What can be done to improve the quality of reporting of research?

The widespread deficiencies of published articles indicate a major system failure. In particular, the fixation on positive findings is a serious blight on the health research literature. The importance of good reporting is seemingly not adequately appreciated by key stakeholders of the research community, including researchers, peer reviewers, editors, and funders of research. It is hard to discern whether the cause is a lack of awareness of the importance of good reporting, a lack of awareness of what information should be included in research reports, an overriding concern of authors to achieve publication at the expense of the (whole) truth [40], an overriding preference of peer reviewers or editors for novel or exciting results, or other reasons. Almost certainly it is a combination of many such factors. Few editors and peer reviewers have received relevant formal training. Similarly, few researchers are trained in a broad range of issues related to scientific writing and publishing, such as publication ethics (http://publicationethics.org/). Indeed, without training, and perhaps quality assurance in the form of certification, it is hard to imagine how the system can improve.

The medical literature is substandard; how can we fix it? [56] Changing behavior or attitude is always a major challenge, rarely amenable to simple solutions. Some aspects offer more hope, both to facilitate good reporting and, preferably, ensure it. Greater quality and value of health research publications could arise from actions by many different stakeholders. Improvements require, as a minimum, wide recognition of the importance of transparent and complete reporting (Box 1.2) and awareness of appropriate guidance to help ensure good reports of research. Numerous reporting guidelines now exist, relating to both broad research types, such as randomized trials or epidemiological studies, and very specific methodological or clinical contexts. The EQUATOR Network website (www.equator-network.org) listed over 200 such guidelines as of February 2014 (see Chapter 9).

Reporting guidelines provide structured advice on the minimum information to be included in an article reporting a particular type of health research. They focus on the scientific content of an article and thus complement journals' instructions to authors, which mostly deal with formatting submitted manuscripts [57]. Some are generic for defined study designs (e.g., RCTs) and should always be observed when reporting this type of study. Most published guidelines are more specific, however, providing guidance relevant to a particular medical specialty or a particular aspect of research (e.g., reporting adverse events or economic evaluations). The content of each of these guidelines was carefully considered by multidisciplinary groups of relevant experts, and there is a strong rationale for each requested information item.

Following internationally accepted generic reporting guidelines helps to ensure that published articles contain all the information that readers need to assess a study's relevance, methodology, validity of its findings and its generalizability. Many medical journals encourage adherence to certain reporting guidelines (see Chapter 4). Later chapters give details of the most widely used reporting guidelines.

Journals have a key role in helping to improve the literature by requiring the full and transparent reporting of research [15]. Much progress has been made in recent years regarding guidelines about what to report in a journal article. Journals have the authority to require authors to comply with these. The power of journals has been illustrated well by the considerable success of the policy of making trial registration a requirement for publication [58], even if adherence is not ideal [59]. It is clear, however, that for journals simply to mention reporting guidelines in their "Instructions to Authors" is insufficient to ensure good reporting [57]. More active enforcement can work, as has been seen for abstracts [60], and some journals have moved in that direction [61]. Journals can also enable and encourage the publication of research protocols [62].

Other groups should also work to ensure that research is reported well. Simera *et al.* presented recommended actions for various groups to improve reporting of research – journals, editorial organizations, research funding organizations, academic and other research institutions, reporting guidelines developers, and (not least) authors of research articles [55]. Young researchers should find reporting guidelines useful when planning their research [63]. Universities and other centers of research activity should play a more active role in promoting complete and transparent reporting of research, particularly the research emanating from their centers. This can take many forms, including teaching courses about issues relating to scientific writing and publishing. There is also a need to consider more seriously how technology can be used to help improve the quality of reporting. Web-enabled reporting guidelines are one possibility as are machine-readable language software to help populate checklists automatically.

References

1 Jordan, K.P. & Lewis, M. (2009) Improving the quality of reporting of research studies. *Musculoskeletal Care*, **7**, 137–142.

2 Zonta, S. & De Martino, M. (2008) Standard requirements for randomized controlled trials in surgery. *Surgery*, **144**, 838–839.

3 DeAngelis, C.D., Drazen, J.M., Frizelle, F.A. *et al.* (2004) Clinical trial registration: a statement from the International Committee of Medical Journal Editors. *JAMA*, **292**, 1363–1364.

4 Simera, I. & Altman, D.G. (2009) Editorial: writing a research article that is "fit for purpose": EQUATOR Network and reporting guidelines. *ACP Journal Club*, **151**, JC2-2–JC2-3.

5 Dechartres, A., Charles, P., Hopewell, S., *et al.* (2011) Reviews assessing the quality or the reporting of randomized controlled trials are increasing over time but raised questions about how quality is assessed. *Journal of Clinical Epidemiology*, **64**, 136–144.

6 Moher, D., Hopewell, S., Schulz, K.F. *et al.* (2010) CONSORT 2010 Explanation and Elaboration: updated guidelines for reporting parallel group randomised trials. *BMJ*, **340**, c869.

7 Mallett, S., Deeks, J.J., Halligan, S., *et al.* (2006) Systematic reviews of diagnostic tests in cancer: review of methods and reporting. *BMJ*, **333**, 413.

8 Mallett, S., Timmer, A., Sauerbrei, W. & Altman, D.G. (2010) Reporting of prognostic studies of tumour markers: a review of published articles in relation to REMARK guidelines. *British Journal of Cancer*, **102**, 173–180.

9 Kilkenny, C., Parsons, N., Kadyszewski, E. *et al.* (2009) Survey of the quality of experimental design, statistical analysis and reporting of research using animals. *PLoS One*, **4**, e7824.

10 Papathanasiou, A.A. & Zintzaras, E. (2010) Assessing the quality of reporting of observational studies in cancer. *Annals of Epidemiology*, **20**, 67–73.

11 Carp, J. (2012) The secret lives of experiments: methods reporting in the fMRI literature. *NeuroImage*, **63**, 289–300.

12 Haidich, A.B., Birtsou, C., Dardavessis, T., *et al.* (2011) The quality of safety reporting in trials is still suboptimal: survey of major general medical journals. *Journal of Clinical Epidemiology*, **64**, 124–135.

13 Mathoulin-Pelissier, S., Gourgou-Bourgade, S., Bonnetain, F. & Kramar, A. (2008) Survival end point reporting in randomized cancer clinical trials: a review of major journals. *Journal of Clinical Oncology*, **26**, 3721–3726.

14 DeMauro, S.B., Giaccone, A., Kirpalani, H. & Schmidt, B. (2011) Quality of reporting of neonatal and infant trials in high-impact journals. *Pediatrics*, **128**, e639–e644.

15 Altman, D.G. (2002) Poor-quality medical research: what can journals do? *JAMA*, **287**, 2765–2767.

16 Chalmers, I. & Glasziou, P. (2009) Avoidable waste in the production and reporting of research evidence. *Lancet*, **374**, 86–89.

17 Glasziou, P., Meats, E., Heneghan, C. & Shepperd, S. (2008) What is missing from descriptions of treatment in trials and reviews? *BMJ*, **336**, 1472–1474.

18 Reveiz, L., Chan, A.W., Krleza-Jeric, K. *et al.* (2010) Reporting of methodologic information on trial registries for quality assessment: a study of trial records retrieved from the WHO search portal. *PLoS One*, **5**, e12484.

19 Milette, K., Roseman, M. & Thombs, B.D. (2011) Transparency of outcome reporting and trial registration of randomized controlled trials in top psychosomatic and behavioral health journals: a systematic review. *Journal of Psychosomatic Research*, **70**, 205–217.

20 Vesterinen, H.M., Egan, K., Deister, A., *et al.* (2011) Systematic survey of the design, statistical analysis, and reporting of studies published in the 2008 volume of the Journal of Cerebral Blood Flow and Metabolism. *Journal of Cerebral Blood Flow and Metabolism*, **31**, 1064–1072.

21 Fleming, P.S., Koletsi, D., Polychronopoulou, A., *et al.* (2012) Are clustering effects accounted for in statistical analysis in leading dental specialty journals? *Journal of Dentistry*, **41**, 265–270.

22 Lang, T. (2004) Twenty statistical errors even you can find in biomedical research articles. *Croatian Medical Journal*, **45**, 361–370.

23 Strasak, A.M., Zaman, Q., Pfeiffer, K.P., *et al.* (2007) Statistical errors in medical research – a review of common pitfalls. *Swiss Medical Weekly*, **137**, 44–49.

24 Dwan, K., Altman, D.G., Arnaiz, J.A. *et al.* (2008) Systematic review of the empirical evidence of study publication bias and outcome reporting bias. *PLoS One*, **3**, e3081.

25 Dwan, K., Altman, D.G., Cresswell, L., *et al.* (2011) Comparison of protocols and registry entries to published reports for randomised controlled trials. *Cochrane Database of Systematic Reviews*, MR000031.

26 Vera-Badillo, F.E., Shapiro, R., Ocana, A., *et al.* (2013) Bias in reporting of end points of efficacy and toxicity in randomized, clinical trials for women with breast cancer. *Annals of Oncology*, **24**, 1238–1244.

27 Chan, A.W., Hrobjartsson, A., Jorgensen, K.J., *et al.* (2008) Discrepancies in sample size calculations and data analyses reported in randomised trials: comparison of publications with protocols. *BMJ*, **337**, a2299.

28 Chowers, M.Y., Gottesman, B.S., Leibovici, L., *et al.* (2009) Reporting of adverse events in randomized controlled trials of highly active antiretroviral therapy: systematic review. *Journal of Antimicrobial Chemotherapy*, **64**, 239–250.

29 Gigerenzer, G. (2008) Psychology and medicine: helping doctors to understand screening tests. *International Journal of Psychology*, **43**, 31.

30 Chan, A.W., Hrobjartsson, A., Haahr, M.T., *et al.* (2004) Empirical evidence for selective reporting of outcomes in randomized trials: comparison of protocols to published articles. *JAMA*, **291**, 2457–2465.

31 Pitkin, R.M., Branagan, M.A. & Burmeister, L.F. (1999) Accuracy of data in abstracts of published research articles. *JAMA*, **281**, 1110–1111.

32 Estrada, C.A., Bloch, R.M., Antonacci, D. *et al.* (2000) Reporting and concordance of methodologic criteria between abstracts and articles in diagnostic test studies. *Journal of General Internal Medicine*, **15**, 183–187.

33 Jannot, A.S., Agoritsas, T., Gayet-Ageron, A. & Perneger, T.V. (2013) Citation bias favoring statistically significant studies was present in medical research. *Journal of Clinical Epidemiology*, **66**, 296–301.

34 Mertens, S. & Baethge, C. (2011) The virtues of correct citation: careful referencing is important but is often neglected/even in peer reviewed articles. *Deutsches Ärzteblatt International*, **108**, 550–552.

35 Boutron, I., Dutton, S., Ravaud, P. & Altman, D.G. (2010) Reporting and interpretation of randomized controlled trials with statistically nonsignificant results for primary outcomes. *JAMA*, **303**, 2058–2064.

36 Ochodo, E.A., de Haan, M.C., Reitsma, J.B., *et al.* (2013) Overinterpretation and misreporting of diagnostic accuracy studies: evidence of "spin". *Radiology*, **267**, 581–588.

37 Mathieu, S., Boutron, I., Moher, D., *et al.* (2009) Comparison of registered and published primary outcomes in randomized controlled trials. *JAMA*, **302**, 977–984.

38 Huic, M., Marusic, M. & Marusic, A. (2011) Completeness and changes in registered data and reporting bias of randomized controlled trials in ICMJE journals after trial registration policy. *PLoS One*, **6**, e25258.

39 Rifai, N., Altman, D.G. & Bossuyt, P.M. (2008) Reporting bias in diagnostic and prognostic studies: time for action. *Clinical Chemistry*, **54**, 1101–1103.

40 Nosek, B.A., Spies, J.R. & Motyl, M. (2012) Scientific utopia II. Restructuring incentives and practices to promote truth over publishability. *Perspectives on Psychological Science*, **7**, 615–631.

41 Song, F., Parekh, S., Hooper, L. *et al.* (2010) Dissemination and publication of research findings: an updated review of related biases. *Health Technology Assessment*, **14**, iii, ix–xi, 1–193.

42 Hopewell, S., Loudon, K., Clarke, M.J., *et al.* (2009) Publication bias in clinical trials due to statistical significance or direction of trial results. *Cochrane Database of Systematic Reviews*, MR000006.

43 Fanelli, D. (2012) Negative results are disappearing from most disciplines and countries. *Scientometrics*, **90**, 891–904.

44 Simes, R.J. (1986) Publication bias: the case for an international registry of clinical trials. *Journal of Clinical Oncology*, **4**, 1529–1541.

45 Eyding, D., Lelgemann, M., Grouven, U. *et al.* (2010) Reboxetine for acute treatment of major depression: systematic review and meta-analysis of published and unpublished placebo and selective serotonin reuptake inhibitor controlled trials. *BMJ*, **341**, c4737.

46 Clarke, M. (2009) Can you believe what you read in the papers? *Trials*, **10**, 55.

47 Devereaux, P.J., Manns, B.J., Ghali, W.A. *et al.* (2001) Physician interpretations and textbook definitions of blinding terminology in randomized controlled trials. *JAMA*, **285**, 2000–2003.

48 Savovic, J., Jones, H.E., Altman, D.G. *et al.* (2012) Influence of reported study design characteristics on intervention effect estimates from randomized, controlled trials. *Annals of Internal Medicine*, **157**, 429–438.

49 Whiting, P., Rutjes, A.W., Reitsma, J.B., *et al.* (2004) Sources of variation and bias in studies of diagnostic accuracy: a systematic review. *Annals of Internal Medicine*, **140**, 189–202.

50 Winslow, E.H. (1996) Failure to publish research: a form of scientific misconduct? *Heart and Lung*, **25**, 169–171.

51 Chalmers, I. (1990) Underreporting research is scientific misconduct. *JAMA*, **263**, 1405–1408.

52 Moher, D. (2007) Reporting research results: a moral obligation for all researchers. *Canadian Journal of Anaesthesia*, **54**, 331–335.

53 Gøtzsche, P. (2011) Why we need easy access to all data from all clinical trials and how to accomplish it. *Trials*, **12**, 249.

54 Savitz, D.A. (2000) Failure to publish results of epidemiologic studies is unethical. *Epidemiology*, **11**, 361–363.

55 Simera, I., Moher, D., Hirst, A., *et al.* (2010) Transparent and accurate reporting increases reliability, utility, and impact of your research: reporting guidelines and the EQUATOR Network. *BMC Medicine*, **8**, 24.

56 Global Alliance of Publication Professionals (GAPP), Woolley, K.L., Gertel, A., Hamilton, C., *et al.* (2012) Poor compliance with reporting research results – we know it's a problem ... how do we fix it? *Current Medical Research and Opinion*. Oct 11 (Epub ahead of print).

57 Schriger, D.L., Arora, S. & Altman, D.G. (2006) The content of medical journal Instructions for authors. *Annals of Emergency Medicine*, **48** 743–749, 749.e1–749.e4.

58 Zarin, D.A., Tse, T. & Ide, N.C. (2005) Trial registration at ClinicalTrials.gov between May and October 2005. *New England Journal of Medicine*, **353**, 2779–2787.

59 Nankervis, H., Baibergenova, A., Williams, H.C. & Thomas, K.S. (2012) Prospective registration and outcome-reporting bias in randomized controlled trials of eczema treatments: a systematic review. *Journal of Investigative Dermatology*, **132**, 2727–2734.

60 Hopewell, S., Ravaud, P., Baron, G. & Boutron, I. (2012) Effect of editors' implementation of CONSORT guidelines on the reporting of abstracts in high impact medical journals: interrupted time series analysis. *BMJ*, **344**, e4178.

61 Roberts, J. (2009) An author's guide to publication ethics: a review of emerging standards in biomedical journals. *Headache*, **49**, 578–589.

62 Altman, D.G., Furberg, C.D., Grimshaw, J.M. & Rothwell, P.M. (2006) Lead editorial: trials – using the opportunities of electronic publishing to improve the reporting of randomised trials. *Trials*, **7**, 6.

63 Rippel RA. Re: Effect of using reporting guidelines during peer review on quality of final manuscripts submitted to a biomedical journal: masked randomised trial. http://www.bmj.com/content/343/bmj.d6783?tab=responses

64 Meuffels, D.E., Reijman, M., Scholten, R.J. & Verhaar, J.A. (2011) Computer assisted surgery for knee ligament reconstruction. *Cochrane Database of Systematic Reviews*, **24**, CD007601.

65 Gordon, M. & Findley, R. (2011) Educational interventions to improve handover in health care: a systematic review. *Medical Education*, **45**, 1081–1089.

66 Nolte, S., Wong, D., Lachford, G. Amphetamines for schizophrenia. *Cochrane Database of Systematic Reviews* 2004:CD004964.

67 Casas, J.P., Kwong, J. & Ebrahim, S. (2010) Telemonitoring for chronic heart failure: not ready for prime time. *Cochrane Database of Systematic Reviews*, **8**, ED000008.

68 Bleakley, C.M., McDonough, S.M. & MacAuley, D.C. (2008) Some conservative strategies are effective when added to controlled mobilisation with external support after acute ankle sprain: a systematic review. *Australian Journal of Physiotherapy*, **54**, 7–20.

69 Yeung CA. New guidelines for trial reporting – CONSORT 2010. *BMJ* 2010; http://www.bmj.com/content/340/bmj.c332/reply.

70 Wager, E., Kleinert, S. *Responsible research publication: International Standards for Authors*. A position statement developed at the 2nd World Conference on Research Integrity, Singapore, July 22–24, 2010. In: Mayer T, Steneck N, eds. *Promoting Research Integrity in a Global Environment*. Singapore: Imperial College Press/World Scientific Publishing, **2011**:309–316.

CHAPTER 2

How to Develop a Reporting Guideline

David Moher[1], Douglas G. Altman[2], Kenneth F. Schulz[3] and Iveta Simera[2]

[1]*Clinical Epidemiology Program, Ottawa Hospital Research Institute, Ottawa, ON, Canada*
[2]*Centre for Statistics in Medicine, University of Oxford, Oxford, UK*
[3]*FHI 360, Durham, and UNC School of Medicine, Chapel Hill, NC, USA*

Deficiencies in reporting health research studies

Globally, no precise estimate exists on the number of health journals publishing articles. In any given month, about 63,000 articles are indexed in PubMed, the US National Library of Medicine's portal for health-related publications. Yet, too many of these articles do not provide a sufficiently clear, accurate, or complete account of what was done and what was found in research studies. This is a scandalous situation that seriously impedes further use of such research and wastes scarce resources.

Chapter 1 provides several examples of the profound deficiencies in published articles. Historically, influential editorial groups, such as the International Committee of Medical Journal Editors, and individual medical journals have produced requirements and recommendations for biomedical publications. These focused mostly on the format of health research articles or provided guidance on the choice of appropriate methods for research conduct and analysis [1, 2], but very little attention was given to advice on how to report research. More recently, some journals have started to take the issue of adequate reporting more seriously and have begun to include more specific guidance in their instructions to authors. A few journals have supported better research reporting by introducing sections within their journals dedicated to issues of research methodology and reporting [e.g., 3, 4]. Although this is a positive development, surveys of journals' instructions to authors [5, 6] suggest that there is still considerable room for improvement.

The role of reporting guidelines in promoting clear and transparent reporting

Over the last 20 years, various multidisciplinary groups of methodologists, medical journal editors, and content experts have developed a series of reporting guidelines to support the improvement of reporting quality of published research articles [7, 8]. Reporting guidelines complement journals' instructions to authors. They usually take the form of a checklist, providing structured advice on how to report research studies. Development of these guidelines has generally followed an explicit methodology; a systematic search for relevant evidence and a consensus process [9] for developing guideline recommendations are crucial parts of this process.

The CONSORT Statement, a 25-item checklist and flow diagram for reporting randomized controlled trials (RCTs), is the first reporting guideline that has been endorsed widely in hundreds of medical journals [10]. The publication of CONSORT inspired the development of many other reporting guidelines. At the time of writing this chapter, more than 200 reporting guidelines are included on the EQUATOR Network's free online Library for Health Research Reporting [www.equator-network.org (cross-reference with EQUATOR chapter)]. Some of the most popular of these guidelines are described in this book.

A recent Cochrane review updated the evidence base as to whether journal endorsement of the 1996 and 2001 CONSORT checklists influences the completeness of reporting of RCTs published in medical journals. Fifty studies evaluating more than 16,000 trial reports were included. Twenty-five of 27 outcomes assessing completeness of reporting in RCTs appeared to favor CONSORT-endorsing journals over nonendorsers, of which five were statistically significant [11]. While these results are promising, there is a paucity of guidance on how to develop a reporting guideline.

Need for harmonization of guideline development methods

A survey of 37 reporting guideline developers (with an 81% response rate, generating 30 responses) asking how they developed, disseminated, and implemented their guidelines indicated that reporting guidelines were developed in various ways with little commonality. The guideline developers called for ways to harmonize methods used in the development of reporting guidelines [12].

This article summarizes the main steps in the development of evidence-based consensus guidelines for reporting health research studies; full details are provided elsewhere [13]. The suggested methodology draws on our collective experience from the development of at least 20 reporting guidelines over the last 17 years. During this period, the processes have evolved considerably, responding to lessons learnt from our own experiences as well as from those of others.

How to develop a guideline for reporting health research articles

Successful development of a reporting guideline requires an executive group of three to five members to facilitate and coordinate the process. Although most of the work can be completed remotely, it is essential to schedule at least one face-to-face meeting during the development process.

We describe developing a reporting guideline in five phases: the *initial steps* of developing a strong rationale for the guidance and ensuring that others have not already done so, the *premeeting activities* that include preparatory work required for a successful meeting, the *face-to-face consensus meeting activities* that enable the collaborative work of a full guideline development group, the *postmeeting activities* that include developing the final guidance and related documents for publication, and *postpublication activities* to support guideline implementation.

The key tasks required to complete all five phases are outlined in 18 steps (see Table 2.1) and briefly described below. A more complete discussion can be found elsewhere [13].

Initial steps

The initial steps involve careful planning of the whole development process and are focused on enabling a productive face-to-face consensus meeting. A clearly defined scope and aim are essential. A comprehensive literature review should be carried out at the beginning of the guideline development to identify any existing guidelines relating to the considered scope, which provide evidence on the current quality of reporting within the domain of interest, and identify key information on the potential sources of bias and other potential deficiencies in such studies.

Securing sufficient funding is important not only for covering costs of the consensus meeting but also for supporting the premeeting and postmeeting activities. Our estimate of the overall cost of developing a guideline (at 2013 prices) is approximately $CAD120,000. In practice, however, key participants may not be paid explicitly for their input.

Premeeting activities

The accumulated information gleaned from the initial steps described above will facilitate identification of stakeholder groups, expert contributors, and a spectrum of items to be considered for inclusion in the reporting guideline checklist. This is an important part of the premeeting activities.

Table 2.1 Checklist of items to consider when developing a guideline for reporting health research [13].

Step	Item number	Detail
Initial steps	1	Identify the need for a guideline
	1.1	Develop new guidance
	1.2	Extend existing guidance
	1.3	Implement existing guidance
	2	Review the literature
	2.1	Identify previous relevant guidance
	2.2	Seek relevant evidence on the quality of reporting in published research articles
	2.3	Identify key information on the potential sources of bias, and other deficiencies, in such study reports
	3	Obtain funding for the guideline initiative
Premeeting activities	4	Identify participants
	5	Conduct a Delphi exercise
	6	Generate a list of items for consideration at the face-to-face meeting
	7[a]	Prepare for the face-to-face meeting
	7.1	Decide size and duration of the face-to-face meeting
	7.2	Develop meeting logistics
	7.3	Develop meeting agenda
	7.3.1	Consider presentations on relevant background topics, including summary of evidence
	7.3.2	Plan to share results of Delphi exercise, if done
	7.3.3	Invite session chairs
	7.4	Prepare materials to be sent to participants prior to meeting
	7.5	Arrange to record the meeting
The face-to-face consensus meeting itself	8[a]	Present and discuss results of premeeting activities and relevant evidence
	8.1[a]	Discuss the rationale for including items in the checklist
	8.2	Discuss the development of a flow diagram
	8.3[a]	Discuss strategy for producing documents; identify who will be involved in which activities; discuss authorship
	8.4	Discuss knowledge translation strategy
Postmeeting activities	9[a]	Develop the guidance statement
	9.1	Pilot test the checklist
	10	Develop an explanatory document (E&E)
	11	Develop a publication strategy
	11.1	Discuss concurrent simultaneous publications with editors
Postpublication activities	12[a]	Seek and deal with feedback and criticism
	13[a]	Encourage guideline endorsement
	14	Support adherence to the guideline
	15	Evaluate the impact of the reporting guidance
	16	Develop website
	17	Translate guideline
	18	Update guideline

[a] Core set of items – see text.

Not all potential contributors will be able to participate in a face-to-face meeting; a Delphi process can help obtain input from a large number of relevant stakeholders and can strengthen the guideline process and recommendations. The development of the initial draft checklist is a complex process that is continued during the face-to-face meeting, the third phase in the reporting guideline development.

Face-to-face consensus meeting

The development of an early draft of the reporting guideline checklist is the most vital outcome of the meeting, which often lasts between one and three days. The substantive meeting begins with formal presentations of background topics, a summary of evidence from the literature, and results of any Delphi exercise. The most detailed and structured discussions revolve around which checklist items to include in the guideline. We have always considered the items included in the final checklist to be a minimum essential set that should be reported. While it is essential to cover the key issues relating to the guideline's scope, the checklist also needs to be short enough to be practical and useful. Editors of journals strongly advise keeping to one journal page.

There is no best way to generate the preliminary list of items for consideration. These will most likely come from various sources, including the Delphi process discussed above and relevant published evidence, and may be informed by how similar issues were handled in other reporting guidelines. Discussions should focus on information content and not precise wording. Ultimately, the views of the meeting participants will usually converge to a consensus, although it may occasionally be necessary to vote on some issues. It is often valuable to revisit the decisions made during this session toward the end of the meeting. We have found that some clarification and simplification is possible, especially when reconsidering topics addressed at the start of the process. For some guidelines, it might be useful to consider developing a flow chart describing the flow of participants or study records through different stages of the research study. These flow charts can bring a further level of clarity and transparency to research reports.

The face-to-face meeting is also a good opportunity for the participants to discuss a strategy for producing guideline documents, identify who will be involved in which activities, discuss authorship, and discuss any proposed knowledge translation strategy.

Postmeeting activities

The postmeeting period is a particularly busy time for the executive group. The most immediate activity is to draft the guideline paper. This will usually consist of a manuscript of about 2000 words describing the guidance, the rationale for its development, and the development process, including a brief description of the meeting and participants involved. It will include the checklist and flow diagram, if developed. Once drafted, the manuscript is circulated for input and feedback to all the consensus meeting participants. This process usually takes several iterations until a final version is agreed to by the named authors. Ideally, reporting guidelines should be accompanied by a detailed explanation and elaboration (E&E) document. However, developing such documents is very time consuming, perhaps taking two to three years to complete, and involves the executive group and several other meeting participants with several face-to-face meetings, so few guidelines include them. E&E papers are valuable as they provide readers with examples of good reporting and the rationale and evidence for the inclusion of each item in the checklist. Like the reporting guideline itself, the E&E paper will usually require several iterations based on input and feedback from the meeting participants.

The postmeeting period is an opportune time to pilot the checklist and flow-diagram, if developed. This period should also be used to implement the publication strategy discussed during the consensus meeting. For a guideline that is relevant to many fields, authors should consider concurrent publications in several relevant journals; therefore, this process should be discussed with journal editors perhaps even prior to drafting the manuscripts to avoid delays. To help gain as wide a readership as possible, the reporting guideline executive group should negotiate open access to the articles even with journals that do not routinely make all their content open access.

Postpublication activities

Postpublication activities support the guideline uptake. Guideline developers need to consider how to encourage accurate translations of their guideline into other languages, how to seek and constructively handle feedback and criticisms, how to support further guideline dissemination, possibly through the development of a dedicated website, and in particular how to ensure a wide endorsement by relevant journals and encourage users' adherence to the guideline. While endorsement by journals and adherence are not strictly part of the development process, they are crucial markers of a guideline's implementation.

Most reporting guideline developers recognize that their guideline will need to be updated requiring regular monitoring of the literature related to the guideline. When considering an update to an existing reporting guideline, developers should give serious consideration to the seven essential items (denoted with an a) in the development steps checklist (see Table 2.1).

Closing comments

Reporting guidelines are currently being used mainly at the end of the research process. However, investigators might benefit from the knowledge of reporting requirements at the beginning of their research (see Chapter 4). Some granting agencies have acted on this concept (e.g., the UK National Institute of Health Research developed a research process flowchart (http://rdinfo.leeds.ac.uk/flowchart/Flowchart.html) to guide researchers through all stages of a research project; the flow chart includes reference to reporting guidelines and encourages researchers to "consult a relevant guideline in the early stages of research planning.") Another example is the SPIRIT initiative aimed at providing guidance for the protocol content of randomized trials (14, 15, also see Chapter 7). Research funders should encourage scientists to use reporting guidelines when preparing new research applications. This might increase the overall quality of the applications to funders and enhance the potential return on research investment. Development and maintenance of robust reporting guidelines can thus significantly contribute to producing more reliable research.

References

1 (1979) Uniform requirements for manuscripts submitted to biomedical journals. International Steering Committee. *Annals of Internal Medicine*, **90** (1), 95–99.
2 Altman, D.G., Gore, S.M., Gardner, M.J. & Pocock, S.J. (1983) Statistical guidelines for contributors to medical journals. *BMJ*, **286** (6376), 1489–1493.
3 Groves, T. (2008) Research methods and reporting. *BMJ*, **337**, 946.
4 The PLoS Medicine Editors (2008) Better reporting, better research: guidelines and guidance in PLoS Medicine. *PLoS Medicine*, **5** (4), e99.
5 Hopewell, S., Altman, D.G., Moher, D. & Schulz, K.F. (2008) Endorsement of the CONSORT Statement by high impact factor medical journals: a survey of journal editors and journal 'Instructions to Authors'. *Trials*, **9**, 20.
6 Schriger, D.L., Arora, S. & Altman, D.G. (2006) The content of medical journal Instructions for authors. *Annals of Emergency Medicine*, **48** (6), 743–749.
7 Moher, D., Weeks, L., Ocampo, M. *et al.* (2011) Describing reporting guidelines for health research: a systematic review. *Journal of Clinical Epidemiology*, **64** (7), 718–742.
8 Simera, I., Moher, D., Hoey, J., *et al.* (2010) A catalogue of reporting guidelines for health research. *European Journal of Clinical Investigation*, **40** (1), 35–53.
9 Murphy, M.K., Black, N.A., Lamping, D.L. *et al.* (1998) Consensus development methods, and their use in clinical guideline development. *Health Technology Assessment*, **2** (3), i–88.
10 Schulz, K.F., Altman, D.G. & Moher, D. (2010) CONSORT 2010 statement: updated guidelines for reporting parallel group randomised trials. *PLoS Medicine*, **7** (3), e1000251.
11 Turner, L., Shamseer, L., Altman, D.G. *et al.* (2012) Consolidated standards of reporting trials [CONSORT] and the completeness of reporting of randomised controlled

trials [RCTs] published in medical journals. *Cochrane Database of Systematic Reviews*, **11**, MR000030.

12 Moher, D., Tetzlaff, J., Tricco, A.C., *et al*. (2007) Epidemiology and reporting characteristics of systematic reviews. *PLoS Medicine*, **4** (3), e78.

13 Moher, D., Schulz, K.F., Simera, I. & Altman, D.G. (2010) Guidance for developers of health research reporting guidelines. *PLoS Medicine*, **7** (2), e1000217.

14 Chan, A.W., Tetzlaff, J.M., Altman, D.G. *et al*. (2013) SPIRIT 2013 statement: defining standard protocol items for clinical trials. *Annals of Internal Medicine*, **158** (3), 200–207.

15 Chan, A.W., Tetzlaff, J.M., Gotzsche, P.C. *et al*. (2013) SPIRIT 2013 explanation and elaboration: guidance for protocols of clinical trials. *BMJ*, **346**, e7586.

CHAPTER 3

Characteristics of Available Reporting Guidelines

David Moher[1], Kenneth F. Schulz[2], Douglas G. Altman[3], John Hoey[4], Jeremy Grimshaw[5], Donald Miller[6], Dugald Seely[7], Iveta Simera[3], Margaret Sampson[8], Laura Weeks[7], and Mary Ocampo[9]

[1] *Clinical Epidemiology Program, Ottawa Hospital Research Institute, Ottawa, ON, Canada*
[2] *FHI 360, Durham, and UNC School of Medicine, Chapel Hill, NC, USA*
[3] *Centre for Statistics in Medicine, University of Oxford, Oxford, UK*
[4] *Queen's University, Kingston, ON, Canada*
[5] *Ottawa Hospital Research Institute and University of Ottawa, Ottawa, ON, Canada*
[6] *Department of Anesthesia, The Ottawa Hospital, Ottawa Hospital Research Institute and University of Ottawa, Ottawa, ON, Canada*
[7] *Ottawa Integrative Cancer Centre, Ottawa, ON, Canada*
[8] *Children's Hospital of Eastern Ontario, Ottawa, ON, Canada*
[9] *Ottawa Hospital Research Institute, Ottawa, ON, Canada*

Evidence points toward considerable waste in medical research, as well as how research results are reported [1]. Many reviews document inadequate reporting across almost every area of health research, specialty, and sub-specialty [2–5].

Readers often find that research reports fail to provide a clear and transparent account of the methods and adequate reporting of the results. If authors do not provide sufficient details of the conduct of their study, readers are left with an incomplete picture of what was done and found. Poorly reported research may result in misinterpretation and inappropriate application in clinical settings. New research projects may also be based on misleading evidence from poorly reported studies. As such, funds devoted to support research may not be used optimally.

Since the early 1990s, research groups consisting primarily of medical journal editors, methodologists, and content experts have developed reporting guidelines as tools to help improve the quality of reporting of health research articles. Carefully developed reporting guidelines provide authors with a minimum set of items that need to be addressed when reporting a study. However, little is known regarding the quality of the guidelines or the process used to develop them.

This chapter focuses mainly on the characteristics of reporting guidelines included in a systematic review [6]. First, we provide a brief description of the methods used. More detailed information can be found elsewhere [7].

Methods

The systematic review sought reporting guidelines of health research. Several electronic databases were searched as was the EQUATOR Network Library for Health Research Reporting. To describe the reporting guidelines, we identified five domains that intuitively appear to be important when developing guidelines: descriptive (e.g., the title, language of publication, name (and affiliations) of the corresponding author), background (e.g., rationale for developing the reporting guidelines, such as a review of the literature to identify previous relevant guidance, relevant evidence on the quality of reporting in published research articles, identification of stakeholders), consensus activities (e.g., whether a Delphi exercise was conducted), face-to-face meeting (e.g., whether the meeting objectives were clarified and whether the meeting involved presentation and/or discussion of any premeeting activities), and postconsensus activities (e.g., details on the drafting of the guidance, how feedback was incorporated, and piloting of the guidance, such as the checklist and diagram).

Results

We identified 2813 records for screening of which 477 full text papers were retrieved for further evaluation. In total, 81 reporting guidelines for health research were included of which 32 (40%) corresponding authors provided additional information, clarification of extracted data, or both.

Descriptive information

A large number of reporting guidelines exist for a broad spectrum of research types, (see Table 3.1). More reporting guidelines were published in recent years than previously. The median publication year was 2005 (range: 1986–2009), with approximately half of the guidelines being published in medical specialty journals ($n=41$; 51%). Working groups contributed to the development of 49 (61%) of the reporting guidelines. Of those guidelines developed by a working group, 31 (63%) reported the number of people participating in the guideline development. Of those that did, 22 (median) people participated in the development (range: 5–66). Twenty (25%) of the reporting guidelines were published in more than one journal. All of the guidelines were reported in English, although translations were available for five reporting guidelines.

Table 3.1 Characteristics of health research reporting guidelines

Characteristic	Number of guidelines	%
Descriptive		
Type of journal		
Medical specialty	41	50.6
General medical	21	25.9
Epidemiology	4	4.9
Other (basic science, education, psychology, health informatics, public health)	15	18.5
Published in more than 1 journal	20	24.7
Working group		
Specific name reported for group	49	60.5
No specific group name reported	32	39.5
Language		
English	81	100.0
French	0	0.0
Translations available	5	6.2
Background		
Guideline classification		
New guidance	47	58.0
Building on existing guidance	24	29.6
Update of existing guidance	10	12.4
Focus of guideline		
Multiple study designs or study design not specified	35	43.2
Randomized controlled trials	16	19.8
Laboratory/preclinical studies	6	7.4
Prospective clinical trials	5	6.2
Observational studies	4	4.9
Economic evaluations	4	4.9
Other specific design or types specified (systematic reviews, diagnostic accuracy studies, qualitative research, quality improvement research)	11	13.6
Checklist included	79	97.5
Flow diagram included	13	16.1
Explanatory document developed	11	13.6
Consensus process		
Stakeholders (can overlap)		
Content experts	69	85.2
Journal editors	26	32.1
Methodologists	41	51.9
Other (clinicians, funders, students, government agencies, professional organizations, publishers)	17	23.5
Not reported	6	7.4
Formal consensus exercises conducted	25	30.9
Delphi conducted	8	32.0

Continued

Table 3.1 (*Continued*)

Characteristic	Number of guidelines	%
Informal consensus exercises conducted	43	53.1
Both formal and informal consensus exercises conducted	7	12.4
Consensus activities not reported	24	28.4
Guideline development process		
Funding obtained		
Full	3	3.7
Partial	13	16.0
Extent not reported	23	28.4
No funding obtained	2	2.5
Funding not reported or unclear	40	49.4
Search for existing reporting guidance conducted	34	42.0
Search for relevant evidence on quality of reporting conducted	45	56.0
Checklist was pilot-tested	11	13.6
Face-to-face meeting was held	45	56.0
Postconsensus activities		
Method of handling feedback reported	25	30.9
Endorsement of guideline encouraged	50	61.7
Through journal instructions to authors	18	36.0
Through compliance by researchers and clinicians	7	14.0

Reprinted with permission from [6].

Background of reporting guidelines

Forty-seven (58%) reporting guidelines were classified as new guidance, while 24 (30%) were extensions of previously published guidelines and 10 (12%) were updates to previous guidelines (see Table 3.1). Many guidelines either did not indicate a specific study design for which they were intended or were intended for multiple study designs ($n = 35$; 43%). Of those particular to a specific design, most relate to reporting randomized controlled trials (RCTs; $n = 16$; 20%). The large majority of guidelines ($n = 76$; 94%) included a checklist of recommended reporting items, with a median of 21 checklist items (range: 5–64 items). Thirteen (16%) of the reporting guidelines had accompanying flow diagrams. Separate explanatory documents were developed for 11 (14%) reporting guidelines, which included evidence to support reporting recommendations, examples of good reporting, or both.

Consensus process

Guideline developers reported involving many stakeholders in the consensus process, most commonly content experts ($n = 69$; 85%), methodologists ($n = 41$; 51%), and journal editors ($n = 26$; 32%). Less commonly reported, however, were the activities the stakeholders engaged in to develop the reporting guidelines and what was discussed during the consensus process.

Formal consensus exercises [8] were reported to have been followed for 25 (31%) guideline initiatives, eight (10%) of which included a modified Delphi process, which is a systematic method to achieve consensus among experts that involves multiple rounds of questioning. Informal exercises, for example, email discussions and telephone conversations were reported to have been followed by 43 (53%) guideline initiatives. The developers of seven (9%) reporting guidelines reported to have followed both formal and informal consensus exercises. In the remaining 24 (30%) guidelines, little or no detail was provided regarding the nature of the consensus process, but these guidelines were included in our review because there was a statement made in the paper that indicated that the guidelines were developed through consensus. Further, for all included reporting guidelines, little detail was provided regarding what was discussed during the consensus process, for example, checklist items, a flow diagram, a document production strategy, or an implementation strategy.

Guideline development process

Reporting guideline developers provided little information about the guideline development process. For example, funding was obtained to assist with the development of at least 39 (48%) reporting guidelines, but this information was not reported or unclearly reported for 40 (49%) reporting guidelines. A variety of groups funded the development of reporting guidelines.

For many guidelines, no information was provided regarding a search for existing reporting guidance or data on the quality of reporting the relevant type of health research. Similarly, details regarding whether the reporting guideline checklist was pilot-tested were poorly reported. Eleven (14%) of the reporting guidelines were reported to have been pilot-tested, for example, by user testing for comprehension and comprehensiveness, but for 58 (72%) of the reporting guidelines this information was not reported or unclear.

A face-to-face meeting was held for 45 (56%) of the reporting guidelines. For 24 (30%) reporting guidelines, it was not reported whether a face-to-face meeting was held, and for one (1%) guideline it was unclear. Eleven (14%) reporting guidelines reported not holding a face-to-face meeting. As with other components of the guideline development process, most details about the face-to-face meetings, for example, the number of participants, length of the meeting, and what was discussed at the meeting were poorly reported. Of those developers who provided some details about their face-to-face meetings, there were 23 (median) meeting participants and the groups met for 2 days (median).

Postconsensus activities

Developers of 25 (31%) reporting guidelines described how they are handling feedback from the guideline audience, most often by inviting comments through a website or an email address, which would be used to refine and update the guidelines in the future. For 46 (57%) guidelines, however, this information was not reported. Only 14 (17%) guideline developers specifically described an intention to formally evaluate their reporting guidelines, for example, to conduct an assessment of reporting quality pre- and postguideline publication. Six guideline developers (7%) reported an intention to not evaluate their guidelines, while this information was not reported for 57 (70%) guidelines and unclear for the remaining four (5%) guidelines.

Developers of 50 (62%) reporting guidelines encouraged endorsement of their guidelines most commonly through journal instructions to authors ($n = 18$; 36%) or by researchers and clinicians following the guidelines when presenting their results ($n = 7$; 14%). The specific mode of endorsement was not reported by five (6%) reporting guideline developers and was unclear for a further 15 (19%) reporting guidelines.

How reporting guidelines were developed

The core items we used to evaluate the methods for the reporting guideline development were generally poorly reported with the exception of providing clear information about face-to-face meeting content ($n = 28$; 62%) and encouraging endorsement of the guidelines ($n = 49$; 61%). Although we were able to judge, based on reported information, that most of the reporting guideline developers used adequate methods to generate checklist items during a consensus process ($n = 52$; 64%), only 15 (33%) discussed the rationale for including items in the checklist and eight (18%) discussed the available evidence at the face-to-face meeting. We judged that most guidelines did not adequately describe how their developers will handle feedback or criticism ($n = 46$; 57%). For most of the items, we were unable to evaluate the methods used to develop the reporting guidelines because of poor reporting. For example, details regarding the organization and logistics of reporting guideline development, a document production strategy and the development of an explanatory (i.e., further explanation and elaboration) document were poorly reported and thus an assessment could not be made.

Overall, because of poor reporting of the guideline development process, the specific methods followed and appropriateness of those methods are unclear.

Comment

There are a large number of reporting guidelines for health research, many of which have been developed in the last few years. An annotated bibliography of reporting guidelines has also been published [9]. Recently a review of reporting guidelines for use in reporting preventive medicine and public health was published [10]. There are more than 200 reporting guidelines indexed on the EQUATOR Network's website (http://www.equator-network.org/). Several more are in active development. They cover a broad spectrum of content areas. The largest concentration of reporting guidelines is for reporting RCTs; the CONSORT Group has produced 12 reporting guidelines. While this is encouraging, the majority of published research uses other study designs [11, 12]. More attention is likely warranted to developing reporting guidelines other than for RCTs.

Although there are a large number of reporting guidelines, big differences exist in how they were developed. A more rigorous approach for developing reporting guidelines is needed. Until very recently, there has been a paucity of literature on how to best approach this task [7]. If reporting guidelines are not developed appropriately, their guidance may be of little use to authors, editors, or readers. As reported above, many guideline developers do not report on several aspects of how their guidelines were developed. As such, it is difficult to determine the quality of the guideline development process. It is possible that lack of reporting on such a large scale may reflect that the guidelines were not appropriately developed. Publishing better descriptions on how reporting guidelines were developed alongside the recommendations will allow potential users to critically assess the robustness of provided recommendations. Reporting guideline developers can learn from other related areas, such as the development of clinical practice guidelines, which has a longer and richer history. Several years ago Woolf [13] described a step-by-step approach for developing clinical practice guidelines. We probably need a similar approach to develop reporting guidelines.

To better appraise the quality of reporting guidelines for health research it is important to identify key guideline attributes that impact on their usability and effectiveness and to develop an assessment tool that could be used by authors and editors to help guide them in creating and evaluating specific reporting guidelines, similar to AGREE II for clinical practice guidelines [14, 15].

Many of the reporting guidelines included in this chapter are silent about their implementation activities, one clear example being whether the guideline developers reported an intention to seek journal endorsement for their guidelines. These results are similar to those of Simera and colleagues. These researchers surveyed 37 (81% response rate; $n = 30$) reporting guideline developers and reported that only 40% of the respondents used any implementation strategies to increase the uptake within journals [16]. Given the length of time taken to develop reporting guidelines, it is unfortunate that in a large proportion of cases only little attention appears to have been given to implementation. For reporting guidelines to be useful, a strategy must be developed to share the results of the development process with those stakeholders for whom the guidelines are intended. This will enhance the credibility of the process in much the same way as meticulous documentation is a desirable attribute of how clinical practice guidelines are developed. One useful strategy is to include journal editors in the development process from the beginning, as a means to develop commitment and improve uptake of the final product; several positive examples exist [7]. Another strategy is accurate translations of reporting guidelines (e.g., [17–19]), particularly checklists. Developing effective implementation requires resources. A collaborative funding approach between journals, publishers, and other stakeholders is worth consideration.

The majority of reporting guidelines included in this chapter neither reported on any evaluation of their guidelines nor had any intention to evaluate them. Similar results have been reported elsewhere [16]. Like many other scientific developments, we see little merit in developing reporting guidelines if they do not effectively address the problems they are designed to solve, namely, improving the quality of reporting for the content area they have been designed to address. Further, evaluation research would help users of reporting guidelines, for example, authors and editors to distinguish between the wide range of reporting guidelines that have emerged in recent years. This being said, we recognize that evaluating reporting guidelines is complicated to perform and execute [20].

Using reporting guidelines to achieve clarity and transparency of the research process might increase the word count of some journal articles. The tension between more lengthy papers and editors' desire to keep articles shorter needs to be managed. Most journals have an online presence and can therefore accommodate the merits of transparency by posting some parts of reports online only. Moreover, editors could decide to include items from a reporting guideline and to exclude more superfluous information from a manuscript, such as descriptions in the methods section of well-known laboratory techniques or subjective comments in the discussion section. In other words, papers following a reporting guideline do not necessarily have to be longer to be better.

References

1 Glaziou P., Altman, D.G., Bossuyt, P., *et al.* (2014) Reducing waste from incomplete or unusable reports of biomedical research. Lancet 383, 267–276.

2 [Chapter 1]. Moher, D., Altman, D., Schulz, K., *et al.* (eds) (2014) *Guidelines for Reporting Health Research: A User's Manual.* Wiley-Blackwell, Oxford.

3 Lai, T.Y., Wong, V.W., Lam, R.F., *et al.* (2007) Quality of reporting of key methodological items of randomized controlled trials in clinical ophthalmic journals. *Ophthalmic Epidemiology,* **14** (6), 390–398.

4 Ma, B., Guo, J., Qi, G. *et al.* (2011) Epidemiology, quality and reporting characteristics of systematic reviews of traditional Chinese medicine interventions published in Chinese journals. *PLoS One,* **6** (5), e20185.

5 Peron, J., Pond, G.R., Gan, H.K. *et al.* (2012) Quality of reporting of modern randomized controlled trials in medical oncology: a systematic review. *Journal of the National Cancer Institute,* **104** (13), 982–989.

6 Moher, D., Weeks, L., Ocampo, M. *et al.* (2011) Describing reporting guidelines for health research: a systematic review. *Journal of Clinical Epidemiology,* **64** (7), 718–742.

7 Moher, D., Schulz, K.F., Simera, I. & Altman, D.G. (2010) Guidance for developers of health research reporting guidelines. *PLoS Medicine,* **7** (2), e1000217.

8 Murphy, M.K., Black, N.A., Lamping, D.L. *et al.* (1998) Consensus development methods, and their use in clinical guideline development. *Health Technology Assessment,* **2** (3), i–88.

9 Simera, I., Moher, D., Hoey, J., *et al.* (2010) A catalogue of reporting guidelines for health research. *European Journal of Clinical Investigation,* **40** (1), 35–53.

10 Popham, K., Calo, W.A., Carpentier, M.Y. *et al.* (2012) Reporting guidelines: optimal use in preventive medicine and public health. *American Journal of Preventive Medicine,* **43** (4), e31–e42.

11 Funai, E.F., Rosenbush, E.J., Lee, M.J. & Del, P.G. (2001) Distribution of study designs in four major US journals of obstetrics and gynecology. *Gynecologic and Obstetric Investigation,* **51** (1), 8–11.

12 Scales, C.D. Jr., Norris, R.D., Peterson, B.L., Preminger, G.M. & Dahm, P. (2005) Clinical research and statistical methods in the urology literature. *Journal of Urology,* **174** (4 Pt 1), 1374–1379.

13 Woolf, S.H. (1992) Practice guidelines, a new reality in medicine. II. Methods of developing guidelines. *Archives of Internal Medicine,* **152** (5), 946–952.

14 Brouwers, M.C., Kho, M.E., Browman, G.P. *et al.* (2010) Development of the AGREE II, part 1: performance, usefulness and areas for improvement. *Canadian Medical Association Journal,* **182** (10), 1045–1052.

15 Brouwers, M.C., Kho, M.E., Browman, G.P. *et al.* (2010) Development of the AGREE II, part 2: assessment of validity of items and tools to support application. *Canadian Medical Association Journal,* **182** (10), E472–E478.

16 Simera, I., Altman, D.G., Moher, D., *et al.* (2008) Guidelines for reporting health research: the EQUATOR network's survey of guideline authors. *PLoS Medicine*, **5** (6), e139.

17 Schulz, K.F., Altman, D.G. & Moher, D. (2010) [CONSORT 2010 statement: updated guidelines for reporting parallel group randomised trials]. [Japanese]. *Japanese Pharmacology and Therapeutics*, **38** (11), 939–947.

18 Urrutia, G. & Bonfill, X. (2010) Declaracio n PRISMA: una propuesta para mejorar la publicacio n de revisiones sistematicas y metaanalisis. *Medicina Clínica (Barcelona)*, **135** (11), 507–511.

19 von Elm, E., Altman, D., Egger, M. *et al.* (2008) Das Strengthening the Reporting of Observational Studies in Epidemiology [STROBE] Statement.[German]. *Der Internist*, **49** (6), 688–693.

20 Turner, L., Shamseer, L., Altman, D.G. *et al.* (2012) Consolidated standards of reporting trials [CONSORT] and the completeness of reporting of randomised controlled trials [RCTs] published in medical journals. *Cochrane Database of Systematic Reviews*, **11**, MR000030.

CHAPTER 4

Using Reporting Guidelines Effectively to Ensure Good Reporting of Health Research

Douglas G. Altman and Iveta Simera
Centre for Statistics in Medicine, University of Oxford, Oxford, UK

"It is the responsibility of everyone involved to ensure that the published record is an unbiased, accurate representation of research." [1]

Inadequate reporting of research is a major concern for several reasons (Chapter 1). If authors do not provide sufficient details about the conduct and findings of their study, readers are unable to judge the reliability of the results and interpret them. There are also ethical and moral reasons for reporting research adequately. Widespread deficiencies in research publications have been extensively documented. In recent years, they have led to the development of reporting guidelines, which outline the key elements of research that should be addressed in a research report and how [2].

The primary role of reporting guidelines is to help researchers write up their research to maximize the value to others. Adherence to reporting guidelines will increase the completeness and transparency of health research publications, thereby providing readers with sufficient details to enable them to critically appraise the study [3]. Improved reporting also has important benefits for systematic reviewers and those developing clinical practice guidelines and improves the efficiency of electronic literature searches. Over time, the use of reporting guidelines may have a beneficial influence on the quality of research by raising general awareness of key methodological issues.

In this chapter, we consider how reporting guidelines can be used by researchers and others to improve the quality of the accumulating research literature and ultimately benefit patients. We also consider whose responsibility it is to ensure good reporting of research.

Guidelines for Reporting Health Research: A User's Manual, First Edition. Edited by David Moher, Douglas G. Altman, Kenneth F. Schulz, Iveta Simera and Elizabeth Wager.
© 2014 John Wiley & Sons, Ltd. Published 2014 by John Wiley & Sons, Ltd.

Reporting guidelines

A reporting guideline lists the minimum set of items (usually as a check-list) that should be included in a research report to provide a clear and transparent account of what was done and what was found. The EQUA-TOR Network's online Library for Health Research Reporting (Chapter 6) currently lists over 200 reporting guidelines. Some of these are generic for specific types of study designs (e.g., randomized trials, systematic reviews, observational studies) and should always be observed when reporting this type of study. Their primary focus is on the description of the study methods and corresponding advice on reporting the study findings. The content of each of these guidelines has been carefully considered by multidisciplinary groups of relevant experts and stakeholders, and there is a strong rationale for each item of requested information. Items range from "simple" requests such as the identification of study design in the title or abstract (neces-sary for the electronic identification of studies) to items focusing on specific aspects that might introduce bias into the research (e.g., details about how participants were selected for inclusion into a study). This book provides an overview of the key methodology guidelines (Chapters 7–24). However, most of the guidelines listed on the EQUATOR website are more specific, providing guidance relevant to a particular medical specialty (e.g., report-ing controlled trials in oncology) or to a particular aspect of research (e.g., reporting of adverse events or particular analyses). Such specific guidelines should, ideally, be used in conjunction with the relevant generic guidelines.

Reporting guidelines do not prescribe how research studies should be conducted. Nevertheless, wider appreciation of what needs to be reported can be expected to feed into improving how future studies are designed and conducted [4]. It is not possible to separate research reporting from research conduct completely, but it is important to be aware of some spe-cific issues arising from the close relationship between these two aspects of the research process (see Chapter 5).

Who benefits from the use of reporting guidelines?

Researchers are the primary target group of most reporting guidelines as they benefit directly from their use both as authors and peer reviewers of research articles. However, many others can indirectly benefit from the use of reporting guidelines: readers of research articles, systematic reviewers, clinical guideline developers, research funders, journal editors and publish-ers, patients, and society at large. All these groups benefit, in various ways, from more completely and accurately reported health research studies.

Research articles are primarily intended to communicate findings to interested parties. Other researchers are one of the most important groups who will read a published article. They may well be working in the same field and likely to be carrying out similar or related research or conducting a review of published articles.

Whether a study's findings support or refute previous research, or the study breaks new ground, fellow researchers who read the article should not simply accept the authors' findings or (especially) their conclusions. Rather, they will wish to understand the methods used, to determine whether the observed findings are relevant to them and are scientifically reliable. Such assessment clearly requires, as a minimum, a full description of the study's methods and transparent reporting of the findings.

For example, from a report of a nonrandomized study to compare two medical treatments, readers will expect to learn about the way in which the treatment was determined for individuals and which statistical analysis methods were employed to try to diminish the effect of confounding. Such key issues are addressed in reporting guidelines, in this case STROBE (Chapter 17).

In principle, other researchers ought to be able to repeat the study from the information given in the article (and perhaps also other referenced study publications). Readers should not have to be "research detectives" [5], yet often that is the reality. This fate applies especially to systematic reviewers who, having struggled to identify studies that are relevant to their review, have to struggle further to extract from publications essential information about study methods and detailed numerical results. It is common in reports of systematic reviews to see comments about the impossibility of extracting information. Box 1.1 in Chapter 1 shows some comments on the impact of reporting on the task of systematic reviewers. Reports that adhere fully to reporting guidelines greatly assist the systematic reviewer. Those that omit key information impede reviews and may lead to studies having to be excluded, which is wasteful and unacceptable [6].

Using reporting guidelines

Researchers

Planning a research study – writing the protocol
Reporting guidelines are primarily intended to aid the clear reporting of a study in a research paper. However, reporting guidelines are also useful when planning a study. Referring to reporting guidelines when writing the protocol will ensure that important details will not be forgotten and may suggest ways in which a study can be strengthened. For example,

certain study methods are especially critical to the validity and value of the research and it is therefore important that the protocol takes account of those elements. Taking reporting requirements into account will also help to structure a protocol method section in a way that can easily be transferred to a manuscript when writing the study up after its completion.

Some guidelines are accompanied by separate, detailed "explanation and elaboration" (E&E) documents, which provide extensive explanations of the rationale behind each checklist item and include illustrative examples of good reporting. These papers can be a particularly valuable resource at the planning stage. Not only do they explain methodological terms (e.g., CONSORT explaining allocation concealment in trials or STROBE describing effect modifiers in observational studies), but they also include examples of good reporting. A reporting guideline might thus provoke thoughts about possible improvements to the study design – for example, how to reduce the risk of bias or improve the reliability of the data being collected. However, E&E papers are neither a substitute for an adequate training in the conduct of such research studies nor for including a methodology expert in the project team.

An excellent example of the link between protocols and reporting guidelines is the SPIRIT guidance for preparing protocols of randomized trials (Chapter 7), which was developed in synergy with the CONSORT statement for reporting trial findings in journal articles (Chapter 9).

Documenting research findings in an article for journal publication

At the writing stage, reporting guidelines provide a useful reminder of fundamental details that should be addressed in the paper. As mentioned above, generic, methodology-focused guidelines such as CONSORT or STROBE suggest minimum sets of reporting requirements that should always be included when reporting this particular type of study. Other guidelines are more specific and recommend additional information that is important, for example, for a particular clinical area.

Researchers, as authors of reports describing their research, have primary responsibility for what is included in research reports. Although many research studies include experienced researchers among the authors, articles will often be drafted by less senior researchers who have little experience of writing articles for publication. Reporting guidelines may be especially valuable for such authors. Without good guidance, inexperienced authors frequently tend to copy the presentation style they see in published articles and thus perpetuate the bad reporting habits that are so prevalent.

The primary purpose of publishing research is to communicate findings to others. Indeed, authors should be aware of the moral responsibility to publish their findings honestly and transparently [7]. Two further general principles are relevant. First, authors should have in mind the possibility that others will want to repeat what they have done, so the information in the article should be detailed enough to allow replication. Second, the study results should be presented in suitable detail to allow them to be included in a meta-analysis. These conditions will be far more likely to be met if authors are aware of, and follow, the relevant reporting guidelines.

Checklists indicate the information that ought to be reported. Although items appear in sequence in the checklist, there are various reasons why the order of presentation may vary from article to article. What matters is that the information is provided somewhere not precisely where it appears. To assist peer review, some journals ask authors to supply a completed checklist indicating the manuscript page on which each item appears. Much more helpfully, authors can also cut and paste key sections of the manuscript text into the boxes [8]. Some journals publish the completed checklist as a web appendix in the interest of transparency. They are most helpful to readers when populated by text rather than page numbers (especially if these refer to the submitted text rather than the published version). It is also possible to indicate in the main text the passages that address each of the checklist items, as is occasionally seen [9]. Even when a journal does not require authors to submit a completed reporting guideline checklist, these checklists are useful when finally checking the manuscript before submission.

Reporting guidelines indicate the *minimum* information that readers would expect to see in a journal article. However, it is a serious error to think that anything not in a checklist need not be mentioned. For example, it is important to document unexpected changes to study methods that occurred when a study was underway. Only CONSORT explicitly mentions reporting if the methods differed from what was planned in the protocol. Not all guidelines ask authors to report the amount of missing data, but this is usually important information. Likewise, it is sensible to report that a study was registered and ethical approval was obtained even if these items are not included in the relevant guidelines.

Some reporting guidelines recommend the inclusion of a diagram showing the flow of participants through the study. Flow diagrams provide a valuable overview of several key aspects of a study's conduct, with a clear statement of critical information about the numbers of participants. The CONSORT flow diagram [10] has been especially widely adopted, and examples are often seen, which imaginatively enhance the basic template with various types of additional information, or extend it to complex study designs. Unfortunately, many published flow diagrams do not adhere fully to the recommended structure, so that important information is missing [11].

Researchers should try to ensure that their article accurately describes the study as done and includes all important information. Readers expect that a study adhered to the prespecified plan except where otherwise indicated, the report should not misrepresent the study. Authors should, therefore, resist attempts by editors or peer reviewers to remove important elements of the study methodology or alter the analysis from what was intended to something suggested by the results. It may, however, sometimes be valuable to include additional analyses suggested by reviewers – it is helpful then to indicate that these additional analyses were not prespecified. As always, readers are best served by full and transparent reporting.

Journal editors

Journal editors can use reporting guidelines in several ways. Perhaps the most common is to include a statement in the journal's instructions for authors about the desirability or, indeed, requirement of manuscripts conforming to specific guidelines. Such statements are quite common, especially for CONSORT [12, 13]. There is evidence that randomized controlled trials reporting is better in journals that have endorsed CONSORT in this way, but the impact is rather modest [14]. That may well be because the language used in journal instructions is often ambiguous or soft [12, 15], and also because there is often no effort to check whether authors have actually followed the guidelines. As a minimum, journals should consider the wording of statements about reporting guidelines in their instruction to authors, preferably strengthening the message about the importance of adherence. The EQUATOR Network (www.equator-network.org) has developed guidance for editors suggesting ways in which their journal can support better reporting of health research.

As noted above, some journals require authors to submit a completed checklist with their submission. As a minimum, that requirement ensures exposure of researchers to the specific reporting guidelines relevant to their study. Some journals use the checklists "in house" (i.e., as part of technical editing) to ensure that submitted manuscripts adhere to the guidelines, often focusing on a subset of the most important methodological issues. While all elements on a checklist are deemed important by their developers, clearly some are especially vital to assess scientific reliability, so it is sensible to focus on those elements in the first instance.

Journals could do much more to ensure that authors and peer reviewers give proper consideration to good reporting. Box 4.1 gives some suggestions for journals.

Peer reviewers

Medical journals ask peer reviewers to assess submitted manuscripts both to assess their suitability for publication and also to suggest ways in which, if published, the article might be improved. Clearly, peer review is a prime opportunity to ensure that published articles include key information about study methods and essential aspects of findings. Despite the high status given to peer review and its ubiquitous use by medical journals, there is surprisingly limited guidance, or even consensus, on exactly what peer reviewers should do [16].

Reporting guidelines are a valuable aid to peer review, providing a reminder to reviewers of key issues that should be addressed in a submitted manuscript. Reviewers may well wish to first consider crucial aspects of methodology, as failure to address these key issues can render review of the remaining manuscript unnecessary. As noted above, some journals ask authors to supply a completed checklist indicating the manuscript page on which each item is addressed; if it is forwarded to the peer reviewers it can aid their task.

The persistent finding of numerous evaluations of published studies of various designs is that reporting of even the most important elements of study methods is poor – for example, fewer than half of the randomized trials give details about the method of randomization [14]. While the faults of the medical literature cannot be laid solely at the door of peer reviewers, it is clear that, currently, peer review is a badly missed opportunity to ensure that manuscripts provide readers with essential information about research studies.

Research funders

In addition to benefiting from the use of reporting guidelines by researchers whose studies they support, research funders are in a unique position to reinforce the requirements for accurate, complete, and transparent reporting. Funders hold one of the biggest incentives for scientists – funds for their future work. Some funders now have statements on their websites supporting the above-described reporting principles as part of their research integrity policies but hardly any of them request adherence to reporting guidelines, despite the fact that this is one of the cheapest and simplest ways to ensure better reporting quality of new research findings. Notable exceptions are the UK Medical Research Council and UK NIHR research program.

Whose responsibility is good reporting of research?

The widespread poor reporting of medical research represents a system failure, in which no one group has primary responsibility. Rather, there is clearly a collective failure across many key groups to appreciate the importance of adequate reporting of research. Why this should be so remains unclear; it is rather remarkable that so many individuals and organizations have persistently failed in this respect over decades.

Changes in behavior by several groups, notably researchers, editors, and peer reviewers, could lead to a rapid, major improvement in the usability of research findings, and a consequent reduction in the waste currently observed [3, 6]. Inertia and the lack of incentives are barriers that must be overcome to maximize the benefit of current research for future patients.

Box 4.1: Recommendations for journal editors

How to support accurate and transparent reporting of health research studies and improve the reporting quality of submitted manuscripts:*

(a) Incorporate an explicit philosophy of transparent, complete and accurate reporting and the use of reporting guidelines into your editorial policy.

(b) Explore the available reporting guidelines on the EQUATOR website (www.equator-network.org); select well-developed guidelines appropriate for the reporting of research studies published in your journal.

(c) Refer to selected guidelines in your 'Instructions to Authors,' ask or instruct authors to adhere to these guidelines, and motivate their use.

(d) Consider including a link to the EQUATOR website as the portal for up to date reporting guidelines and other related resources. This will ensure that your links to instructions are current without additional effort for your journal.

(e) Publish editorials to widen awareness of the importance of good reporting and the use of reporting guidelines by authors and peer reviewers, and indicate that your editorial policies will be incorporating them.

(f) Consider strategies and actions to ensure (and verify) that authors realise and assume full responsibility for the reporting quality of their studies and adhere to reporting guidelines.

How to improve the peer review of submitted manuscripts:**

(a) Increase transparency of your peer review process by providing your instructions to peer reviewers openly on your website. Ideally instructions should be collated in one place, made available as a printable pdf and include the date of their last revision. Consider linking to these from your instructions to authors to give your authors an indication of how their manuscript will be evaluated.

(b) Alert your peer reviewers to the importance of good reporting and the availability of reporting guidelines which can act as an *aide memoire* for items indicating complete reporting. Provide or link to relevant guidelines/checklists and ask peer reviewers to use them during their manuscript assessment. This will make the review more helpful for authors in revising their manuscripts.

(c) If you provide training for peer reviewers consider a module on reporting guidelines and how they can be used in manuscript assessment. Link to other available resources [17, 18].

(d) Where provided, journals should link to resources for peer reviewers provided by their publishers.

Slightly modified from *[3] and **[16].

References

1 PLoS Medicine Editors. (2009) An unbiased scientific record should be everyone's agenda. *PLoS Medicine*, **6**, e1000038.
2 Simera, I., Moher, D., Hoey, J., *et al.* (2010) A catalogue of reporting guidelines for health research. *European Journal of Clinical Investigation*, **40**, 35–53.
3 Simera, I., Moher, D., Hirst, A., *et al.* (2010) Transparent and accurate reporting increases reliability, utility, and impact of your research: reporting guidelines and the EQUATOR Network. *BMC Medicine*, **8**, 24.
4 Moher, D., Hopewell, S., Schulz, K.F. *et al.* (2010) CONSORT 2010 Explanation and Elaboration: updated guidelines for reporting parallel group randomised trials. *BMJ*, **340**, c869.
5 Gøtzsche, P.C. (2009) Readers as research detectives. *Trials*, **10**, 2.
6 Chalmers, I. & Glasziou, P. (2009) Avoidable waste in the production and reporting of research evidence. *Lancet*, **374**, 86–89.
7 Moher, D. (2007) Reporting research results: a moral obligation for all researchers. *Canadian Journal of Anesthesia*, **54**, 331–335.
8 Haien, Z., Yong, J., Baoan, M., *et al.* (2013) Post-operative auto-transfusion in total hip or knee arthroplasty: a meta-analysis of randomized controlled trials. *PLoS One*, **8**, e55073.
9 Rupinski, M., Zagorowicz, E., Regula, J. *et al.* (2011) Randomized comparison of three palliative regimens including brachytherapy, photodynamic therapy, and APC in patients with malignant dysphagia (CONSORT 1a) (Revised II). *American Journal of Gastroenterology*, **106**, 1612–1620.
10 Schulz, K.F., Altman, D.G. & Moher, D. (2010) CONSORT 2010 Statement: updated guidelines for reporting parallel group randomized trials. *Annals of Internal Medicine*, **152**, 726–732.
11 Hopewell, S., Hirst, A., Collins, G.S., *et al.* (2011) Reporting of participant flow diagrams in published reports of randomized trials. *Trials*, **12**, 253.
12 Hopewell, S., Altman, D.G., Moher, D. & Schulz, K.F. (2008) Endorsement of the CONSORT Statement by high impact factor medical journals: a survey of journal editors and journal 'Instructions to Authors'. *Trials*, **9**, 20.
13 Schriger, D.L., Arora, S. & Altman, D.G. (2006) The content of medical journal instructions for authors. *Annals of Emergency Medicine*, **48** 743–749, 749.e1–749.e4.
14 Turner, L., Shamseer, L., Altman, D.G. *et al.* (2012) Consolidated standards of reporting trials (CONSORT) and the completeness of reporting of randomised controlled trials (RCTs) published in medical journals. *Cochrane Database of Systematic Reviews*, **11**, MR000030.
15 Altman, D.G. (2005) Endorsement of the CONSORT statement by high impact medical journals: survey of instructions for authors. *BMJ*, **330**, 1056–1057.
16 Hirst, A. & Altman, D.G. (2012) Are peer reviewers encouraged to use reporting guidelines? A survey of 116 health research journals. *PLoS One*, **7**, e35621.
17 Garmel, G.M. (2010) Reviewing manuscripts for biomedical journals. *The Permanent Journal*, **14**, 32–40.
18 Winck, J.C., Fonseca, J.A., Azevedo, L.F. & Wedzicha, J.A. (2011) To publish or perish: how to review a manuscript. *Revista Portuguesa de Pneumologia*, **17**, 96–103.

CHAPTER 5

Ambiguities and Confusions Between Reporting and Conduct

Kenneth F. Schulz[1], David Moher[2] and Douglas G. Altman[3]

[1] *FHI 360, Durham, and UNC School of Medicine, Chapel Hill, NC, USA*
[2] *Clinical Epidemiology Program, Ottawa Hospital Research Institute, Ottawa, ON, Canada*
[3] *Centre for Statistics in Medicine, University of Oxford, Oxford, UK*

Theoretically, the reporting and conduct of research should be in harmony. Indeed, we argue that good reporting is an essential part of good conduct. In practice, however, while good reporting promotes enlightenment and clarity, poor reporting creates ambiguities and confusions. In addition, further confusion arises because a study can be excellently reported but poorly conducted or poorly reported but excellently conducted.

The primary goal of reporting guidelines is clarity, completeness, and transparency of reporting (see Chapter 1) [1, 2]. This allows readers to judge the validity of the methods and results, enabling them to develop an informed, enlightened interpretation and, for those interested researchers, to replicate the methods. Indeed, most reporting guidelines, such as the CONSORT 2010 Statement [3], do not incorporate requirements or recommendations for designing and conducting research. Reporting guidelines focus solely on a research report describing what was done and what was found [1, 2]. Obviously, reporting properly does not directly improve the design or conduct of a study, and adherence to a reporting guideline does not confer any stamp of quality on the research conduct.

Most developers of reporting guidelines embrace an intense interest in improving the design and conduct of health research. Nonetheless, they must relegate that interest to a secondary, indirect goal of their guideline. They hope that better design and conduct will materialize as a byproduct of proper reporting, which forces investigators who design and conduct deficient studies to divulge those deficiencies when they publish. Thus, good reporting in this instance provides enlightenment and clarity to readers while producing unease in authors. That unease, however, is encouraged by guideline developers as a constructive path to improve design and conduct in the future.

A further confusion between reporting and conduct emanates from the misuse of reporting guidelines. This misuse often takes the form of researchers using a guideline to develop a quality score for conduct of studies. Such a process is not advocated in most reporting guidelines, as stated in the CONSORT 2010 statement:

> Moreover, the CONSORT 2010 statement does not include recommendations for designing and conducting randomized trials. The items should elicit clear pronouncements of how and what the authors did, but do not contain any judgments on how and what the authors should have done. Thus, CONSORT 2010 is not intended as an instrument to evaluate the quality of a trial. Nor is it appropriate to use the checklist to construct a "quality score." [2]

Still, some researchers have misused CONSORT as a basis for a quality score. CONSORT only states what to report but does not offer any judgment as to what is good and what is bad. Certainly, if authors report according to CONSORT, readers have the information needed to make their own judgments on the quality of design and conduct, but CONSORT does not indicate how they should make those judgments. CONSORT specifically, and reporting guidelines in general, were not conceived to serve as a springboard to a quality score. Moreover, the entire industry of quality scores is suspect [3]. This misuse of reporting guidelines creates confusion in the assessments of conduct.

Examples of item-specific scenarios

Some individual items in reporting guidelines elicit clear, unambiguous information on conduct. For example, Item 1a in CONSORT 2010 asks for "identification as a randomized trial in the title."

However, other items can engender ambiguities and confusions between reporting and conduct that complicate the use of reporting guidelines. For most of us, those item-specific difficulties are hard to grasp abstractly, but examples are more easily understood.

Allocation concealment from the CONSORT 2010 statement

As examples, we use conduct and reporting of an envelope method of allocation concealment in a randomization scheme, under different scenarios. As stated by some authors, an adequate envelope method would at a minimum use sequentially numbered, opaque, sealed envelopes

[4–6]. This represents a quality criterion for this item. If the description of allocation concealment reported in an article meets that quality criterion, a reader would likely judge the trial to be of good quality on the allocation concealment item in CONSORT 2010. With this as a baseline quality criterion, we present a few item-specific scenarios that serve as examples.

Scenario 1: Excellent reporting of excellent conduct

In this scenario, the authors have harmonized reporting and conduct. A superb example is the following:

> . . .The allocation sequence was concealed from the researcher (JR) enrolling and assessing participants in sequentially numbered, opaque, sealed and stapled envelopes. Aluminium foil inside the envelope was used to render the envelope impermeable to intense light. To prevent subversion of the allocation sequence, the name and date of birth of the participant was written on the envelope and a video tape made of the sealed envelope with participant details visible. Carbon paper inside the envelope transferred the information onto the allocation card inside the envelope and a second researcher (CC) later viewed video tapes to ensure envelopes were still sealed when participants' names were written on them. Corresponding envelopes were opened only after the enrolled participants completed all baseline assessments and it was time to allocate the intervention [7].

This description includes the quality criterion of sequentially numbered, opaque, sealed envelopes but also incorporates many other methods that greatly strengthen allocation concealment. This excellent reporting of excellent conduct leaves little room for confusion or ambiguity.

Scenario 2: Incomplete, ambiguous reporting of excellent conduct

If investigators actually conducted a trial following the methods described in Scenario 1 but described their allocation approach as simply "sequentially numbered, opaque, sealed envelopes," that description would be true but incomplete. Moreover, the apparent reporting would be considered adequate reporting by many readers because it meets the sequentially numbered, opaque, sealed envelope quality criterion. Even so, the actual reporting is incomplete and ambiguous because it does not convey the true strength of this allocation concealment approach.

Scenario 3: Poor, ambiguous reporting of excellent conduct

Investigators actually conducted a trial following the methods described in Scenario 1 but described their allocation approach as simply "sealed, opaque envelopes." That description would be true but distinctively incomplete. Generally, a reader would classify this description, based on the quality criterion, as ambiguous because the investigators might have only used sealed, opaque envelopes that were not sequentially numbered.

In actuality, just reporting the excellent conduct described in Scenario 1 as simply "sealed, opaque envelopes" is poor, incomplete reporting. Readers of articles face enormous ambiguity when they are confronted with that incomplete description because they have no concrete idea whether the conduct was poor or excellent.

Scenario 4: Poor, ambiguous reporting of excellent conduct

Investigators actually conducted a trial following the methods described in Scenario 1, but they failed to provide any details of their approach to allocation concealment, that is, no mention of envelopes, let alone adjectives. Generally, readers would consider this apparent reporting as unclear. This unclear, obscure reporting could represent anything from poor to excellent conduct. In this case, poor reporting camouflages excellent conduct.

Scenario 5: Excellent reporting of inadequate conduct

Assume that investigators used sealed, opaque envelopes that were not sequentially numbered, which would be considered inadequate conduct. If authors reported that they used "sealed, opaque envelopes" and explicitly stated that "the envelopes were not sequentially numbered," we would classify this description as excellent reporting of inadequate conduct. Owing to adequate, clear, and transparent reporting, no confusion or ambiguity would exist, even though the conduct was inadequate.

Scenario 6: Ambiguous reporting of inadequate conduct

Again assume that investigators used sealed, opaque envelopes that were not sequentially numbered. If authors reported that they simply used "sealed, opaque envelopes," this reporting is unclear because the authors may have used envelopes that were also sequentially numbered but just failed to report that fact. Scenarios 5 and 6 represent similar situations except that the authors in Scenario 5 have made it clear that sequentially numbered envelopes were not used. That led to the reporting being excellent in Scenario 5, whereas in Scenario 6 the reporting is unclear. Admittedly, these judgments are nuanced, but this illustrates the ambiguities between reporting and conduct. Whenever authors report simply "sealed, opaque envelopes" without clarifying information, ambiguity and confusion are created. Scenario 6 is, to a reader, indistinguishable from Scenario 3 above. Readers are confused whether this represents good reporting of inadequate conduct or poor reporting of adequate conduct.

Scenario 7: Inadequate, fallacious reporting of inadequate conduct

Authors reported that they used sequentially numbered, opaque, sealed envelopes, but they actually only used opaque, sealed envelopes that were not sequentially numbered. This form of fabricated, misleading reporting to give the appearance of having met some quality criterion (which in fact was not met) worries many of us who develop reporting guidelines. A quality criterion should be a goal by which investigators adjust conduct and not by which they adjust reporting. This scenario is particularly pernicious because it falsely describes inadequate conduct as adequate.

Sequence generation from the CONSORT 2010 statement

As another example of less obvious ambiguities, we shall use conduct and reporting of a sequence generation method in a randomization scheme under different scenarios. As stated in some publications, an adequate sequence generation method would, at a minimum, use a specified method of randomization, such as a random number table or a reasonable computer random number generator [4−6]. This represents the quality criterion for this item. If that is reported in an article, a reader might judge the trial to be of good quality on the sequence generation item in CONSORT 2010. However, ambiguities and confusions can occur between reporting and conduct.

Assume that investigators used a computer random number generator to select random permuted blocks of size 6. In some instances, this might be considered adequate sequence generation, such as in trials where everyone is totally blinded [8, 9]. However, the trial in this example is unblinded (open-label), meaning everyone knows the treatment assigned to a participant after randomization. Thus, fixed block sizes may be discerned by the pattern of past assignments, with the obvious consequence being that some future assignments can be accurately anticipated [8, 9]. Scenarios 8 and 9 depict scenarios of reporting this form of inadequate conduct of sequence generation.

Scenario 8: Poor, ambiguous reporting of inadequate conduct

Authors used the approach just discussed but reported their sequence generation approach as using a computer random number generator. In the absence of clarifying information, this description would be interpreted by many readers as implying a simple randomization scheme, which is adequate randomization to prevent bias under virtually all circumstances. By the quality criterion for sequence generation, many readers would judge this as apparently adequate reporting of adequate conduct. However, more astute readers, knowing this was an unblinded trial and that the authors did not explicitly state that simple randomization was used, might consider the reporting to be unclear. In any case, however, ambiguities exist between reporting and conduct. We would consider this actually poor (incomplete) reporting of inadequate conduct.

Scenario 9: Excellent reporting of inadequate conduct

In this scenario, the actual conduct was the same as that in Scenario 8. However, in Scenario 9 the authors completely and transparently reported that they used a computer random number generator to select random permuted blocks of size 6. We view this as excellent reporting of inadequate conduct in this instance. Under this scenario, ambiguities and confusions dissipate.

Discussion

Owing to the lack of complete and transparent reporting, ambiguities and confusions abound in the medical research literature. It is no wonder that peer reviewers and readers become uneasy and perplexed over manuscripts, whether submitted or already published. A medical epidemiologist friend terms this unease "dumbfounding." Without adequate reporting, an ensuing knowledge abyss overwhelms readers, peer reviewers, and systematic reviewers. Indeed, for systematic reviewers, incomplete reports of studies enormously complicate the entire review process.

We hope our use of scenarios gives some clue as to the difficulties created by inadequate reporting. We rely on scenarios involving the CONSORT 2010 statement [2, 10] because it is the most familiar reporting guideline to readers and presents, arguably, the most complicated reporting issues. Nevertheless, analogous misuses and ambiguities arise from other reporting guidelines, such as STROBE [11].

What also should be clear from the scenarios presented is that ambiguities and confusions dissipate with adequate reporting. Granted, reporting guidelines may breed some unease in authors of poorly conducted studies, but this is constructive unease that encourages better study conduct in the longer term. Most importantly, complete, clear and transparent reporting eliminates ambiguities and confusions.

Reporting guidelines form part of the solution to inadequate reporting. Nevertheless, guidelines by themselves offer meager assistance if they are not used by authors, peer reviewers, and editors [12]. Additional emphasis on knowledge translation should unleash more of the benefits from existing reporting guidelines.

References

1 Moher, D., Schulz, K.F., Simera, I. & Altman, D.G. (2010) Guidance for developers of health research reporting guidelines. *PLoS Medicine*, **7**, e1000217.

2 Schulz, K.F., Altman, D.G. & Moher, D. (2010) CONSORT 2010 statement: updated guidelines for reporting parallel group randomised trials. *BMJ*, **340**, c332.

3 Jüni, P., Witschi, A., Bloch, R. & Egger, M. (1999) The hazards of scoring the quality of clinical trials for meta-analysis. *JAMA*, **282**, 1054–1060.

4 Altman, D.G. & Doré, C.J. (1990) Randomisation and baseline comparisons in clinical trials. *Lancet*, **335**, 149–153.

5 Schulz, K.F., Chalmers, I., Hayes, R.J. & Altman, D.G., (1995) Empirical evidence of bias. Dimensions of methodological quality associated with estimates of treatment effects in controlled trials. *JAMA*, **273**, 408–412.

6 Schulz, K.F., Chalmers, I., Grimes, D.A. & Altman, D.G. (1994) Assessing the quality of randomization from reports of controlled trials published in obstetrics and gynecology journals. *JAMA*, **272**, 125–128.

7 Radford, J.A., Landorf, K.B., Buchbinder, R. & Cook, C. (2006) Effectiveness of low-dye taping for the short-term treatment of plantar heel pain: a randomised trial. *BMC Musculoskeletal Disorders*, **7**, 64.

8 Schulz, K.F. & Grimes, D.A. (2002) Unequal group sizes in randomised trials: guarding against guessing. *Lancet*, **359**, 966–970.

9 Schulz, K.F. & Grimes, D.A. (2002) Generation of allocation sequences in randomised trials: chance, not choice. *Lancet*, **359**, 515–519.

10 Moher, D., Hopewell, S., Schulz, K.F. *et al.* (2010) CONSORT 2010 Explanation and Elaboration: updated guidelines for reporting parallel group randomised trials. *Journal of Clinical Epidemiology*, **63**, e1–e37.

11 da Costa, B.R., Cevallos, M., Altman, D.G., *et al.* (2011) Uses and misuses of the STROBE statement: bibliographic study. *BMJ Open*, **1**, e000048.

12 Simera, I., Moher, D., Hirst, A., *et al.* (2010) Transparent and accurate reporting increases reliability, utility, and impact of your research: reporting guidelines and the EQUATOR Network. *BMC Medicine*, **8**, 24.

CHAPTER 6

The EQUATOR Network: Helping to Achieve High Standards in the Reporting of Health Research Studies

Iveta Simera[1], Allison Hirst[2] and Douglas G. Altman[1]

[1] *Centre for Statistics in Medicine, University of Oxford, Oxford, UK*
[2] *Nuffield Department of Surgical Sciences, University of Oxford, Oxford, UK*

Previous chapters have shown why transparent, accurate, complete, and timely reporting of research studies is important (Chapter 1) and how well-developed reporting guidelines (Chapter 2) can help in producing high-quality research publications (Chapters 3 and 4).

Over the past 15 years, we have seen a proliferation of published guidance on how to report a research study or some particular aspect of it [1]. Probably the first systematically developed reporting guideline was the CONsolidated Standards Of Reporting Trials (CONSORT) Statement for reporting randomized controlled trials [2], and numerous extensions have been published for specific study designs and types of intervention [3]. CONSORT has influenced the development of many other reporting guidelines well beyond the trials area.

As of January 2014, we have identified over 200 reporting guidelines published since 1996 [4]. The existence of such a large number and variety of published guidelines inevitably creates challenges: identification of all guidance relevant to a particular study is difficult and time consuming; the scope and development methods of available guidelines vary greatly, making it difficult for users to judge the robustness of their recommendations; and occasionally guidelines are not very clear in their scope or duplicate guidance exists for the same topic. Also, many potential users are not aware that so much helpful guidance exists. All these issues have contributed to an underuse of reporting guidelines by researchers writing up their studies as well as by journals instructing their authors on manuscript requirements.

Guidelines for Reporting Health Research: A User's Manual, First Edition. Edited by David Moher, Douglas G. Altman, Kenneth F. Schulz, Iveta Simera and Elizabeth Wager.
© 2014 John Wiley & Sons, Ltd. Published 2014 by John Wiley & Sons, Ltd.

The benefits of adhering to reporting guidelines are self-evident, and promoting their use to increase the number of usable and unbiased research reports is of utmost importance [5].

EQUATOR Network

The Enhancing the QUAlity and Transparency Of health Research (EQUATOR) Network program was launched in 2008 to promote the responsible reporting of health research studies and to tackle the slow uptake of reporting guidelines. EQUATOR is an international collaborative initiative led by experts in the area of research methodology, reporting, and editorial work. The team collaborates closely with key parties involved in the conduct and publication of research (academic and clinical researchers, journal editors, peer reviewers and technical staff, publishers, scientists developing reporting guidelines, educators, and research funders) all of whom share the responsibility for the quality of research publications. EQUATOR provides free online resources supported by education and training activities and assists in the development of robust reporting guidelines. Box 6.1 lists the major goals of the Network.

Box 6.1: Major goals of the EQUATOR Network

- Develop and maintain a comprehensive online resource center providing up-to-date information, tools, and other materials related to health research reporting
- Assist in the development, dissemination, and implementation of robust reporting guidelines
- Actively promote the use of reporting guidelines and good research reporting practices through an education and training program
- Conduct regular assessments of how journals implement and use reporting guidelines
- Conduct regular audits of reporting quality across the health research literature
- Set up a global network of local EQUATOR "centers" to facilitate the improvement of health research reporting on a worldwide scale
- Develop a general strategy for translating principles of responsible research reporting into practice

---

EQUATOR resources

The EQUATOR website (http://www.equator-network.org) provides a unique, single portal for scientists, editors and peer reviewers, funders, and anybody interested in responsible research reporting. The online *Library for Health Research Reporting* (Figure 6.1) hosts a comprehensive collection of reporting guidelines published since 1996; this collection is kept up-to-date through regular systematic literature searches. The guidelines are organized by broad study type to allow users to find guidelines

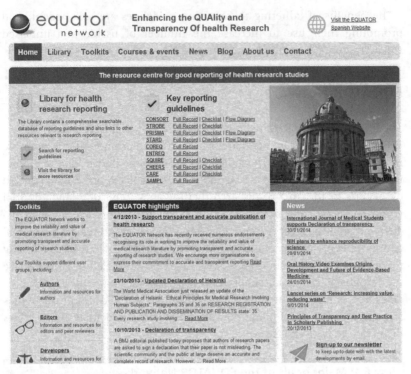

Figure 6.1 EQUATOR website.

relevant to their needs. The website also contains other guidance relevant to reporting: guidance on scientific writing, ethical conduct in research and publication, resources related to the development of robust reporting guidelines, examples of good research reporting, and highlights from new methodology literature.

The EQUATOR website is a useful resource not only for the later stages of the research process, when preparing manuscripts for publication but it can also help researchers planning a new study. Well-designed and conducted research is a prerequisite for a good publication. It is important for researchers to be aware of reporting expectations at the planning stage of the research process and think about reporting during the study to avoid mistakes that might later compromise the quality of their study publication.

The EQUATOR website is also a valuable reference point for journals who wish to implement effective policies and processes to aid accurate and transparent research reporting in their journals. The website provides links to guidance from influential editorial organizations, examples of good practices shared with us by journal editors, and editorials introducing reporting policies. In collaboration with editorial organizations, such as the International Society of Managing and Technical Editors [6], EQUATOR has developed education and training materials and practical tools to aid the implementation of reporting guidelines in editorial offices. In order to help journal editors to choose the most suitable guidelines for implementation in their journal and request an appropriate level of compliance from authors, we initiated the development of a reporting guideline assessment tool that will allow evaluation of available guidelines against identified criteria of importance.

Guideline development

Robustness of the methodology used to develop reporting guidelines is an important factor in the reliability and usefulness of reporting recommendations. At present, there is no one universally accepted "best" approach for such development. However, there is a wealth of collective experience from the last 15 years of the reporting guideline development "boom"; we have harnessed some of this experience [7] and have compiled useful resources for scientists who have identified a gap in guidance and wish to develop a robust reporting guideline [8].

Global reach

English is the language most used for the international communication of science; however, we recognize the challenges experienced by non-native English speakers in communicating their new research findings. The EQUATOR team is actively seeking collaborations to extend the reach of resources beyond English-speaking countries. Learning the principles of research methodology and reporting in one's native language is likely to improve the understanding of concepts and definitions. One of the first EQUATOR efforts in this direction has been the collaboration with the Pan American Health Organization (PAHO) to raise the standards of research reporting in South and Central America and the Caribbean. The EQUATOR website, including the whole *Library*, has been translated into Spanish. The site also contains a brief online English/Spanish glossary of methodological terminology [9].

  The provision of free resources, a wide geographical reach, and collaboration across different types of organizations (e.g., research institutions, professional organizations, funders, journals, publishers, etc.) are not the only important factors facilitating the improvement of quality of research reporting. Educational and hands-on training activities targeting all parties involved in research publishing are crucial to support effective implementation of responsible reporting and available tools. The EQUATOR team is currently directing educational activities to editors, peer reviewers, and researchers. However, targeting research students and early career research professionals will be key to ingraining good reporting habits early in their scientific careers.

EQUATOR future

The EQUATOR program is still at a relatively early stage, and there are many important areas that we plan to address in our future work [10]. These include

- strengthening the methodology for the development and assessment of reporting guidelines,
- investigating barriers to and facilitators of the use of reporting guidelines by various stakeholders,
- assessing the implementation of reporting guidelines and its impact on the quality of published research,
- increasing awareness of the EQUATOR Network and available resources worldwide and supporting activities leading to better reporting of health research.

The work of EQUATOR aims to increase the usability and value of available research evidence. An overview of scientific and scholarly journal publishing indicates that although readers read more articles per year they spend much less time on each article [11]. Scientific publications are being read, assessed, and used for a variety of reasons: from informing research or clinical practice to inclusion in systematic reviews and clinical practice guidelines. Published research articles must ideally satisfy the needs of all types of reader. This requires clarity, a well-structured format, and logical flow of the key information that should be reported. Adherence to robust reporting guidelines helps to produce articles that can withstand rigorous scrutiny and makes a real difference to their usability in future research or decisions relating to patients' care. The EQUATOR resources and activities are here to help achieve high standards in research publications and in health research itself.

Funding

The EQUATOR program is jointly funded by the UK National Institute for Health Research, UK Medical Research Council, Scottish Chief Scientist Office, Canadian Institutes of Health Research, and PAHO.

References

1 Simera, I., Moher, D., Hoey, J., *et al.* (2010) A catalogue of reporting guidelines for health research. *European Journal of Clinical Investigation*, **40**, 35–53.

2 Schulz, K.F., Altman, D.G. & Moher, D. (2010) for the CONSORT Group. CONSORT 2010 Statement: updated guidelines for reporting parallel group randomised trials. *PLoS Medicine*, **7** (3), e1000251.

3 CONSORT Statement website. http://www.consort-statement.org/ [accessed on 4 April 2011].

4 EQUATOR Network website, Library for Health Research Reporting. http://www. equator-network.org/library/ [accessed 3 February 2014].

5 Chalmers, I. & Glasziou, P. (2009) Avoidable waste in the production and reporting of research evidence. *Lancet*, **374**, 86–89.

6 International Society of Managing and Technical Editors. http://www.ismte.org/ [accessed on 4 April 2011].

7 Moher, D., Schulz, K.F., Simera, I. & Altman, D.G. (2010) Guidance for developers of health research reporting guidelines. *PLoS Medicine*, **7**, e1000217.

8 EQUATOR Network, Resources for Reporting Guidelines Developers. http://www. equator-network.org/toolkits/developers/ [accessed 3 February 2014]

9 EQUATOR Network, Spanish version. http://www.espanol.equator-network.org/ [accessed on 4 April 2011].

10 Simera, I., Moher, D., Hirst, A., *et al.* (2010) Transparent and accurate reporting increases reliability, utility, and impact of your research: reporting guidelines and the EQUATOR Network. *BMC Medicine*, **8** (1), 24.

11 Ware, M. & Mabe, M. (2009) The STM report: an overview of scientific and scholarly journals publishing. http://www.stm-assoc.org/news.php?id=255&PHPSESSID =3c5575d0663c0e04a4600d7f04afe91f [accessed on 30 March 2011].

PART II

Specific Reporting Guidelines

CHAPTER 7

SPIRIT (Standard Protocol Items: Recommendations for Interventional Trials)

David Moher[1] and An-Wen Chan[2,3,4]

[1] *Clinical Epidemiology Program, Ottawa Hospital Research Institute, Ottawa, ON, Canada*
[2] *Women's College Research Institute, Toronto, ON, Canada*
[3] *ICES@UofT, Toronto, ON, Canada*
[4] *Department of Medicine, Women's College Hospital, University of Toronto, Toronto, ON, Canada*

Name of guideline

The SPIRIT 2013 Statement (Standard Protocol Items: Recommendations for Interventional Trials) [1] contains guidance for authors of protocols for randomized and nonrandomized clinical trials. Funding agencies, institutional review boards (IRB), journals, and regulators can also use SPIRIT as their standard guidance for the content of submitted protocols.

At its core, the SPIRIT 2013 Statement is a 33-item checklist defining minimum content for a clinical trial protocol. The 33 items are divided into five sections, covering administrative information (5 items), the introduction (3 items), methods (15 items), ethics and dissemination (8 items), and appendices (2 items). SPIRIT also recommends that protocols include a diagram depicting the proposed schedule of enrollment, interventions, and assessments.

Where possible, SPIRIT 2013 checklist items mirror those in CONSORT 2010 to enable authors to convert protocol text efficiently to a trial report based on CONSORT 2010.

The SPIRIT initiative also includes a comprehensive Explanation and Elaboration (E&E) paper [2]. This document provides information to promote a more complete understanding of the checklist recommendations. For each checklist item, the SPIRIT 2013 E&E paper provides a rationale, detailed description, examples from actual protocols, and relevant

Guidelines for Reporting Health Research: A User's Manual, First Edition. Edited by David Moher, Douglas G. Altman, Kenneth F. Schulz, Iveta Simera and Elizabeth Wager.
© 2014 John Wiley & Sons, Ltd. Published 2014 by John Wiley & Sons, Ltd.

references supporting its importance. We strongly recommend that the
E&E paper be used in conjunction with the SPIRIT 2013 Statement.

When to use this guideline (what types of studies it covers)

SPIRIT defines a protocol as a document that enables readers to understand,
in sufficient detail, the background, rationale, objectives, study population,
interventions, methods, statistical analyses, ethical considerations, dissemination plans, and administration of a proposed trial; replicate key aspects
of trial methods and conduct; and appraise the trial's scientific and ethical
rigor. SPIRIT 2013 can be used by investigators developing any type of clinical trial protocol, regardless of topic, intervention type, or study design. It
is relevant for any research study that prospectively assigns human participants to one or more interventions in order to measure the effects on
health-related outcomes.

Current version

The SPIRIT 2013 statement is published in the *Annals of Internal Medicine*
[1], and the SPIRIT 2013 (E&E) paper is published in the *BMJ* [2]. Both
papers are open access. The checklist and explanatory text are also available
on the SPIRIT website (www.spirit-statement.org), along with resources to
facilitate implementation.

Extensions or implementations

No extensions or implementations of SPIRIT 2013 have been published to
date. However, a similar initiative is under development for protocols of
systematic reviews – the PRISMA-P statement [3]. The PRISMA-P statement aims to help authors draft protocols of systematic reviews (item 5,
PRISMA checklist) and to facilitate their registration – PROSPERO [4, 5].

Related activities

The SPIRIT Group is exploring opportunities for collaboration with other
groups involved in promoting protocol standards – such as IRBs, trial
registries, the Clinical Data Interchange Standards Consortium (CDISC)

Protocol Representation Group, and Pragmatic Randomized Controlled Trials in HealthCare (PRACTIHC).

How best to use the guideline

By providing guidance for protocol content, SPIRIT 2013 aims to facilitate protocol development for clinical trial investigators. The explanatory paper also serves as an educational resource to promote understanding of each recommended checklist item.

It is hoped that improvements in protocol completeness will improve the conduct, efficiency, and external review of trials [6]. Better protocols can help trial personnel to implement the trial in a robust manner. High-quality protocols should also be easier for IRBs and funders to review and reduce the number of avoidable amendments, which can help prevent costly delays. If investigators adequately address all of the SPIRIT items, there will likely be fewer queries from the IRB to the investigators, thereby reducing the overall time for approval.

Development process

Several stakeholder groups (clinical trial investigators and coordinators, health care professionals, methodologists and statisticians, IRBs, ethicists, pharmaceutical industry and government funders, regulatory agencies, and medical journal editors) involving more than 100 individuals helped to develop SPIRIT 2013.

As with the development of other reporting guidelines, SPIRIT 2013 included two systematic reviews which characterized existing guidance for reporting clinical trial protocols [7] and identified empirical evidence relating to the relevance of specific protocol items for trial conduct or risk of bias [8]. An extensive Delphi process [9] involving 96 participants, and two in-person consensus meetings (2007 and 2009), were also conducted. The initial checklist of 59 potential items evolved into 33 items by the end of the development process.

The SPIRIT 2013 Statement was drafted, discussed, and refined over email by the SPIRIT group. A similar process was used by a subset of SPIRIT group members to draft the SPIRIT 2013 explanatory paper [2]. To identify examples for each checklist item, the SPIRIT group obtained protocols from public websites, journals, trial investigators, and industry sponsors. Finally, the checklist was pilot tested with graduate students from two Masters level courses on clinical trials.

Evidence of effectiveness of guideline

No evaluations of SPIRIT 2013 have been published. We are aware of one ongoing and one planned evaluation of protocol adherence to SPIRIT. We encourage others to consider such an evaluation [Adrienne Stevens, systematic review underway, personal communication].

Endorsement and adherence

By endorsing SPIRIT, stakeholders with enforcement capability can help to achieve the intended impact of improving the completeness of protocols as well as the quality and efficiency of their review. IRBs, funders, journals, and regulators can encourage investigators to ensure that submitted protocols adhere to SPIRIT. Several journals advise authors to develop their protocols using SPIRIT. A list of supporters is available on the SPIRIT website (www.spirit-statement.org).

Cautions and limitations (including scope)

SPIRIT 2013 is not a tool to help readers assess the quality of clinical trial protocols as investigators could fully address all SPIRIT checklist items and yet describe inadequate methods. Using the checklist to construct a quality score is not advised. SPIRIT 2013 is also not intended to be used for reporting a completed clinical trial; authors should instead use CONSORT 2010 [10] or one of the extensions for this purpose (see Chapters 8–14).

SPIRIT 2013 is designed to be a minimum standard that is broadly applicable to all types of clinical trials regardless of study design, intervention, or topic. There may be specific issues that are important to a particular protocol but are not covered in SPIRIT, such as carryover effects in analyzing crossover trials. Authors are encouraged to address additional protocol items as needed.

Creators' preferred bits

Outcomes

Outcomes are central to all clinical trial protocols (item 12). Outcomes are fundamental to the objectives, sample size, analysis, and interpretation of the planned trial. The choice of outcomes should reflect measures that are valid, reproducible, responsive, and patient centered. SPIRIT 2013 recommends that protocol authors detail four components of each proposed primary and secondary outcome: the measurement variable (e.g., serum hemoglobin A1c, all-cause mortality), the value to be used from each trial participant for analysis (e.g., change from baseline, final value), the method used to aggregate each participant's response to produce a summary measure for each study group (e.g., mean, scoring above a prespecified threshold), and the specific measurement time point of interest for analysis.

Sample size

The planned number of participants included in a clinical trial is important not only from a statistical sense but also in terms of its relevance to the trial budget and feasibility. The method of determining the planned sample size, whether through a statistical or nonstatistical process, needs to be explicitly described in the protocol in order to facilitate transparency and assessment of the trial's ability to achieve its objectives. When derived through a formal calculation, the sample size estimate is generally dependent on the expected values for the primary outcome, the statistical analysis plan, the desired power, and the anticipated amount of missing data. If protocol authors document the sample size information recommended by SPIRIT, then this will make it easier to transparently describe the sample size considerations in the final trial report in adherence to CONSORT 2010.

Administrative information

This section includes five items enshrining several important administrative elements of trial protocol development and conduct, including the title, protocol version, trial registration, funding, and the roles and responsibilities of the sponsor and key members of the protocol development team. A descriptive title and the protocol version help to identify the trial and most recent protocol document and amendments. Having a trial registration section in the protocol serves as a trial summary and a reminder to update the registry record whenever this section is modified. Relevant information can simply be copied from this protocol section into the registry, which may improve the quality of registry records. Finally, an explicit description of the roles of the sponsor, funders, protocol contributors, and key trial groups provides accountability, transparency, and identification of potential competing interests.

Future plans

The SPIRIT group is implementing a comprehensive strategy to maximize uptake across a broad spectrum of stakeholders. The strategy includes dissemination, endorsement, and evaluation. Various implementation resources, including a web-based protocol authoring tool, are being developed to help investigators draft their protocol based on the SPIRIT 2013 recommendations.

References

1 Chan, A.W., Tetzlaff, J.M., Altman, D.G. *et al.* (2013) SPIRIT 2013 Statement: defining standard protocol items for clinical trials. *Annals of Internal Medicine*, **158**, 200–207.

2 Chan, A.W., Tetzlaff, J.M., Gøtzsche, P.C. *et al.* (2013) SPIRIT 2013 explanation and elaboration: guidance for protocols of clinical trials. *BMJ*, **346**, e7586.

3 Moher, D., Shamseer, L., Clarke, M. *et al. Reporting Guidelines for Systematic Review Protocols*. 10th Annual Cochrane Canada Symposium. Winnipeg, Canada. May 9–10, 2012.

4 Booth, A., Clarke, M., Dooley, G. *et al.* (2012) The nuts and bolts of PROSPERO: an international prospective register of systematic reviews. *Systematic Reviews*, **1**, 2.

5 Booth, A., Clarke, M., Dooley, G. *et al.* (2013) PROSPERO at one year: an evaluation of its utility. *Systematic Reviews*, **2**, 4.

6 Chan, A.W., Tetzlaff, J., Altman, D., *et al.* (2013) SPIRIT: new guidance for content of clinical trial protocols. *Lancet*, **381**, 91–92.

7 Tetzlaff, J.M., Chan, A.W., Kitchen, J., *et al.* (2012) Guidelines for randomized clinical trial protocol content: a systematic review. *Systematic Reviews*, **1**, 43.

8 Tetzlaff, J.M. (2010) *Developing an evidence-based reporting guideline for randomized controlled trial protocols: the SPIRIT Initiative*. ProQuest Dissertations and Theses, 1–183. University of Ottawa, Canada.

9 Tetzlaff, J.M., Moher, D. & Chan, A.W. (2012) Developing a guideline for clinical trial protocol content: Delphi consensus survey. *Trials*, **13**, 176.

10 Schulz, K.F., Altman, D.G. & Moher, D. (2010) CONSORT 2010 statement: updated guidelines for reporting parallel group randomized trials. *Annals of Internal Medicine*, **152**, 726–732.

SPIRIT 2013 checklist: recommended items to address in a clinical trial protocol and related documents*

Section/item	Item No	Description
Administrative information		
Title	1	Descriptive title identifying the study design, population, interventions, and, if applicable, trial acronym
Trial registration	2a	Trial identifier and registry name. If not yet registered, name of intended registry
	2b	All items from the World Health Organization Trial Registration Data Set
Protocol version	3	Date and version identifier
Funding	4	Sources and types of financial, material, and other support
Roles and responsibilities	5a	Names, affiliations, and roles of protocol contributors
	5b	Name and contact information for the trial sponsor
	5c	Role of study sponsor and funders, if any, in study design; collection, management, analysis, and interpretation of data; writing of the report; and the decision to submit the report for publication, including whether they will have ultimate authority over any of these activities
	5d	Composition, roles, and responsibilities of the coordinating centre, steering committee, endpoint adjudication committee, data management team, and other individuals or groups overseeing the trial, if applicable (see Item 21a for data monitoring committee)
Introduction		
Background and rationale	6a	Description of research question and justification for undertaking the trial, including summary of relevant studies (published and unpublished) examining benefits and harms for each intervention
	6b	Explanation for choice of comparators
Objectives	7	Specific objectives or hypotheses
Trial design	8	Description of trial design including type of trial (eg, parallel group, crossover, factorial, single group), allocation ratio, and framework (eg, superiority, equivalence, noninferiority, exploratory)

(*continued*)

Section/item	Item No	Description
Methods: Participants, interventions, and outcomes		
Study setting	9	Description of study settings (eg, community clinic, academic hospital) and list of countries where data will be collected. Reference to where list of study sites can be obtained
Eligibility criteria	10	Inclusion and exclusion criteria for participants. If applicable, eligibility criteria for study centres and individuals who will perform the interventions (eg, surgeons, psychotherapists)
Interventions	11a	Interventions for each group with sufficient detail to allow replication, including how and when they will be administered
	11b	Criteria for discontinuing or modifying allocated interventions for a given trial participant (eg, drug dose change in response to harms, participant request, or improving/worsening disease)
	11c	Strategies to improve adherence to intervention protocols, and any procedures for monitoring adherence (eg, drug tablet return, laboratory tests)
	11d	Relevant concomitant care and interventions that are permitted or prohibited during the trial
Outcomes	12	Primary, secondary, and other outcomes, including the specific measurement variable (eg, systolic blood pressure), analysis metric (eg, change from baseline, final value, time to event), method of aggregation (eg, median, proportion), and time point for each outcome. Explanation of the clinical relevance of chosen efficacy and harm outcomes is strongly recommended
Participant timeline	13	Time schedule of enrolment, interventions (including any run-ins and washouts), assessments, and visits for participants. A schematic diagram is highly recommended (see Figure)
Sample size	14	Estimated number of participants needed to achieve study objectives and how it was determined, including clinical and statistical assumptions supporting any sample size calculations
Recruitment	15	Strategies for achieving adequate participant enrolment to reach target sample size

Section/item	Item No	Description

Methods: Assignment of interventions (for controlled trials)

Allocation:

Sequence generation	16a	Method of generating the allocation sequence (eg, computer-generated random numbers), and list of any factors for stratification. To reduce predictability of a random sequence, details of any planned restriction (eg, blocking) should be provided in a separate document that is unavailable to those who enrol participants or assign interventions
Allocation concealment mechanism	16b	Mechanism of implementing the allocation sequence (eg, central telephone; sequentially numbered, opaque, sealed envelopes), describing any steps to conceal the sequence until interventions are assigned
Implementation	16c	Who will generate the allocation sequence, who will enrol participants, and who will assign participants to interventions
Blinding (masking)	17a	Who will be blinded after assignment to interventions (eg, trial participants, care providers, outcome assessors, data analysts), and how
	17b	If blinded, circumstances under which unblinding is permissible, and procedure for revealing a participant's allocated intervention during the trial

Methods: Data collection, management, and analysis

Data collection methods	18a	Plans for assessment and collection of outcome, baseline, and other trial data, including any related processes to promote data quality (eg, duplicate measurements, training of assessors) and a description of study instruments (eg, questionnaires, laboratory tests) along with their reliability and validity, if known. Reference to where data collection forms can be found, if not in the protocol
	18b	Plans to promote participant retention and complete follow-up, including list of any outcome data to be collected for participants who discontinue or deviate from intervention protocols
Data management	19	Plans for data entry, coding, security, and storage, including any related processes to promote data quality (eg, double data entry; range checks for data values). Reference to where details of data management procedures can be found, if not in the protocol

(continued)

Section/item	Item No	Description
Statistical methods	20a	Statistical methods for analysing primary and secondary outcomes. Reference to where other details of the statistical analysis plan can be found, if not in the protocol
	20b	Methods for any additional analyses (eg, subgroup and adjusted analyses)
	20c	Definition of analysis population relating to protocol non-adherence (eg, as randomised analysis), and any statistical methods to handle missing data (eg, multiple imputation)
Methods: Monitoring		
Data monitoring	21a	Composition of data monitoring committee (DMC); summary of its role and reporting structure; statement of whether it is independent from the sponsor and competing interests; and reference to where further details about its charter can be found, if not in the protocol. Alternatively, an explanation of why a DMC is not needed
	21b	Description of any interim analyses and stopping guidelines, including who will have access to these interim results and make the final decision to terminate the trial
Harms	22	Plans for collecting, assessing, reporting, and managing solicited and spontaneously reported adverse events and other unintended effects of trial interventions or trial conduct
Auditing	23	Frequency and procedures for auditing trial conduct, if any, and whether the process will be independent from investigators and the sponsor
Ethics and dissemination		
Research ethics approval	24	Plans for seeking research ethics committee/institutional review board (REC/IRB) approval
Protocol amendments	25	Plans for communicating important protocol modifications (eg, changes to eligibility criteria, outcomes, analyses) to relevant parties (eg, investigators, REC/IRBs, trial participants, trial registries, journals, regulators)
Consent or assent	26a	Who will obtain informed consent or assent from potential trial participants or authorised surrogates, and how (see Item 32)
	26b	Additional consent provisions for collection and use of participant data and biological specimens in ancillary studies, if applicable

Section/item	Item No	Description
Confidentiality	27	How personal information about potential and enrolled participants will be collected, shared, and maintained in order to protect confidentiality before, during, and after the trial
Declaration of interests	28	Financial and other competing interests for principal investigators for the overall trial and each study site
Access to data	29	Statement of who will have access to the final trial dataset, and disclosure of contractual agreements that limit such access for investigators
Ancillary and post-trial care	30	Provisions, if any, for ancillary and post-trial care, and for compensation to those who suffer harm from trial participation
Dissemination policy	31a	Plans for investigators and sponsor to communicate trial results to participants, healthcare professionals, the public, and other relevant groups (eg, via publication, reporting in results databases, or other data sharing arrangements), including any publication restrictions
	31b	Authorship eligibility guidelines and any intended use of professional writers
	31c	Plans, if any, for granting public access to the full protocol, participant-level dataset, and statistical code
Appendices		
Informed consent materials	32	Model consent form and other related documentation given to participants and authorised surrogates
Biological specimens	33	Plans for collection, laboratory evaluation, and storage of biological specimens for genetic or molecular analysis in the current trial and for future use in ancillary studies, if applicable

CHAPTER 8

CONSORT for Abstracts

Sally Hopewell[1,2,3,4] *and Mike Clarke*[5]

[1] *Centre for Statistics in Medicine, University of Oxford, Oxford, UK*
[2] *INSERM, U738, Paris, France*
[3] *AP-HP (Assistance Publique des Hôpitaux de Paris), Hôpital Hôtel Dieu,*
Centre d'Epidémiologie Clinique, Paris, France
[4] *Univ. Paris Descartes, Sorbonne Paris Cité, Paris, France*
[5] *All-Ireland Hub for Trials Methodology Research, Centre for Public Health,*
Queens University Belfast, Belfast, Northern Ireland

Timetable

Name of reporting guideline initiative	Notes	Consensus meeting date	Reporting guideline publication
CONSORT for reporting randomized trials in journal and conference abstracts	Extension incorporated into main CONSORT checklist in 2010	January 2007	January 2008 1. Statement [1] 2. Explanation and Elaboration paper [2]

Name of guideline

CONsolidated Standards Of Reporting Trials (CONSORT) for reporting randomized trials in journal and conference abstracts was developed as an extension of the CONSORT statement to provide a list of essential items that authors should include when reporting the main results of a randomized trial in the abstract of a journal article or in a conference abstract. In this chapter, we refer to this extension as CONSORT for Abstracts.

History

Clear, transparent, and sufficiently detailed abstracts of conference presentations and journal articles reporting randomized trials are important

Guidelines for Reporting Health Research: A User's Manual, First Edition. Edited by David Moher, Douglas G. Altman, Kenneth F. Schulz, Iveta Simera and Elizabeth Wager.
© 2014 John Wiley & Sons, Ltd. Published 2014 by John Wiley & Sons, Ltd.

because readers will often base their initial assessment of a trial on the content of the abstract. In some cases, health practitioners will have access only to the abstract, and may, therefore, make health care decisions based solely on the information in that abstract [3]. Where a trial is reported only as a conference abstract, this may provide the only permanent record of a study and the only way its findings can be accessed by most readers [4].

The CONSORT Statement was first published in 1996 [5] and was updated in 2001 [6] and 2010 [7] (see Chapter 8). The 2001 CONSORT Statement provided limited guidance about reporting the results of a randomized trial in the abstract. It encouraged the use of a structured format, but this was not a formal requirement. Before 2008, the International Committee of Medical Journal Editors (ICMJE) Uniform Requirements also provided limited guidance on the format of abstracts for reports of randomized trials in journal articles [8]. A study published in 2006 that examined 35 journals' "Instructions to Authors" found that only 4% of the instructional text was devoted to the content or format of the abstract [9].

In response to these limitations and in the belief that journals and conference organizers should do more to provide specific instructions about the key elements of a trial that authors should report, within the space limitations of an abstract (typically 250–300 words), we began to develop an extension to the CONSORT Statement. The CONSORT for Abstracts checklist and accompanying explanatory document was published in January 2008 [1, 2]. Since publication, the checklist was incorporated into the recently revised main CONSORT Statement in March 2010 [7, 10]. In October 2008, the ICMJE also recommended that "all articles on clinical trials should contain abstracts that include the items that the CONSORT Group has identified as essential" (www.icmje.org).

When to use this guideline (what types of studies it covers)

CONSORT for Abstracts provides guidance for reporting the main results (i.e., the prespecified primary outcomes) of parallel group randomized trials in journals or conference abstracts.

Because the Ad Hoc Working Group for Critical Appraisal of the Medical Literature [11] first published recommendations for the adoption of structured abstracts in 1987, many journals have promoted their use and many different structures now exist. We therefore recognized that many journals have developed their own set of headings for abstracts, which they feel are of most help to their readers. CONSORT for Abstracts therefore does not suggest how an abstract should be structured (i.e., what the headings should be) but, rather, it recommends what information should be reported within them when describing a randomized trial.

It is important to note that space limitations mean that it will only be possible to provide a limited amount of information about a trial within an abstract, so the available words need to be used carefully to maximize the transfer of knowledge about the trial. CONSORT for Abstracts provides guidance on the key information that should be reported within these constraints.

Development process

CONSORT for Abstracts was developed in collaboration with the CONSORT Group, and the process was led by a small steering committee. To develop the checklist, we generated a list of potential items from existing quality assessment and reporting tools, including the CONSORT Statement itself [6] and other guidance for the structured reporting of journal abstracts and short reports [11–14]. We then used a modified Delphi consensus method to select and reduce the number of possible checklist items. A total of 109 people with an interest in trial reporting or the structure of abstracts, participated in a web-based survey to rate the importance of suggested checklist items [2]. Respondents included journal editors, health care professionals, methodologists, statisticians, and trialists. During three rounds of the survey, participants were asked to rate the relative importance of the possible checklist items.

The results of the survey were presented at a one-day meeting in January 2007, in Montebello, Canada, attended by 26 participants several of whom had participated in the Delphi survey. The meeting began with a review of the checklist items proposed as a result of the Delphi process. Participants then discussed whether these items should be included, excluded, or modified in the final checklist. Following the meeting, the checklist was revised and circulated to the steering committee and meeting participants to ensure that it reflected the discussions. The steering committee also developed an explanation and elaboration document, which was iterated several times among the authors.

Current version compared with the previous versions

The CONSORT for Abstracts checklist and explanatory document were published in January 2008 [1, 2]. While this remains the current version, the guidance has also been incorporated into the recently revised CONSORT

Statement 2010 [7], with guidance included in its accompanying explanation and elaboration document [10].

Extensions and/or implementations

There are two recently published extensions to the CONSORT for Abstracts checklist – one for the reporting of abstracts of cluster randomized trials [15] and the other for abstracts of noninferiority and equivalence trials [16]. However, there may be other instances where different types of trial information, such as composite outcomes, different designs, or different areas of health care will require additional information. Therefore, additional extensions or adaptions to the checklist may be warranted, as has been done for the CONSORT Statement for full reports [17–21].

How best to use the guideline

The CONSORT for Abstracts checklist for reporting an abstract of a randomized trial recommends including information about the objectives, design (e.g., method of allocation, blinding), participants (i.e., description, numbers randomized and analyzed), interventions intended for each randomized group and their effect on primary efficacy outcomes and harms, conclusions, registration name and number, and source of funding [1, 2].

We recommended using the CONSORT for Abstracts checklist in conjunction with its explanatory document which includes a description of each checklist item, a recent example of good reporting of the item, an explanation including the rationale and scientific background and, where available, the evidence for including the item as it relates to trials reported in journal or conference abstracts [2].

Journals and conference organizers should provide specific instructions about the key elements of a trial that authors should report. In developing CONSORT for Abstracts, preparatory work showed that all the checklist items can be accommodated within the typical 250 to 300 word limit of an abstract.

Evidence of effectiveness of guideline

Journal and conference abstracts should contain sufficient information about a trial to provide an accurate record of its conduct and findings, providing optimal information about the trial within the space constraints of the abstract format. A properly constructed and written abstract should enable readers to assess quickly the validity and applicability of the findings and in the case of abstracts of journal articles, aid the identification of reports within electronic databases [22]. Conference abstracts, in particular, can provide valuable information for systematic reviewers about studies not otherwise published, the exclusion of which from the review might introduce bias [23].

A number of studies have highlighted poor reporting in conference and journal abstracts presenting the results of randomized trials [24]. There are concerns over the accuracy and quality of trial reports published in the proceedings of scientific meetings, including lack of information about the trial and the robustness of the presented results [25–27]. Studies have also shown that trial information reported in conference abstracts may differ from that reported in subsequent full publications of the same study [28–30].

The abstracts of journal articles have similar limitations to conference abstracts. Studies comparing the accuracy of information in journal abstracts with that found in the main text have found claims that are inconsistent with, or missing from, the body of the full article [31–33]. Conversely, omitting important contrary results from the abstract, such as those concerning side effects, could seriously mislead someone's interpretation of the trial findings [34].

CONSORT for Abstracts addresses some of these problems of poor reporting. Several studies [35–41] have assessed the impact of CONSORT for Abstracts and suggest some improvements in reporting following publication of the guideline; however, the overall adherence to specific checklist items remains poor. A recent study [42] investigated the effect of different journal editorial policies to implement the CONSORT for Abstracts guideline on the reporting quality of 944 abstracts of randomized trials published between 2006 and 2009. This study found that the two journals (*Annals of Internal Medicine* and *The Lancet*) that had an active policy to implement the guideline showed a significant increase in the number of checklist items reported following publication of CONSORT for Abstracts in 2008. However, there was no improvement in the number of checklist items reported in the three journals (*BMJ*, *JAMA*, and *New England Journal of Medicine*) that did not have a policy to actively implement the guideline.

Endorsement and adherence

In October 2008, the ICMJE formally endorsed CONSORT for Abstracts. They stated that "all articles on clinical trials should contain abstracts that include the items that the CONSORT Group has identified as essential" (www.icmje.org).

On a broader level, the main CONSORT Statement from 2010, in which the CONSORT for Abstracts checklist is incorporated [7, 10], has been widely endorsed by organizations such as the World Association of Medical Editors, the ICMJE, the Council of Science Editors, and more than four hundred journals and editorial groups worldwide. The main CONSORT Statement has also been translated into many different languages. It is hoped that incorporation of the CONSORT for Abstracts checklist within the main CONSORT Statement will assist in promoting its endorsement and ultimately improve adherence to the guidance.

Journals and conference organizers should endorse the use of CONSORT for Abstracts by modifying their "Instructions to Authors" and drawing attention to the checklist through an editorial in their journal or, in the case of conference organizers, by making it a requirement for abstract submission and including a link to the checklist on the conference website. They should also institute procedures to check that authors and presenters follow the guidance.

Cautions and limitations (including scope)

As with the main CONSORT Statement, CONSORT for Abstracts urges completeness, clarity, and transparency of reporting, to reflect accurately the trial design and its conduct. However, as with any other reporting guideline there is a danger that authors might report fictitiously the information required in the guideline rather than what was actually done in the trial [10]. The prospective registration of trials and access to trial protocols is one way to help researchers, editors, and peer reviewers safeguard against this potential for fraud.

The CONSORT for Abstracts checklist is principally designed as a reporting guideline and therefore should not be used as a tool for assessing the quality of abstracts of randomized trials. There are many examples in the literature where the main CONSORT Statement has been used as an instrument to assess the quality of reports of randomized trials and an overall quality assessment score assigned. Such practices should be discouraged as CONSORT was designed to encourage transparency in reporting how and what authors did and not to make judgments about how and what authors should have done.

Mistakes and/or misconceptions

A common misconception is that the current word limit for abstracts in journals and conferences is not long enough to report all items required in the CONSORT for Abstracts checklist. In the past, MEDLINE truncated journal abstracts at 250 words [43] and this resulted in many journals imposing a limit of 250 words for their abstracts. However, since 2000 the National Library of Medicine increased the word limit for an abstract appearing in MEDLINE to 10,000 characters which is sufficient for more than 1000 words. While most abstract reports will not come close to 1000 words, such a word length will be sufficient to report even the most complex of trials in abstract form. In developing the checklist, 250 to 300 words were found to be sufficient to address all of the items in the checklist for typical trials. Worked examples of using the CONSORT for Abstracts checklist are available on the CONSORT website at www.consort-statement.org.

Creators' preferred bits

These recommendations arise from both the importance of internal validity (minimising bias) and the need to improve the general level of reporting in the literature. We have selected items that are important but are frequently inadequately reported, for our "creators' top three preferred bits" list:

State how participants were allocated to interventions

The method used to allocate participants to an intervention is the principal way of reducing bias within a randomized trial. Allocation concealment is generally poorly reported in conference and journal abstracts [26, 44, 45]. For example, in a review of 494 abstracts presented at an oncology conference in 1992 and 2002, only nine abstracts reported the method of allocation concealment [26].

For the primary outcome, a result for each group and the estimated effect size and its precision should be stated

For the primary outcome, authors should report trial results as a summary of the outcome in each group (e.g., the number of participants with or without the event or the mean and standard deviation of measurements), together with the contrast between groups known as the effect size and its precision. Studies have identified deficiencies in the reporting of statistical results in journal abstracts [46–48] and found that journal abstracts of randomized trials tended to overemphasize statistically significant outcomes compared with the full journal article, leading to problems in interpretation of the results. Poor reporting of results is also a problem for trials presented in conference abstracts [27, 49].

Include the registration number and name of trial register

Registration information is particularly important for conference abstracts, as a large proportion of these are not subsequently published [4]. Information on the trial's registration provides readers with a way to obtain more information about the trial and makes it easier to link abstracts with subsequent full publications (or multiple abstracts from the same trial).

Future plans

As with any reporting guideline, CONSORT for Abstracts is an evolving document built around the best available evidence. The evidence for what is important in reporting the findings from randomized trials is dynamic and as the evidence base evolves so does the need to update these guidelines. Regular monitoring of the scientific literature will help ensure that CONSORT for Abstracts remains current and up-to-date.

Work to promote the endorsement and adherence of the CONSORT for Abstracts checklist by journals has been greatly helped by its endorsement by the ICMJE and its inclusion in the newly revised CONSORT Statement 2010. There is a need to continue to monitor its impact and, as with the main CONSORT Statement, emphasis is now on promoting endorsement and doing more to try and ensure adherence by authors and journal editors.

Progress in promoting endorsement and ensuring adherence of CONSORT for Abstracts at scientific conferences have been more problematic and, while there have been some successes, more work is needed in this area. Implementation is made more difficult because unlike journal editors, members of scientific conference committees often change from year to year so it can be difficult to know who to target. More work is needed in targeting clinical societies to get endorsement of the CONSORT for Abstracts guidelines, which would then be filtered down to the committees of individual scientific conferences.

Acknowledgments

We would like to acknowledge the work of David Moher, Liz Wager, and Philippa Middleton who contributed to the CONSORT for Abstracts explanation and elaboration document on which this chapter is based.

Checklist: items to include when reporting a randomized trial in a journal or conference abstract

Item	Description
Title	Identification of the study as randomized
Authors[a]	Contact details for the corresponding author
Trial design	Description of the trial design (e.g., parallel, cluster, noninferiority)
Methods	
Participants	Eligibility criteria for participants and the settings where the data were collected
Interventions	Interventions intended for each group
Objective	Specific objective or hypothesis
Outcome	Clearly defined primary outcome for this report
Randomization	How participants were allocated to interventions
Blinding (masking)	Whether participants, care givers, and those assessing the outcomes were blinded to group assignment
Results	
Numbers randomized	Number of participants randomized to each group
Recruitment	Trial status
Numbers analysed	Number of participants analysed in each group
Outcome	For the primary outcome, a result for each group and the estimated effect size and its precision
Harms	Important adverse events or side effects
Conclusions	General interpretation of the results
Trial registration	Registration number and name of trial register
Funding	Source of funding

[a]This item is specific to conference abstracts.

References

1 Hopewell, S., Clarke, M., Moher, D. *et al.* (26 January 2008) CONSORT for reporting randomised trials in journal and conference abstracts. *Lancet*, **371** (9609), 281–283.
2 Hopewell, S., Clarke, M., Moher, D. *et al.* (22 January 2008) CONSORT for reporting randomized controlled trials in journal and conference abstracts: explanation and elaboration. *PLoS Medicine*, **5** (1), e20.
3 The PLoS Medicine Editors. (May 2006) The impact of open access upon public health. *PLoS Med*, **3** (5), e252.

4 Scherer, R.W., Langenberg, P., von Elm, E. Full publication of results initially pre-sented in abstracts. *Cochrane Database of Methodology Reviews* 2007, MR00005. doi:10 1002/14651858.

5 Begg, C., Cho, M., Eastwood, S. *et al.* (1996) Improving the quality of reporting of randomized controlled trials. The CONSORT statement. *JAMA*, **28** (276), 637–639.

6 Moher, D., Schulz, K.F. & Altman, D.G. (2001) The CONSORT statement: revised recommendations for improving the quality of reports of parallel-group randomised trials. *Lancet*, **357** (9263), 1191–1194.

7 Schulz, K.F., Altman, D.G. & Moher, D. (2010) CONSORT 2010 statement: updated guidelines for reporting parallel group randomized trials. *Annals of Internal Medicine*, **152** (11), 726–732.

8 International Committee of Medical Journal Editors. Uniform requirements for manuscripts submitted to biomedical journals: writing and editing for biomedical publication [updated February 2006]. Available from www.icmje.org [Accessed on 1 December 2006; 1996].

9 Schriger, D.L., Arora, S. & Altman, D.G. (2006) The content of medical journal instructions for authors. *Annals of Emergency Medicine*, **48** (6), 743–748.

10 Moher, D., Hopewell, S., Schulz, K.F. *et al.* (2010) CONSORT 2010 Explanation and Elaboration: Updated guidelines for reporting parallel group randomised trials. *Journal of Clinical Epidemiology*, **63** (8), e1–e37.

11 Ad Hoc Working Group for Critical Appraisal of the Medical Literature (1987) A proposal for more informative abstracts. *Annals of Internal Medicine*, **106**, 598–604.

12 Haynes, R.B., Mulrow, C.D., Huth, E.J., *et al.* (1996) More informative abstracts revisited. *Cleft Palate-Craniofacial Journal*, **33** (1), 1–9.

13 Haynes, R.B., Mulrow, C.D., Huth, E.J., *et al.* (1990) More informative abstracts revised. *Annals of Internal Medicine*, **113** (1), 69–76.

14 Deeks, J.J. & Altman, D.G. (1998) Inadequate reporting of controlled trials as short reports. *Lancet*, **318** (7177), 193–194.

15 Campbell, M.K., Piaggio, G., Elbourne, D.R. & Altman, D.G. (2012) Consort 2010 statement: extension to cluster randomised trials. *BMJ*, **345**, e5661.

16 Piaggio, G., Elbourne, D.R., Pocock, S.J., *et al.* (2012) Reporting of noninferiority and equivalence randomized trials: extension of the CONSORT 2010 statement. *JAMA*, **308** (24), 2594–2604.

17 Ioannidis, J.P., Evans, S.J., Gotzsche, P.C. *et al.* (2004) Better reporting of harms in randomized trials: an extension of the CONSORT statement. *Annals of Internal Medicine*, **141** (10), 781–788.

18 Zwarenstein, M., Treweek, S., Gagnier, J.J. *et al.* (2008) Improving the reporting of pragmatic trials: an extension of the CONSORT statement. *BMJ*, **337**, a2390.

19 Gagnier, J.J., Boon, H., Rochon, P., *et al.* (2006) Reporting randomized, controlled trials of herbal interventions: an elaborated CONSORT statement. *Annals of Internal Medicine*, **144** (5), 364–367.

20 Boutron, I., Moher, D., Altman, D.G. *et al.* (2008) Extending the CONSORT statement to randomized trials of nonpharmacologic treatment: explanation and elaboration. *Annals of Internal Medicine*, **148** (4), 295–309.

21 MacPherson, H., Altman, D.G., Hammerschlag, R. *et al.* (2010) Revised STandards for Reporting Interventions in Clinical Trials of Acupuncture (STRICTA): extending the CONSORT statement. *PLoS Medicine*, **7** (6), e1000261.

22 Harbourt, A.M., Knecht, L.S. & Humphreys, B.L. (1995) Structured abstracts in MEDLINE, 1989–1991. *Bulletin of the Medical Library Association*, **83** (2), 190–195.

23 Hopewell, S., McDonald, S., Clarke, M. & Egger, M. (2007) Grey literature in meta-analyses of randomized trials of health care interventions. *Cochrane Database of Systematic Reviews*, **2**, MR000010.

24 Hopewell, S., Eisinga, A. & Clarke, M. (2008) Better reporting of randomized trials in biomedical journal and conference abstracts. *Journal of Information Science*, **34**, 162–173.

25 Herbison, P. (2005) The reporting quality of abstracts of randomised controlled trials submitted to the ICS meeting in Heidelberg. *Neurourology and Urodynamics*, **21** (1), 21–24.

26 Hopewell, S. & Clarke, M. (2005) Abstracts presented at the American Society of Clinical Oncology conference: how completely are trials reported? *Clinical Trials*, **2** (3), 265–268.

27 Krzyzanowska, M.K., Pintilie, M. & Tannock, I.F. (2003) Factors associated with failure to publish large randomized trials presented at an oncology meeting. *JAMA*, **290** (4), 495–501.

28 Toma, M., McAlister, F.A., Bialy, L., *et al.* (2006) Transition from meeting abstract to full-length journal article for randomized controlled trials. *JAMA*, **295** (11), 1281–1287.

29 Dundar, Y., Dodd, S., Dickson, R., *et al.* (2006) Comparison of conference abstracts and presentations with full-text articles in the health technology assessments of rapidly evolving technologies. *Health Technology Assessment*, **10** (5):iii–iv, ix–145.

30 Chokkalingam, A., Scherer, R. & Dickersin, K. (1998) Agreement of data abstracts compared to full publications. *Controlled Clinical Trials*, **19**, 61S–62S.

31 Froom, P. & Froom, J. (July 1993) Deficiencies in structured medical abstracts. *Journal of Clinical Epidemiology*, **46** (7), 591–594.

32 Pitkin, R.M., Branagan, M.A. & Burmeister, L.F. (1999) Accuracy of data in abstracts of published research articles. *JAMA*, **281** (12), 1110–1111.

33 Ward, L.G., Kendrach, M.G. & Price, S.O. (2004) Accuracy of abstracts for original research articles in pharmacy journals. *Annals of Pharmacotherapy*, **38** (7–8), 1173–1177.

34 Ioannidis, J.P. & Lau, J. (2001) Completeness of safety reporting in randomized trials: an evaluation of 7 medical areas. *JAMA*, **285** (4), 437–443.

35 De, S.M., Yakoubi, R., De, N.C. *et al.* (2012) Reporting quality of abstracts presented at the European Association of Urology meeting: a critical assessment. *Journal of Urology*, **188** (5), 1883–1886.

36 Faggion, C.M. Jr. & Giannakopoulos, N.N. (2012) Quality of reporting in abstracts of randomized controlled trials published in leading journals of periodontology and implant dentistry: a survey. *Journal of Periodontology*, **83** (10), 1251–1256.

37 Fleming, P.S., Buckley, N., Seehra, J., *et al.* (2012) Reporting quality of abstracts of randomized controlled trials published in leading orthodontic journals from 2006 to 2011. *American Journal of Orthodontics and Dentofacial Orthopedics*, **142** (4), 451–458.

38 Ghimire, S., Kyung, E., Kang, W. & Kim, E. (2012) Assessment of adherence to the CONSORT statement for quality of reports on randomized controlled trial abstracts from four high-impact general medical journals. *Trials*, **13**, 77.

39 Can, O.S., Yilmaz, A.A., Hasdogan, M. *et al.* (2011) Has the quality of abstracts for randomised controlled trials improved since the release of Consolidated Standards of Reporting Trial guideline for abstract reporting? A survey of four high-profile anaesthesia journals. *European Journal of Anaesthesiology*, **28** (7), 485–492.

40 Knobloch, K., Yoon, U., Rennekampff, H.O. & Vogt, P.M. (2011) Quality of reporting according to the CONSORT, STROBE and Timmer instrument at the American Burn

Association (ABA) annual meetings 2000 and 2008. *BMC Medical Research Methodology,* **11**, 161.

41 Chen, Y., Li, J., Ai, C. *et al.* (2010) Assessment of the quality of reporting in abstracts of randomized controlled trials published in five leading Chinese medical journals. *PLoS One,* **5** (8), e11926.

42 Hopewell, S., Ravaud, P., Baron, G. & Boutron, I. (2012) Effect of editors' implementation of CONSORT guidelines on the reporting of abstracts in high impact medical journals: interrupted time series analysis. *BMJ,* **344**, e4178.

43 National Library of Medicine. MEDLINE/PubMed data element (field) descriptions. Available from www.nlm.nih.gov [Accessed on 10 August 2010; 2007].

44 Scherer, R.W. & Crawley, B. (1998) Reporting of randomized clinical trial descriptors and use of structured abstracts. *JAMA,* **280** (3), 269–272.

45 Burns, K.E., Adhikari, N.K., Kho, M. *et al.* (2005) Abstract reporting in randomized clinical trials of acute lung injury: an audit and assessment of a quality of reporting score. *Critical Care Medicine,* **33** (9), 1937–1945.

46 Pocock, S.J., Hughes, M.D. & Lee, R.J. (1987) Statistical problems in the reporting of clinical trials. *New England Journal of Medicine,* **317** (7), 426–432.

47 Dryver, E. & Hux, J.E. (2002) Reporting of numerical and statistical differences in abstracts: improving but not optimal. *Journal of General Internal Medicine,* **17** (3), 203–206.

48 Gotzsche, P.C. (2006) Are relative risks and odds ratios in abstracts believable? *Ugeskrift for Laeger,* **168** (33), 2678–2680.

49 Bhandari, M., Devereaux, P.J., Guyatt, G.H. *et al.* (2002) An observational study of orthopaedic abstracts and subsequent full-text publications. *Journal of Bone and Joint Surgery,* **84-A** (4), 615–621.

CHAPTER 9

CONSORT

Kenneth F. Schulz[1], David Moher[2] and Douglas G. Altman[3]

[1] *FHI 360, Durham, and UNC School of Medicine, Chapel Hill, NC, USA*
[2] *Clinical Epidemiology Program, Ottawa Hospital Research Institute, Ottawa, ON, Canada*
[3] *Centre for Statistics in Medicine, University of Oxford, Oxford, UK*

CONSORT timetable

Reporting guideline	Notes	Meeting date	Publication date
CONSORT	For randomized trials – brought together two reporting guideline groups to produce the CONSORT Statement	September 1995	1996
CONSORT 2001	Updated the CONSORT Statement and also produced the first explanation and elaboration paper	May 1999	2001
CONSORT 2010	Updated both the statement and the explanation and elaboration paper	January 2007	2010

Name of guideline

The Consolidated Standards of Reporting Trials (CONSORT) is a guidance for authors reporting a randomized controlled trial (RCT). Such trials when appropriately designed, conducted, and reported represent the gold standard in evaluating healthcare interventions. However, this lofty position in the medical research hierarchy does not mean that readers should uncritically accept the results of all RCTs. Indeed, randomized trials can yield biased results if they lack methodological rigor [1]. To assess a trial accurately, readers of a published report need complete, clear, and transparent

Guidelines for Reporting Health Research: A User's Manual, First Edition. Edited by David Moher, Douglas G. Altman, Kenneth F. Schulz, Iveta Simera and Elizabeth Wager.
© 2014 John Wiley & Sons, Ltd. Published 2014 by John Wiley & Sons, Ltd.

information on its methodology and findings. Unfortunately, attempted assessments frequently fail because authors of many trial reports neglect to provide lucid and complete descriptions of that critical information [2–4].

The updated CONSORT Statement, the CONSORT 2010 Statement, is designed to elicit clear and complete information on RCTs. It was published in nine journals with eight providing direct citations [5–12]. It comprises explicit text, a 25-item checklist (Table 9.1), and a flow diagram (Figure 9.1). Along with the statement, we have updated the explanation and elaboration (E&E) article, published in two journals [16, 17], that explains the inclusion of each checklist item, provides methodological background, and illustrates published examples of transparent reporting.

When to use CONSORT

CONSORT provides guidance for reporting all RCTs, in which investigators allocate the healthcare interventions, such as a comparison of two drugs, to participants, or the participants to interventions, by some random process. CONSORT focuses on the most common design type, individually randomized two-group parallel trials.

Current version compared with previous versions

The most recent version, the CONSORT 2010 Statement [5–12] updated the statement published in 2001. CONSORT 2010 was initially published in nine journals. We added several new items asking authors to describe the trial design they used (e.g., parallel) and the allocation ratio (item 3a); address any important changes to methods after trial commencement, with a discussion of reasons (item 6); report any changes to the primary and secondary outcome (endpoint) measures after the trial commenced (item 6); describe why the trial ended or was stopped (subitem 14.b); inform about their trial's registration (item 23); the availability of the trial's protocol (item 24); and inform about the trial's funding (item 25).

We modified several items: we encouraged greater specificity by stating that descriptions of interventions (formerly item 4 from CONSORT 2001) should include "sufficient details to allow replication" (item 5); we added the specification of how blinding was done and also, if relevant, a description of the similarity of interventions and procedures while eliminating text on "how the success of blinding (masking) was assessed" because of a lack of empirical evidence supporting the practice as well as theoretical concerns about the validity of any such assessment (item 11); we replaced mention of "intention-to-treat" analysis, a widely misused term, with a

Table 9.1 CONSORT 2010 checklist of information to include when reporting a randomized trial[a].

Section/topic	Item #	Checklist item	Reported on page #
Title and abstract	1a	Identification as a randomized trial in the title	
	1b	Structured summary of trial design, methods, results, and conclusions; for specific guidance, see Chapter 8 [13, 14]	
Introduction			
Background and objectives	2a	Scientific background and explanation of rationale	
	2b	Specific objectives or hypotheses	
Methods			
Trial design	3a	Description of trial design (e.g., parallel, factorial) including allocation ratio	
	3b	Important changes to methods after trial commencement (e.g., eligibility criteria) with reasons	
Participants	4a	Eligibility criteria for participants	
	4b	Settings and locations where the data were collected	
Interventions	5	The interventions for each group with sufficient details to allow replication, including how and when they were actually administered	
Outcomes	6a	Completely defined prespecified primary and secondary outcome measures, including how and when they were assessed	
	6b	Any changes to trial outcomes after the trial commenced with reasons	
Sample size	7a	How sample size was determined	
	7b	When applicable, explanation of any interim analyses and stopping guidelines	
Randomization			
Sequence generation	8a	Method used to generate the random allocation sequence	
	8b	Type of randomization; details of any restriction (e.g., blocking and block size)	
Allocation concealment mechanism	9	Mechanism used to implement the random allocation sequence (e.g., sequentially numbered containers), describing any steps taken to conceal the sequence until interventions were assigned	
Implementation	10	Who generated the random allocation sequence, who enrolled participants, and who assigned participants to interventions	
Blinding	11a	If done, who was blinded after assignment to interventions (e.g., participants, care providers, those assessing outcomes) and how	
	11b	If relevant, description of the similarity of interventions	

Table 9.1 (*Continued*)

Section/topic	Item #	Checklist item	Reported on page #
Statistical methods	12a	Statistical methods used to compare groups for primary and secondary outcomes	
	12b	Methods for additional analyses, such as subgroup analyses and adjusted analyses	
Results			
Participant flow (A diagram is strongly recommended)	13a	For each group, the numbers of participants who were randomly assigned, received intended treatment, and analyzed for the primary outcome	
	13b	For each group, losses and exclusions after randomization, together with reasons	
Recruitment	14a	Dates defining the periods of recruitment and follow-up	
	14b	Why the trial ended or was stopped	
Baseline data	15	A table showing baseline demographic and clinical characteristics for each group	
Numbers analyzed	16	For each group, number of participants (denominator) included in each analysis and whether the analysis was by original assigned groups	
Outcomes and estimation	17a	For each primary and secondary outcome, results for each group, and the estimated effect size and its precision (e.g., 95% confidence interval)	
	17b	For binary outcomes, presentation of both absolute and relative effect sizes is recommended	
Ancillary analyses	18	Results of any other analyses performed, including subgroup analyses and adjusted analyses, distinguishing prespecified from exploratory	
Harms	19	All important harms or unintended effects in each group; for specific guidance, see CONSORT for Harms [15] (see Chapter 10)	
Discussion			
Limitations	20	Trial limitations, addressing sources of potential bias, imprecision, and, if relevant, multiplicity of analyses	
Generalizability	21	Generalizability (external validity, applicability) of the trial findings	
Interpretation	22	Interpretation consistent with results, balancing benefits and harms, and considering other relevant evidence	
Other information			
Registration	23	Registration number and name of trial registry	
Protocol	24	Where the full trial protocol can be accessed, if available	
Funding	25	Sources of funding and other support (e.g., supply of drugs), role of funders	

[a]We strongly recommend reading this statement in conjunction with the CONSORT 2010 E&E [16, 17] for important clarifications on all the items. If relevant, we also recommend reading CONSORT extensions for cluster randomized trials [18], noninferiority and equivalence trials [19], nonpharmacologic treatments [20], herbal interventions [21], and pragmatic trials [22]. Moreover, additional extensions are forthcoming. For those and also for up-to-date references relevant to this checklist, see www.consort-statement.org.

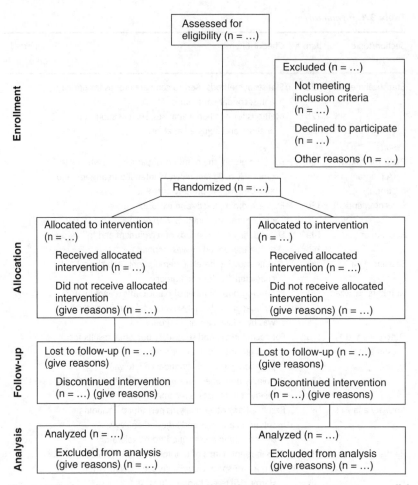

Figure 9.1 Flow diagram of the progress through the phases of a two-group parallel randomized trial (i.e., enrollment, intervention allocation, follow-up, and data analysis).

more explicit request for information about retaining participants in their original assigned groups (item 16); for appropriate clinical interpretability, we added the wording "For binary outcomes, presentation of both relative and absolute effect sizes is recommended" (subitem 17.b); we changed the topic from "Interpretation" to "Limitations" and supplanted the prior text with a sentence focusing on the reporting of sources of potential bias and imprecision (item 20); and we changed the topic from "Overall evidence" to "Interpretation," because concerns in the CONSORT Group emerged that too frequently conclusions in papers misrepresented the actual analytical results and that harms were ignored or marginalized; therefore, we changed the checklist item to include the concepts of results matching interpretations and of benefits being balanced with harms (item 22).

Extensions and implementations of CONSORT

The main CONSORT Statement is based on the "standard" two-group par-allel design. Extensions of CONSORT have been developed for randomized trials that have different designs, data, and interventions (Figure 9.2). Examples for different designs include the extensions for cluster random-ized trials [18], noninferiority and equivalence trials [19], abstracts [13], and pragmatic trials [22]. Examples for different interventions include extensions for nonpharmacologic treatments [20], herbal interventions [21], and acupuncture [23]. An example for different data is the extension for harms [15].

CONSORT is primarily defined by trial aims, type of intervention, and methodology. This allows for leeway in illustrating its implementation in particular specialties. As an example, an implementation of CONSORT was done for behavioral medicine [24], although it was not done in cooperation with the CONSORT Group. Such implementations will generally include a generous amount of topic-specific information.

A number of authors have developed reporting guidelines based on CONSORT but have done it without our knowledge and without the partic-ipation of anyone from the CONSORT Executive. The topics are varied from evidence-based behavioral medicine to homeopathic treatments. Those

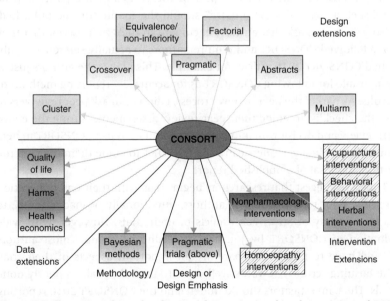

Figure 9.2 Illustration of actual and potential extensions and implementations of CON-SORT.

unofficial extensions and implementations that have been brought to our attention, along with the official, can be found on the CONSORT website.

How best to use the guideline

When authors use CONSORT, we suggest that the format of the articles should abide by journal style, editorial directions, the traditions of the research field addressed, and, where possible, author preferences. We do not wish to standardize the structure of reporting. Authors should simply address checklist items somewhere in the article, with ample detail and lucidity. That stated, we think that manuscripts benefit from frequent subheadings within the major sections, especially the methods and results sections. Diligent adherence by authors to the checklist items facilitates clarity, completeness, and transparency of reporting. Explicit descriptions, not ambiguity or omission, best serve the interests of all readers. Of note, the statement does not include recommendations for designing, conducting, and analyzing trials. It solely addresses reporting – what was done and what was found.

We propose several ways in which CONSORT can be used by editors. During the manuscript submission process, editors can ask authors to complete the CONSORT checklist and include it as part of the submission process. The checklist can then become part of the corpus of the paper and be published as part of a "web extra" should the manuscript be published. Also, editors can ask that authors document in their manuscript that they have followed CONSORT and require authors to actually reference a published CONSORT 2010 article, for example. This makes the authors just as responsible for following CONSORT as for accurately reporting methods or results. As part of the peer review process, editors can ask peer reviewers to use the checklist to guide their peer review assessment. During the editorial review and decision-making process, editors can use CONSORT to help guide them. Finally, readers can use CONSORT to guide them through the critical appraisal of a published report.

Thus, we suggest that researchers begin trials with their end publication in mind. Poor reporting allows authors, intentionally or inadvertently, to escape scrutiny of any weak aspects of their trials. However, with wide adoption of CONSORT by journals and editorial groups, most authors should have to report transparently all important aspects of their trial. The ensuing scrutiny rewards well-done trials and penalizes poorly done trials. Thus, investigators should understand the CONSORT 2010 reporting guidelines before beginning a trial as a further incentive to design and conduct their trials according to rigorous standards. We strongly recommend using the E&E in conjunction with the checklist to foster complete, clear, and transparent reporting and aid appraisal of published trial reports.

Development process

Efforts to improve the reporting of RCTs accelerated in the mid-1990s, spurred partly by methodological research. Although researchers had shown for many years that authors poorly report RCTs, empirical evidence began to accumulate that some poorly conducted or poorly reported aspects of trials were associated with bias [25]. Two initiatives, Standards Of Reporting Trials and Asilomar, aimed at developing reporting guidelines culminated in the first CONSORT Statement in 1996 [26]. Further methodological research on similar topics reinforced earlier findings [27] and fed into the revision of 2001 [28–30]. The experience gained with CONSORT since 2001 and the expanding body of methodological research informed the refinement of CONSORT. More than 700 studies comprise the CONSORT Database (located on the CONSORT website), which provides the empirical evidence to underpin the CONSORT initiative. Consequently, we organized a CONSORT Group meeting to update the 2001 CONSORT Statement.

Thirty-one members of the 2010 CONSORT Group met in Montebello, Canada, in January 2007 to update the 2001 CONSORT Statement. Prior to the meeting, some participants were given primary responsibility for aggregating and synthesizing the relevant evidence on a particular checklist item of interest. On the basis of that evidence, the group deliberated the value of each item. As in prior CONSORT versions, we kept only those items deemed absolutely fundamental to reporting an RCT. Moreover, an item may be fundamental to a trial but not included, such as approval by an institutional ethical review board, because funding bodies strictly enforce ethical review, and medical journals usually address reporting ethical review in their instructions for authors. Other items may seem desirable, such as reporting on whether on-site monitoring was done, but a lack of empirical evidence, or any consensus on their value, cautions against inclusion at this point. The statement thus addresses the minimum criteria, although that should not deter authors from including other information if they consider it important.

After the meeting, the CONSORT Executive convened teleconferences and in-person meetings to revise the checklist. After seven major iterations, a revised checklist was distributed to the larger group for feedback. With that feedback, the executive met twice in person to consider all the comments and to produce a penultimate version. This served as the basis for writing the first draft of this paper, which was then distributed to the group for feedback. After consideration of their comments, the executive finalized the CONSORT 2010 Statement [5–12].

The CONSORT Executive then drafted an updated E&E manuscript, with assistance from other members of the larger group. The substance of the 2007 CONSORT meeting provided the material for the update. The updated E&E was distributed to the entire group for additions, deletions, and changes. This final iterative process converged to the CONSORT 2010 E&E [16, 17].

Evidence of effectiveness of guideline

Several studies have evaluated whether the use of CONSORT is associated with improvements in the quality of reporting randomized trials. A systematic review of eight studies was published in 2006. The authors observed that the use of CONSORT was associated with improvements in the quality of reporting randomized trials [31]. This review has recently been updated [32].

Endorsement and adherence

More than 600 journals, published around the world and in many languages, have explicitly supported the statement. Many other healthcare journals support it without our knowledge. Moreover, thousands more have implicitly supported it with the endorsement of the statement by the International Committee of Medical Journal Editors (www.icmje.org). Other prominent editorial groups, the Council of Science Editors and the World Association of Medical Editors, officially support CONSORT.

Although this endorsement is substantial, many more journals should endorse CONSORT and encourage adherence to it. In examining the "Instructions to Authors" of 165 high-impact journals, only 38% mentioned CONSORT in their instructions, and, moreover, only 37% of those stated that adhering was a requirement [33]. In a survey of those same 165 journals, only 64 (39%) responded. Of those that responded, only 62% said they required adherence to the CONSORT Statement, only 41% reported incorporating the statement into their peer review process, and only 47% reported incorporating it into their editorial process [33].

CONSORT 2010 supplants the prior version published in 2001. If a journal supports or endorses CONSORT 2010, it should cite one of the original versions of CONSORT 2010, the E&E, and the CONSORT website in their "Instructions to Authors." We suggest that authors who wish to cite

CONSORT should cite one of the original journal versions of CONSORT 2010 [5–12], and, if appropriate, the E&E [16, 17].

Cautions and limitations

CONSORT urges completeness, clarity, and transparency of reporting, which simply reflects the actual trial design and conduct. However, as a potential drawback, a reporting guideline might encourage some authors to report fictitiously the information suggested by the guidance rather than what was actually done. Authors, peer reviewers, and editors should vigilantly guard against that potential drawback and refer to, for example, trial protocols, information on trial registers, and regulatory agency websites.

Moreover, the statement does not include recommendations for designing and conducting RCTs. The items should elicit clear pronouncements of how and what the authors did but do not contain any judgments on how and what the authors should have done. Thus, CONSORT 2010 is neither intended as an instrument to evaluate the quality of an RCT nor is it appropriate to use the checklist to construct a "quality score."

Creators' preferred bits

We make our recommendations based on a combination of importance to internal validity (minimizing bias) and general current level of reporting in the literature.

An item that is important, but frequently inadequately reported in the literature, reflects the type of item that made our "creators' preferred bits" list:

Randomization (items 8–10) Randomization is the principal bias-reducing technique in a controlled trial. Elimination of selection bias in a trial depends on proper randomization. By randomization, we mean the sequence generation, allocation concealment mechanism, and implementation items in the checklist, items 8–10.

Participant flow (item 13) Randomization eliminates selection bias at baseline, but to maintain that elimination of bias, investigators have to analyze all the originally assigned participants in the intervention groups to which they were originally assigned. Without adequate retention of participants and proper analysis in the originally assigned groups, bias creeps into the trial. Thus, this participant flow item is critical for readers to assess the extent to which the properties of randomization have been maintained in the analysis of results.

Blinding (item 11) Proper blinding of all those involved in a trial, usually called double-blinding, can reduce bias in the assessment of outcome, as well as aid retention (lessen lost to follow-up) and minimize cointerventions. Even if total blinding of everyone involved in the trial is impossible, investigators may attempt to blind assessments of outcome.

Future plans

We updated the CONSORT Statement in 2010, so we do not have plans to update it in the next 12–24 months. Likely, the next major update will occur around 2016 or shortly thereafter. However, we are planning to develop extensions for multiarm trials, crossover trials, N-of-1 trials, and factorial trials.

Our current emphasis is on improving the implementation of CONSORT within key user groups. Our focus is on endorsement by journals and adherence by trial authors. Trials published in journals that endorse CONSORT have been shown to be more completely reported than those in non-endorsing journals or those published prior to endorsement [34]. We plan on understanding the barriers to implementing CONSORT in biomedical journals and developing a knowledge translation (KT) strategy to overcome those barriers. We have developed a prototype for an electronic tool to facilitate seamless checklist completion and adherence by authors submitting trial manuscripts to journals. We anticipate piloting it in a small number of journals in 2014 with plans for subsequent widespread implementation. We are also planning to quantify and characterize the use of CONSORT during the journal peer review process to help target areas for implementation improvement.

Lastly, a redesign, update and modernization of the CONSORT website (www.consort-statement.org) will be launched in 2014. This update provides further clarification of the nuances of the checklist, and a more in-depth explanation of items for the main CONSORT checklist as well as extensions. The update also provides additional resources for users such as a library of examples of good reporting in trials and sample text that journals may wish to include in their instructions to authors.

References

1 Jüni, P., Altman, D.G. & Egger, M. (2001) Systematic reviews in health care: assessing the quality of controlled clinical trials. *BMJ*, **323**, 42–46.
2 Chan, A.W. & Altman, D.G. (2005) Epidemiology and reporting of randomised trials published in PubMed journals. *Lancet*, **365**, 1159–1162.
3 Glasziou, P., Meats, E., Heneghan, C. & Shepperd, S. (2008) What is missing from descriptions of treatment in trials and reviews? *BMJ*, **336**, 1472–1474.

4 Dwan, K., Altman, D.G., Arnaiz, J.A. *et al.* (2008) Systematic review of the empirical evidence of study publication bias and outcome reporting bias. *PLoS ONE*, **3** (8), e3081.

5 Schulz, K.F., Altman, D.G. & Moher, D. (2010) CONSORT 2010 statement: updated guidelines for reporting parallel group randomised trials. *PLoS Medicine*, **7** (3), e1000251.

6 Schulz, K.F., Altman, D.G., Moher, D. (2010) CONSORT 2010 Statement: updated guidelines for reporting parallel group randomised trials. *J Clin Epidemiol*, **63** (8), 834–40.

7 Schulz, K.F., Altman, D.G. & Moher, D. (2010) CONSORT 2010 Statement: updated guidelines for reporting parallel group randomized trials. *Annals of Internal Medicine*, **152** (11), 726–32.

8 Schulz, K.F., Altman, D.G., Moher, D., CONSORT Group. (2010) CONSORT 2010 Statement: updated guidelines for reporting parallel group randomised trials. *BMC Medicine*, **8** (1), 18.

9 Schulz, K.F., Altman, D.G., Moher, D., CONSORT Group. (2010) CONSORT 2010 Statement: updated guidelines for reporting parallel group randomised trials. *Trials*, **11** (1), 32.

10 Schulz, K.F., Altman, D.G. & Moher, D. (2010) CONSORT 2010 statement: updated guidelines for reporting parallel group randomised trials. *BMJ*, **340**, c332c.

11 Schulz, K.F., Altman, D.G., Moher, D. & CONSORT Group. (2010) CONSORT 2010 statement: updated guidelines for reporting parallel group randomized trials. *Obstetrics & Gynecology*, **115** (5), 1063–70.

12 Schulz, K.F., Altman, D.G., Moher, D. & CONSORT Group. (2010) CONSORT 2010 statement: updated guidelines for reporting parallel group randomized trials. *Open Medicine*, **4** (1), e60–8.

13 Hopewell, S., Clarke, M., Moher, D. *et al.* (2008) CONSORT for reporting randomised trials in journal and conference abstracts. *Lancet*, **371**, 281–283.

14 Hopewell, S., Clarke, M., Moher, D. *et al.* (2008) CONSORT for reporting randomized controlled trials in journal and conference abstracts: explanation and elaboration. *PLoS Medicine*, **5** (1), e20.

15 Ioannidis, J.P., Evans, S.J., Gotzsche, P.C. *et al.* (2004) Better reporting of harms in randomized trials: an extension of the CONSORT statement. *Annals of Internal Medicine*, **141** (10), 781–788.

16 Moher, D., Hopewell, S., Schulz, K.F. *et al.* (2010) CONSORT 2010 Explanation and Elaboration: updated guidelines for reporting parallel group randomised trials. *Journal of Clinical Epidemiology*.

17 Moher, D., Hopewell, S., Schulz, K.F. *et al.* (2010) CONSORT 2010 explanation and elaboration: updated guidelines for reporting parallel group randomised trials. *BMJ*, **340**, c869.

18 Campbell, M.K., Piaggio, G., Elbourne, D.R., Altman, D.G. for the CONSORT Group. (2012) CONSORT 2010 statement: extension to cluster randomised trials. *BMJ*, **345**, e5661.

19 Piaggio, G., Elbourne, D.R., Pocock, S.J. *et al.* (2012) Reporting of noninferiority and equivalence randomized trials. An extension of the CONSORT 2010 statement. *JAMA*, **308** (24), 2594–2604.

20 Boutron, I., Moher, D., Altman, D.G. *et al.* (2008) Extending the CONSORT statement to randomized trials of nonpharmacologic treatment: explanation and elaboration. *Annals of Internal Medicine*, **148** (4), 295–309.

21 Gagnier, J.J., Boon, H., Rochon, P. *et al.* (2006) Reporting randomized, controlled trials of herbal interventions: an elaborated CONSORT statement. *Annals of Internal Medicine*, **144** (5), 364–367.

22 Zwarenstein, M., Treweek, S., Gagnier, J.J. *et al.* (2008) Improving the reporting of pragmatic trials: an extension of the CONSORT statement. *BMJ*, **337**, a2390.

23 MacPherson, H., Altman, D.G., Hammerschlag, R. *et al.* (2010) Revised STandards for Reporting Interventions in Clinical Trials of Acupuncture (STRICTA): Extending the CONSORT statement. *J Evidence Based Medicine*, **3** (3), 140–55.

24 Davidson, K.W., Goldstein, M., Kaplan, R.M. *et al.* (2003) Evidence-based behavioral medicine: what is it and how do we achieve it? *Annals of Behavioral Medicine*, **26** (3), 161–171.

25 Schulz, K.F., Chalmers, I., Hayes, R.J. & Altman, D.G. (1995) Empirical evidence of bias. Dimensions of methodological quality associated with estimates of treatment effects in controlled trials. *JAMA*, **273** (5), 408–412.

26 Begg, C., Cho, M., Eastwood, S. *et al.* (1996) Improving the quality of reporting of randomized controlled trials. The CONSORT statement. *JAMA*, **276** (8), 637–639.

27 Moher, D., Pham, B., Jones, A. *et al.* (1998) Does quality of reports of randomised trials affect estimates of intervention efficacy reported in meta-analyses? *Lancet*, **352** (9128), 609–613.

28 Moher, D., Schulz, K.F. & Altman, D. (2001) The CONSORT statement: revised recommendations for improving the quality of reports of parallel-group randomized trials. *JAMA*, **285** (15), 1987–1991.

29 Moher, D., Schulz, K.F. & Altman, D.G. (2001) The CONSORT statement: revised recommendations for improving the quality of reports of parallel-group randomized trials. *Annals of Internal Medicine*, **134** (8), 657–662.

30 Moher, D., Schulz, K.F. & Altman, D.G. (2001) The CONSORT statement: revised recommendations for improving the quality of reports of parallel-group randomised trials. *Lancet*, **357** (9263), 1191–1194.

31 Plint, A.C., Moher, D., Morrison, A. *et al.* (2006) Does the CONSORT checklist improve the quality of reports of randomised controlled trials? A systematic review. *Medical Journal of Australia*, **185** (5), 263–267.

32 Moher, D., Plint, A.C., Altman, D.G. *et al.* (2010) Consolidated standards of reporting trials (CONSORT) and the quality of reporting of randomized controlled trials. *Cochrane Database of Systematic Reviews*, (**3**):MR000030. doi:10.1002/ 14651858.MR000030.

33 Hopewell, S., Altman, D.G., Moher, D. & Schulz, K.F. (2008) Endorsement of the CONSORT statement by high impact factor medical journals: a survey of journal editors and journal 'Instructions to Authors'. *Trials*, **9**, 20.

34 Turner, L., Shamseer L., Altman, D.G. *et al.* (2012) Does use of the CONSORT Statement impact the completeness of reporting of randomised controlled trials published in medical journals?. *A Cochrane review. Systematic Reviews*, **1**, 60.

CHAPTER 10

CONSORT Extension for Better Reporting of Harms

John P.A. Ioannidis

Stanford Prevention Research Center, Department of Medicine and Division of Epidemiology, Department of Health Research and Policy, Stanford University School of Medicine, and Department of Statistics, Stanford University School of Humanities and Sciences, Stanford, CA, USA

Timetable

Name of reporting guideline initiative	Notes	Consensus meeting date	Reporting guideline publication
CONSORT extension for harms		May 2003	November 2004

Name of guideline

The extension of the CONSORT statement for better reporting of harms in randomized trials is a guidance document for authors reporting randomized trials, with emphasis on how to best report aspects of harm-related data. The extension can be used by authors who wish to improve the quality of information that they include in a trial report, by peer reviewers and editors reviewing a submitted report of a randomized trial, and by readers who want to understand the completeness and validity of harm-related information in a randomized trial report.

The guideline extension adds 10 recommendations to the standard CONSORT list. The recommendations address the title/abstract, introduction, methods, results, and discussion of randomized trial publications. In the guidance, there is also accompanying explanation and examples to highlight specific aspects of proper reporting.

Guidelines for Reporting Health Research: A User's Manual, First Edition. Edited by David Moher, Douglas G. Altman, Kenneth F. Schulz, Iveta Simera and Elizabeth Wager.
© 2014 John Wiley & Sons, Ltd. Published 2014 by John Wiley & Sons, Ltd.

History/development

The guidance for reporting of harms was first contemplated in 2001, when it was realized by accumulating empirical evidence that reporting of adverse events in randomized trials (including clinical adverse events, laboratory-documented toxicity, and withdrawals due to toxicity) was suboptimal. A meeting in Montebello, Canada in 2003 set the foundations for developing this guidance as an extension building on the existing items of the CONSORT statement.

When to use this guideline (what types of studies it covers)

The extension for better reporting of harms is aimed at those reporting randomized controlled trials. It relates to all randomized trials regardless of the type of intervention being studied and it is thus pertinent to both pharmacological and nonpharmacological interventions.

Previous version

None; for previous versions of CONSORT, see Chapter 9.

Current version

The extension for harms has been published in the Annals of Internal Medicine [1].

Extensions and/or implementations

Not applicable (this is an extension itself).

Related activities

None.

How best to use the guideline

Authors

Harms are often considered to be of secondary importance in randomized trials; however, this is a grave misconception because decisions about interventions depend on the balance between benefits and harms. Several empirical studies on pharmacological and nonpharmacological interventions (summarized in references [2–4]) have shown that reporting of harms in randomized trials is suboptimal. The CONSORT extension for harms aims to remedy this deficiency by highlighting specific steps that need attention in presenting results. Even though most trials will have inconclusive results regarding adverse events (as they are generally not powered to detect relatively rare events), this is another reason why reporting should be comprehensive and transparent, to allow the incorporation of findings in future reviews of the evidence and avoid adding selective reporting bias on top of stochastic uncertainty.

Peer reviewers

Peer reviewers often pay limited attention to harms when appraising a randomized trial for publication. The provided guidance may help remedy this deficiency by focusing attention on the important aspects that need to be conveyed in the final published paper.

Editors

Editors can use the checklist as a routine adjunct to the CONSORT statement to encourage authors to report trials fully. In this regard, the uses of the extension are similar to the uses of the main CONSORT statement (see Chapter 9) because harms are pertinent to all trials.

Development process

A three-day meeting was held in Montebello, Canada, in May 2003 with participants including methodologists, clinical epidemiologists, statisticians, FDA representatives, medical editors, industry representatives, and a consumer. Before the meeting, the team leader completed a systematic review of studies examining the quality of reporting of harms and a comprehensive literature search to identify methodological and other articles that might inform the meeting, in particular, relating to the epidemiology and reporting of harms in randomized trials. This evidence was communicated to the wider team during the meeting. Then, each CONSORT checklist item was discussed as to whether it should be elaborated and supplemented with aspects especially related to harms. Only items deemed essential were retained or added to the extension checklist. A strategy for producing the extension along with incorporated examples and explanation was also discussed.

Shortly after the meeting, a draft of the extension checklist was circulated to the group, including those invited to the meeting but unable to attend.

After several iterations, the checklist was approved by the working group. Simultaneously, the manuscript was drafted by the writing team of seven authors and after several iterations was approved by the group.

Evidence of effectiveness of guideline

We are unaware of any evaluations of whether the use of the CONSORT extension for harms is associated with improved quality of reporting of harms in randomized trials. Several studies have addressed reporting of harms in samples of trials [2–5] and some modest improvement of reporting over time is possible. However, it is difficult to say whether this can be attributed in part to the CONSORT extension or other forces that improved sensitization to harms over time. Moreover, these empirical studies have addressed different types of trials, so confounding cannot be excluded, especially in cross-study comparisons.

Endorsement and adherence

The extension for harms follows the endorsement trajectory of the main CONSORT document (see Chapter 9 for details).

Cautions and limitations (including scope)

The CONSORT extension for harms is not intended as an instrument to evaluate the quality of a randomized trial, although investigators and peer reviewers may check which of the items are included in a published or submitted paper. It would not be appropriate to use the checklist to construct an aggregate quality score as such a score has unknown operational properties and lacks interval scaling.

The extension was developed to cover any type of intervention that may be tested in a randomized trial. However, it is conceivable that special issues may arise with other study designs.

Creators' preferred bits

Definition of adverse events

It is often unclear in most trial reports whether the reported adverse events encompass all the recorded adverse events or a selected sample, although one can often infer that the latter is the case. If some selection filter has been used, authors should explain how, why, and who selected adverse events for reporting. Authors should also be explicit about separately reporting anticipated and unexpected adverse events. Expectation may influence the incidence of reported or ascertained adverse events. For example, making participants aware in the consent form of the possibility of a specific adverse event ("priming") may increase the reporting rate of the event. Authors should report whether they used standardized and validated measurement instruments for adverse events. Several medical fields have developed standardized scales, but use of nonvalidated scales is still very common. The source document for well-established definitions and scales should be referenced. New definitions for adverse events should be explicit and clear. Given the plethora of existing scales, the development of new scales should have a rationale and authors should describe how they developed and validated new scales. Definitions should explicitly deal with the grading of the collected harms events. For interventions that target healthy individuals (e.g., preventive interventions), any harm, however minor, may be important to capture and report because the balance of harms and benefits may easily lean toward harms in a low-risk population. For other populations and for interventions that improve major outcomes (e.g., survival), severe and life-threatening adverse events may be the only ones that are important in the balance of benefits and harms.

Withdrawals due to harms

Discontinuations and withdrawals due to adverse events reflect the ultimate decision of the participant and/or physician to discontinue treatment. This constitutes important clinical information about any tested intervention and it should be presented separately for each treatment arm. Treatment may occasionally be discontinued for mild or moderate adverse events, and attribution of discontinuation to a specific reason may sometimes be difficult as the decision to stop treatment may reflect an array of multiple reasons that include both perceptions of effectiveness and tolerability. However, information about withdrawal reasons can be valuable for understanding the treatment experience.

Deaths in particular are very important to report in each study group during a trial, regardless of whether death is an end point and whether attribution to a specific cause is possible.

Trials with prolonged follow-up should ideally report the timing of allocated treatment received, dose reductions and discontinuations, and study withdrawals. Early withdrawals may be due to different reasons than late withdrawals.

Absolute risks per arm and per adverse event type, grade, and seriousness

Authors should present results separately for each arm of the trial, otherwise the comparative information is lost. For each type of adverse event, they should offer appropriate metrics of absolute risk (e.g., frequency or incidence), with separate information about the severity grade of the event, if relevant. Information merging different types, different grades, or different levels of seriousness for harms is often presented in trial reports, but this conveys little insight and such mergers should be avoided. Serious events in particular should be reported separately for each type of event. Recurrent events and timing of events also need appropriate reporting.

Future plans

No revision of the extension is planned in the near future, but as for other CONSORT checklists, the team is welcoming suggestions for improvements.

References

1 Ioannidis, J.P.A., Evans, S.J.W., Goetzsche, P.C. *et al.* (2004) Better reporting of harms in randomized trials: an extension of the CONSORT statement. *Annals of Internal Medicine*, **141**, 781–788.
2 Ioannidis, J.P. (2009) Adverse events in randomized trials: neglected, restricted, distorted, and silenced. *Archives of Internal Medicine*, **169**, 1737–1739.
3 Ioannidis, J.P. & Lau, J. (2002) Improving safety reporting from randomised trials. *Drug Safety*, **25**, 77–84.
4 Ioannidis, J.P. & Lau, J. (2001) Completeness of safety reporting in randomized trials: an evaluation of 7 medical areas. *JAMA*, **285**, 437–443.
5 Golder, S., Loke, Y.K. & Zorzela, L. (2013) Some improvements are apparent in identifying adverse effects in systematic reviews from 1994 to 2011. *Journal of Clinical Epidemiology*, **66** (3), 253–260.

Checklist of items to include when reporting harms in randomized, controlled trials*

Standard CONSORT Checklist: Paper Section and Topic	Standard CONSORT Checklist: Item Number	Descriptor	Reported on Page Number
Title and abstract	1	If the study collected data on harms and benefits, the title or abstract should so state.	
Introduction			
Background	2	If the trial addresses both harms and benefits, the introduction should so state	
Methods			
Participants	3		
Interventions	4		
Objectives	5		
Outcomes	6	List addressed adverse events with definitions for each (with attention, when relevant, to grading, expected vs. unexpected events, reference to standardized and validated definitions, and description of new definitions). Clarify how harms-related information was collected (mode of data collection, timing, attribution methods, intensity of ascertainment, and harms-related monitoring and stopping rules, if pertinent)	
Sample size	7		
Randomization			
Sequence generation	8		
Allocation concealment	9		
Implementation	10		
Blinding (masking)	11		
Statistical methods	12	Describe plans for presenting and analyzing information on harms (including coding, handling of recurrent events, specification of timing issues, handling of continuous measures, and any statistical analyzes).	
Results			
Participant flow	13	Describe for each arm the participant withdrawals that are due to harms and their experiences with the allocated treatment.	
Recruitment	14		
Baseline data	15		

(continued)

Standard CONSORT Checklist: Paper Section and Topic	Standard CONSORT Checklist: Item Number	Descriptor	Reported on Page Number
Numbers analyzed	16	Provide the denominators for analyzes on harms.	
Outcomes and estimation	17	Present the absolute risk per arm and per adverse event type, grade, and seriousness, and present appropriate metrics for recurrent events, continuous variables, and scale variables, whenever pertinent.[†]	
Ancillary analyzes	18	Describe any subgroup analyzes and exploratory analyzes for harms.[†]	
Adverse events	19		
Discussion			
Interpretation	20	Provide a balanced discussion of benefits and harms with emphasis on study limitations, generalizability, and other sources of information on harms.[‡]	
Generalizability	21		
Overall evidence	22		

*This proposed extension for harms includes 10 recommendations that correspond to the original CONSORT checklist.
[†]Descriptors refer to items 17, 18, and 19.
[‡]Descriptor refers to items 20, 21, and 22.

CHAPTER 11

CONSORT for Nonpharmacologic Treatments

Isabelle Boutron[1,2] and Philippe Ravaud[1,2]

[1] *Centre d'Epidémiologie Clinique, Assistance Publique-Hôpitaux de Paris, Paris, France*
[2] *Centre Cochrane Français, INSERM U738, Université Paris Descartes, Paris, France*

CONSORT development path

Reporting guideline	Notes	Meeting date	Publication date
Extension of the CONSORT Statement for nonpharmacologic treatments	For randomized trials assessing nonpharmacologic treatments such as surgery, technical intervention, devices, rehabilitation, psychotherapy, education	February 2006	2008

Name of guideline

Nonpharmacologic treatments include a wide range of interventions such as surgery, technical operations, rehabilitation, behavioral therapy, psychotherapy, and medical devices. The number of published reports of randomized controlled trials assessing nonpharmacologic treatments is increasing [1]. In a sample of randomized controlled trials with results published in 2006, 21% assessed surgical or procedural interventions, 18% participative interventions such as counseling or lifestyle interventions, and 3% equipment or devices. Assessing nonpharmacologic treatments raises specific methodological issues [2, 3]. In fact, nonpharmacologic treatments are frequently complex interventions involving several components, all having a possible influence on the success of

Guidelines for Reporting Health Research: A User's Manual, First Edition. Edited by David Moher, Douglas G. Altman, Kenneth F. Schulz, Iveta Simera and Elizabeth Wager.
© 2014 John Wiley & Sons, Ltd. Published 2014 by John Wiley & Sons, Ltd.

the treatment. The interventions are consequently difficult to describe, standardize, and administer consistently to all patients. Furthermore, there may be differences between the planned intervention and the intervention actually delivered. Another important issue when assessing nonpharmacologic treatments is the possible influence of care providers' and centers' expertise on the treatment effect. Finally, in trials assessing nonpharmacologic treatments, blinding of patients and care providers is frequently not feasible, which raises concerns about the risk of bias.

Several studies have shown that these methodological issues are inadequately reported in publications for randomized controlled trials assessing nonpharmacologic treatments. For example, in a sample of randomized controlled trials assessing surgical procedures with results published in 2004, details on the surgical procedure were reported in 87% of the articles, anesthetic management in 35%, preoperative care in 15%, and postoperative care in 49%. The setting and the center volume were reported in less than 1% of the articles [4]. The number of care providers performing the intervention was given in 32% of the articles. In another study, nonpharmacologic treatments were adequately described in less than one-third of published reports [5].

To overcome the inadequate reporting for studies of nonpharmacologic treatments, the CONSORT group developed an extension of the CONSORT Statement for nonpharmacologic treatments. This extension was published with an explanation and elaboration document in *Annals of Internal Medicine* in 2008 [6, 7]. In this extension, 11 items of the CONSORT Statement were modified, and one new item was added. The flow diagram was also modified. The extension was published along with the 22 items of the 2001 CONSORT Statement. In this article, we discuss the extension in relation to the recently updated CONSORT Statement (i.e., with the 25 items of the CONSORT 2010 Statement).

When to use the extension of the CONSORT Statement for nonpharmacologic treatments

The extension of the CONSORT Statement for nonpharmacologic treatments provides guidance for reporting the results of randomized controlled trials assessing nonpharmacologic treatments. The box shown in the next page describes the different types of interventions that this extension covers. Depending on the trial design used, this extension should be used with the relevant extension for cluster randomized controlled trials, noninferiority and equivalence trials or pragmatic trials (Figure 11.1).

> **Nonpharmacologic treatments**
>
> *Definition*: treatments that do not mainly involve the use of pharmaceuticals
>
> *Different categories and examples*:
>   Therapist interventions such as surgery and angioplasty: the success depends highly on the care providers' skill.
>   Participative interventions such as rehabilitation, physiotherapy, behavioral therapy, and psychotherapy involving collaboration between patients and care providers.
>   Devices such as ultrasound treatment and orthoses.

Development process

A steering committee was responsible for the development of this extension. The extension was developed according to the accepted strategy for developing reporting guidelines [8]. First, a literature review was performed to identify the specific issues involved in assessing nonpharmacologic treatments that should be taken into account when reporting results of randomized controlled trials. Then the steering committee identified expert participants for the consensus meeting: 37 were invited and 30 attended. The 30 attendees included methodologists ($n = 14$), surgeons ($n = 6$), medical journal editors ($n = 5$), clinicians involved in rehabilitation ($n = 1$), psychotherapy ($n = 2$), education ($n = 1$), and implantable devices ($n = 1$).

Before the meeting, the steering group surveyed meeting invitees, using a web-based interface, to identify the specific issues that should be discussed. Invitees were asked to suggest which of the 22 CONSORT 2001 checklist items might need modification for the proposed extension. Respondents were also asked whether they believed the following items should be added to the CONSORT checklist:

In the Methods section
- eligibility criteria for care providers (surgeons, physiotherapists, psychologists, etc.) included in the trial
- center volume for the procedure or similar procedures (as a proxy for experience)

In the Results section
- the number of care providers performing the treatment in each group
- the number of participants receiving treatment from each care provider
- participants' expectancies or preference for the treatments at baseline
- baseline data on care providers
- care providers' compliance with the planned procedure

Invitees were also asked to identify additional items they felt were important when evaluating nonpharmacologic treatments.

When more than one-third of the respondents stated that an item needed to be modified or that another item should be added, that item was selected for further discussion during the consensus meeting.

A three-day consensus meeting was held in February 2006 in Paris, France. The meeting began with several presentations on specific topics that allowed for discussion of the specific methodological issues relevant to reporting results of trials of nonpharmacologic treatment.

Each CONSORT checklist item proposed for modification or as an addition to the checklist was then introduced and discussed by the participants. These discussions were moderated by at least one member of the steering group. The remaining CONSORT checklist items were then considered to determine whether additional modifications were needed.

After the meeting, a draft of the CONSORT extension for nonpharmacologic treatment was circulated to all meeting participants. A "disposition file" containing comments and suggested revisions from each respondent was created. The modified statement was revised to ensure that it accurately represented the decisions made during the meeting. After the revisions, the group approved the checklist, the flow diagram, and the articles arising from the meeting.

Extension compared with the CONSORT checklist

The consensus was that 11 items on the CONSORT checklist needed some modifications for trials of nonpharmacologic treatments: the items dedicated to the title and abstract, participants, interventions, sample size, randomization, blinding, statistical methods, participant flow, baseline data, discussion – interpretation, and discussion – generalizability were modified and clarified in the context of assessing nonpharmacologic treatments. In addition, one item related to implementation of the intervention was added.

The modifications focused on the specific issues involved in assessing nonpharmacologic treatments. The statement requests that authors provide a clear description of the intervention and the comparator with a description of all the components of the intervention intended, the procedure for tailoring the intervention to patients, how the intervention was standardized, and how adherence was assessed. A new item for the results section was dedicated to the description of the intervention as it was actually administered. In fact, because nonpharmacologic treatments are complex interventions, the intervention planned and described in the protocol and the intervention actually administered to patients may differ.

The extension also encourages authors to provide more details of study centers, settings, and care providers' expertise. Publications should describe eligibility criteria for care providers and centers and also the care providers and centers that actually participated. Finally, the statement clarifies the need to consider the clustering of patients treated in the same center by the same care provider.

The flow diagram was also modified, with a specific box added to indicate the number of care providers and centers performing the intervention in each arm and the number of patients treated by each care provider and in each center in each arm.

The item dedicated to blinding was slightly modified to clarify the need to indicate the blinding status for all care providers: those administering the intervention and those administering cointerventions. The discussions and modifications proposed for the item related to blinding were included in the recently updated 2010 CONSORT Statement that specified "if relevant, description of the similarity of interventions."

How best to use the extension guidelines

The CONSORT extension for nonpharmacologic treatments should be used by authors when reporting results of trials assessing nonpharmacologic treatments and by editors and reviewers when evaluating such manuscripts. We encourage readers to use the elaboration and explanation document of the extension [6]. Although the extension of the CONSORT Statement for nonpharmacologic treatment was not developed to improve the planning and conducting of randomized controlled trials, we recommend reading the statement when writing the trial protocol and when conducting the trial. In fact, adequate reporting supposes that the relevant data were collected. For example, the statement indicates that authors should provide a *"description of the different components of the interventions and, when applicable, descriptions of the procedure for tailoring the interventions to individual participants."* This text implies that authors adequately described their intervention in the trial protocol. Similarly, the statement indicates that *"the number of care providers or centers performing the intervention in each group and the number of patients treated by each care provider or in each center"* should be reported. Again, this implies that investigators systematically registered which care provider treated which patient.

Evidence of effectiveness of the extension guidelines

To our knowledge, no study has specifically evaluated the impact of the extension for nonpharmacologic treatments on the quality of reporting.

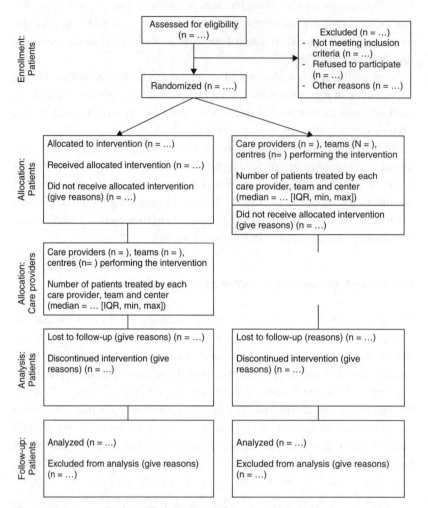

Figure 11.1 Example of modified CONSORT flow chart for individual randomized controlled trials of nonpharmacologic treatments with an extra box per intervention group relating to care providers. For cluster randomized controlled trials, authors should refer to the extension related to such trials. IQR, interquartile range.

Endorsement and adherence

The specific endorsement of the extension of the CONSORT Statement for nonpharmacologic treatments has not been evaluated; however, the extension is on the CONSORT website (http://www.consort-statement.org/?%20=1190), which is supported and endorsed by the International Committee of Medical Journal Editors (http://www.icmje.org).

Cautions and limitations

The extension of the CONSORT Statement for nonpharmacologic treatments is designed to improve the transparency of reporting randomized nonpharmacologic trials. This extension implies that authors, editors, and reviewers accept that a transparent report highlighting an imperfect methodology has a greater chance to be published than a report with lack of transparency, hiding a possibly imperfect methodology. Another important issue is that the extension should be used in conjunction with other statements such as the 2010 CONSORT Statement but also other specific extensions related to the design (e.g., cluster randomized controlled trials, pragmatic trials, etc.) and data (harm). However, following multiple statements may pose difficulties for authors [9].

Creators' preferred items

Precise details of both the experimental treatment and comparator.

   For readers to adequately translate trial findings into clinical practice, the description of the intervention should be sufficiently detailed to be reproduced. This recommendation suggests describing all the steps used to standardize the intervention during the trial and to highlight what intervention was actually administered to patients.

Participant flow

The flow diagram is essential for readers to appraise internal and external validity. Several studies have demonstrated the impact of care providers' expertise and centers' volume of care on the success of treatments [10–12]. The suggested flow diagram has consequently been modified and now includes the number of patients and centers in each arm and the number of patients treated by each care provider in each center. Therefore, the reader can appraise the applicability of the trial results.

Blinding

Blinding is essential to limit the risk of performance bias and detection bias [13] but is more difficult to achieve and maintain in trials of nonpharmacologic treatments [3]. For example, to avoid detection bias in a surgical trial, the patients, the surgeons, the anesthesiologists, the surgical team, the nurses, or the care providers administering cointerventions could be blinded. Because the methods of blinding are often complex [14], the methods used should be clearly described and discussed. If blinding is not feasible, the risk of bias should be discussed taking into consideration the subjectivity of the primary outcome.

Future plans

The CONSORT Statement has been updated in 2010, whereas the extension for nonpharmacologic treatments was published in 2008. For the purpose of this article, we updated the extension according to the 2010 CONSORT Statement (see Table 11.1).

The main issue related to this extension is probably the lack of endorsement and adherence. To improve endorsement of this and other extensions, we plan to develop a CONSORT web tool, which will be available on the CONSORT website and will provide an individualized checklist that links all the checklists. For example, for a pragmatic, cluster-randomized trial evaluating nonpharmacologic treatments, the 2010 CONSORT Statement will be linked to the three relevant extensions and a merged checklist provided

Table 11.1 Extension of the CONSORT Statement for reporting the results of randomized trials assessing nonpharmacologic treatments[a].

Section/topic	Item #[b]	CONSORT 2010 checklist items	Extension for trials of nonpharmacologic treatments
Title and abstract	1a	Identification as a randomized trial in the title	In the abstract, description of the experimental treatment, comparator, care providers, centers, and blinding status
	1b	Structured summary of trial design, methods, results, and conclusions; for specific guidance, see CONSORT for Abstracts	
Introduction			
Background and objectives	2a	Scientific background and explanation of rationale	
	2b	Specific objectives or hypotheses	
Methods			
Trial design	3a	Description of trial design (e.g., parallel, factorial) including allocation ratio	
	3b	Important changes to methods after trial commencement (e.g., eligibility criteria), with reasons	
Participants	4a	Eligibility criteria for participants	When applicable, eligibility criteria for centers and those performing the interventions
	4b	Settings and locations where the data were collected	
Interventions	5	The interventions for each group with sufficient details to allow replication, including how and when they were actually administered	Precise details of both the experimental treatment and comparator

Table 11.1 (*Continued*)

Section/topic	Item #	CONSORT 2010 checklist items	Extension for trials of nonpharmacologic treatments
	5a		Description of the different components of the interventions and, when applicable, descriptions of the procedure for tailoring the interventions to individual participants
	5b		Details of how the interventions were standardized
	5c		Details of how adherence of care providers with the protocol was assessed or enhanced
Outcomes	6a	Completely defined pre-specified primary and secondary outcome measures, including how and when they were assessed	
	6b	Any changes to trial outcomes after the trial commenced with reasons	
Sample size	7a	How sample size was determined	When applicable, details of whether and how the clustering by care providers or centers was addressed
	7b	When applicable, explanation of any interim analyses and stopping guidelines	
Randomization: Sequence generation	8a	Method used to generate the random allocation sequence	When applicable, how care providers were allocated to each trial group
	8b	Type of randomization; details of any restriction (e.g., blocking and block size)	
Allocation concealment mechanism	9	Mechanism used to implement the random allocation sequence (e.g., sequentially numbered containers), describing any steps taken to conceal the sequence until interventions were assigned	
Implementation	10	Who generated the random allocation sequence, who enrolled participants, and who assigned participants to interventions	

(*continued*)

Table 11.1 (*Continued*)

Section/topic	Item #	CONSORT 2010 checklist items	Extension for trials of nonpharmacologic treatments
Blinding	11a	If done, who was blinded after assignment to interventions (e.g., participants, care providers, those assessing outcomes) and how	Whether or not those administering cointerventions were blinded to group assignment
	11b	If relevant, description of the similarity of interventions	If blinded, method of blinding and description of the similarity of interventions
Statistical methods	12a	Statistical methods used to compare groups for primary and secondary outcomes	When applicable, details of whether and how the clustering by care providers or centers was addressed
	12b	Methods for additional analyses, such as subgroup analyses and adjusted analyses	
Results			
Participant flow (A diagram is strongly recommended)	13a	For each group, the numbers of participants who were randomly assigned, received intended treatment, and were analyzed for the primary outcome	The number of care providers or centers performing the intervention in each group and the number of patients treated by each care provider or in each center
	13b	For each group, losses and exclusions after randomization, together with reasons	
Implementation of intervention	New item		Details of the experimental treatment and comparator as they were implemented
Recruitment	14a	Dates defining the periods of recruitment and follow-up	
	14b	Why the trial ended or was stopped	
Baseline data	15	A table showing baseline demographic and clinical characteristics for each group	When applicable, a description of care providers (case volume, qualification, expertise, etc.) and centers (volume) in each group
Numbers analyzed	16	For each group, number of participants (denominator) included in each analysis and whether the analysis was by original assigned groups	
Outcomes and estimation	17a	For each primary and secondary outcome, results for each group, and the estimated effect size and its precision (e.g., 95% confidence interval)	

Table 11.1 (*Continued*)

Section/topic	Item #	CONSORT 2010 checklist items	Extension for trials of nonpharmacologic treatments
	17b	For binary outcomes, presentation of both absolute and relative effect sizes is recommended	
Ancillary analyses	18	Results of any other analyses performed, including subgroup analyses and adjusted analyses, distinguishing pre-specified from exploratory	
Harms	19	All important harms or unintended effects in each group; for specific guidance, see CONSORT for Harms	
Discussion			
Limitations	20	Trial limitations, addressing sources of potential bias, imprecision, and, if relevant, multiplicity of analyses	
Generalizability	21	Generalizability (external validity, applicability) of the trial findings	Generalizability (external validity) of the trial findings according to the intervention, comparators, patients, and care providers and centers involved in the trial
Interpretation	22	Interpretation consistent with results, balancing benefits and harms, and considering other relevant evidence	In addition, take into account the choice of the comparator, lack of or partial blinding, and unequal expertise of care providers or centers in each group
Other information			
Registration	23	Registration number and name of trial registry	
Protocol	24	Where the full trial protocol can be accessed, if available	
Funding	25	Sources of funding and other support (e.g., supply of drugs); role of funders	

[a]We strongly recommend reading this Statement in conjunction with the CONSORT explanation and elaboration nonpharmacologic treatments [6] and the 2010 CONSORT explanation and elaboration [15].
[b]Item numbers were modified according to the 2010 CONSORT Statement.

to authors. We will evaluate the impact of this tool on compliance with the CONSORT Statement in a randomized controlled trial.

References

1   Hopewell, S., Dutton, S., Yu, L.M. *et al.* (2010) The quality of reports of randomised trials in 2000 and 2006: comparative study of articles indexed in PubMed. *BMJ*, **340**, c723.

2   Boutron, I., Tubach, F., Giraudeau, B. & Ravaud, P. (2003) Methodological differences in clinical trials evaluating nonpharmacological and pharmacological treatments of hip and knee osteoarthritis. *JAMA*, **290** (8), 1062–1070.

3   Boutron, I., Tubach, F., Giraudeau, B. & Ravaud, P. (2004) Blinding was judged more difficult to achieve and maintain in nonpharmacologic than pharmacologic trials. *Journal of Clinical Epidemiology*, **57** (6), 543–550.

4   Jacquier, I., Boutron, I., Moher, D. *et al.* (2006) The reporting of randomized clinical trials using a surgical intervention is in need of immediate improvement: a systematic review. *Annals of Surgery*, **244** (5), 677–683.

5   Glasziou, P., Meats, E., Heneghan, C. & Shepperd, S. (2008) What is missing from descriptions of treatment in trials and reviews? *BMJ*, **336** (7659), 1472–1474.

6   Boutron, I., Moher, D., Altman, D.G. *et al.* (2008) Extending the CONSORT statement to randomized trials of nonpharmacologic treatment: explanation and elaboration. *Annals of Internal Medicine*, **148** (4), 295–309.

7   Boutron, I., Moher, D., Altman, D.G. *et al.* (2008) Methods and processes of the CONSORT Group: example of an extension for trials assessing nonpharmacologic treatments. *Annals of Internal Medicine*, **148** (4), W60–W66.

8   Moher, D., Schulz, K.F., Simera, I. & Altman, D.G. (2010) Guidance for developers of health research reporting guidelines. *PLoS Medicine*, **7** (2), e1000217.

9   Plint, A.C., Moher, D., Morrison, A. *et al.* (2006) Does the CONSORT checklist improve the quality of reports of randomised controlled trials? A systematic review. *Medical Journal of Australia*, **185** (5), 263–267.

10 Halm, E.A., Lee, C., Chassin, M.R. (2002) Is volume related to outcome in health care? A systematic review and methodologic critique of the literature. *Annals of Internal Medicine*, **137** (6), 511–520.

11 Biau, D.J., Halm, J.A., Ahmadieh, H. *et al.* (2008) Provider and center effect in multicenter randomized controlled trials of surgical specialties: an analysis on patient-level data. *Annals of Surgery*, **247** (5), 892–898.

12 Khuri, S.F., Daley, J., Henderson, W. *et al.* (1999) Relation of surgical volume to outcome in eight common operations: results from the VA National Surgical Quality Improvement Program. *Annals of Surgery* **230**, 414–432.

13 Juni, P., Altman, D.G. & Egger, M. (2001) Systematic reviews in health care: assessing the quality of controlled clinical trials. *BMJ*, **323** (7303), 42–46.

14 Boutron, I., Guittet, L., Estellat, C. *et al.* (2007) Reporting methods of blinding in randomized trials assessing nonpharmacological treatments. *PLoS Medicine*, **4** (2), e61.

15 Moher, D., Hopewell, S., Schulz, K.F. *et al.* (2010) CONSORT 2010 Explanation and Elaboration: updated guidelines for reporting parallel group randomised trials. *BMJ*, **340**, c869.

CHAPTER 12
CONSORT for Pragmatic Trials

Merrick Zwarenstein
Schulich School of Medicine and Dentistry, Western University, London, ON, Canada

Timetable

Name of reporting guideline initiative	Notes	Consensus meeting date	Reporting guideline publication
Practihc		January 2005 and March 2008	December 2008

Practihc (Pragmatic Randomized Controlled Trials in Health Care)

The Pragmatic Randomized Controlled Trials in Health Care extension to the CONSORT [1] Statement is a guidance document for authors reporting randomized trials of interventions directly aimed at improving health status, or healthcare processes or outcomes, under real-world conditions, that is, under the conditions of healthcare settings as usually organized, resourced, and run. The Practihc guideline for reporting pragmatic randomized controlled trials is a 22-item checklist covering the design, methods, results, and discussion of a completed randomized trial. It is an extension of the 2001 CONSORT Statement [2]. Practihc may be useful for peer reviewers and editors reviewing reports of randomized trials, for authors wishing to provide a full report oriented toward decision makers, and for readers wanting to gauge the relevance of a randomized trial conducted elsewhere, to the care setting in which they might wish to use the evaluated intervention.

Guidelines for Reporting Health Research: A User's Manual, First Edition. Edited by David Moher, Douglas G. Altman, Kenneth F. Schulz, Iveta Simera and Elizabeth Wager.
© 2014 John Wiley & Sons, Ltd. Published 2014 by John Wiley & Sons, Ltd.

History/development

In 2005 and in 2008, two meetings of an informal group of trialists (the Practihc group) were held to discuss ways to increase the contribution of randomized controlled trials to healthcare decision making. Participants included clinicians, trialists, research commissioners, clinical practice guideline developers, and experts on research reporting.

One of the principal stimuli for the work and a key document circulated to meeting participants was a paper from 1969, titled "Pragmatic and explanatory attitudes in therapeutical trials," by two French statisticians [3]. This paper was one of the first to explain the differences between randomized trials conducted under idealized circumstances and those conducted under conditions designed to replicate real-world healthcare settings and to clarify the implications of these two kinds of approaches to the usefulness of the trial results for healthcare decision making. After the 2005 meeting, a draft checklist for extension of the 2001 CONSORT Statement was circulated to a writing group, and after several revisions this group produced a draft summary paper. At the 2008 meeting, the draft was discussed and modified. It was circulated to the CONSORT Group for feedback, modified, and submitted for publication.

The Practihc statement offers extensions of eight items in the 2001 CONSORT Statement, in order to more fully capture those details of trial conduct that can influence whether findings will apply in usual healthcare settings.

When to use this guideline (what types of studies it covers)

The Practihc statement can be used when reporting randomized controlled trials of health and healthcare interventions (including drugs, devices, educational, and organizational interventions) that are intended to be used in usual care settings. The Practihc statement is particularly useful when findings are claimed to be directly relevant to usual clinical care or health service settings, and immediate implementation is being recommended.

Previous version

None.

Current version

The Practihc statement consists of some brief text explaining the development of the reporting guideline, a 22-item checklist and a standard

CONSORT flow diagram. Eight of the 22 items from the 2001 CONSORT Statement have been extended. These are described below: the original text is shown in *italics*, followed by the text that has been added to the item.

Item 2: introduction, background

Scientific background and explanation of rationale

Extension for pragmatic trials: Describe the health or health service problem that the intervention is intended to address and other interventions that may commonly be aimed at this problem.

Item 3: methods, participants

Eligibility criteria for participants and the settings and the locations where the data were collected.

Extension for pragmatic trials: Eligibility criteria should be explicitly framed to show the degree to which they include typical participants and, where applicable, typical providers (e.g., nurses), institutions (e.g., hospitals), communities (or localities, e.g., towns), and settings of care (e.g., different healthcare financing systems).

Item 4: methods, interventions

Precise details of the interventions intended for each group and how and when they were actually administered.

Extension for pragmatic trials: Describe extra resources added to (or resources removed from) usual settings in order to implement the intervention. Indicate if efforts were made to standardize the intervention or if the intervention and its delivery were allowed to vary between participants, practitioners, or study sites. Describe the comparator in similar detail to the intervention.

Item 6: methods, outcomes

Clearly defined primary and secondary outcome measures, and, when applicable, any methods used to enhance the quality of measurements (e.g., multiple observations, training of assessors)

Extension for pragmatic trials: Explain why the chosen outcomes and, when relevant, the length of follow-up are considered important to those who will use the results of the trial.

Item 7: methods, sample size

How sample size was determined; when applicable, explanation of any interim analyses and stopping rules

Extension for pragmatic trials: If calculated using the smallest difference considered important by the target decision maker audience (the minimally important difference), then report where this difference was obtained.

Item 11: methods, blinding (masking)

Whether participants, those administering the interventions, and those assessing the outcomes were blinded to group assignment

   Extension for pragmatic trials: If blinding was not done, or was not possible, explain why.

Item 13: results, participant flow

Flow of participants through each stage (a diagram is strongly recommended). Specifically, for each group report the number of participants randomly assigned, receiving intended treatment, completing the study protocol, and analyzed for the primary outcome. Describe protocol deviations from study as planned, together with reasons

   Extension for pragmatic trials: The number of participants or units approached to take part in the trial, the number which were eligible, and reasons for nonparticipation should be reported.

Item 21: generalizability (applicability, external validity)

Generalizability of the trial findings

   Extension for pragmatic trials: Describe key aspects of the setting that determined the trial results. Discuss possible differences in other settings where clinical traditions, health service organization, staffing, or resources may vary from those of the trial.

Extensions and/or implementations

The Practihc extension has been published in one journal where it is freely accessible. There is no elaboration and explanation paper, but the published Practihc extension does include illustrative examples of good descriptions, extracted from published randomized trials for each item where extra information is sought and an explanation of the justification for seeking this extra information.

   No extensions of the Practihc work have been published.

Related activities

The work described in the Practihc extension of the CONSORT Statement has been extended to the design stage of randomized trials. We have published a guide to help trial teams consider, at the design stage of their trial, where their key design choices lie on the spectrum between pragmatic and explanatory [4]. This is in order to help the teams make consistent and explicit choices in their design, so that the trial serves its intended purpose on a spectrum extending from confirming a physiological hypothesis (explanatory) to assisting in making a program decision between two interventions aimed at the same problem (pragmatic).

This extension of the Practihc work could also help reviewers of randomized trials submitted for funding or for methodological review to consider whether the design of the trial matches the stated intents of the designers.

The Practihc group was established originally to increase the number of randomized trials directly relevant to decision makers. With this in mind, the Practihc group has developed and made available for download the Trial Protocol Tool, a web-based resource that is free for nonprofit users [5]. This resource contains a large library of pragmatic trial protocols, text describing pragmatic trials, templates that can be used for designing such trials, and a library of PowerPoint slides, which could be used in teaching on pragmatic trial design. This library of resources and templates for the design of a pragmatic randomized trial is available at www.practihc.org. A paper describing the Trial Protocol Tool has been published.

How best to use the guideline

Authors
The Practihc extension has been developed to help authors who evaluate interventions with the goal of using their published results to influence decisions on "real-world" use of the intervention that they have evaluated. It is intended to help them accurately and transparently report the design choices they made in their trial to decision makers. It should particularly assist authors in fully reporting the items most relevant to decision makers, without omitting any details that might be important to those who will use the results for decisions on implementation, funding, or adaptation of the intervention evaluated in the trial.

Peer reviewers
The Practihc extension is designed to help peer reviewers assess whether a potentially important intervention that has undergone a randomized trial is reported in a way that decision-making users would find useful.

Editors
Editors can use the checklist is many ways. By asking authors to complete and include a populated checklist as part of the submission process, editors can gauge the level of detail provided by the authors, especially for those areas that are of particular interest to decision makers who will directly use the trial results to purchase (or not), implement (or not), or recommend (or not) the evaluated intervention. This will help editors to commission and frame editorials to accompany the article, thereby helping readers to

judge both the validity of the trial results and their relevance to their own decision making.

Development process

In January 2005 and in March 2008, we held two-day meetings in Toronto, Canada, to discuss ways to increase the contribution of randomized controlled trials to healthcare decision making, focusing on pragmatic trials. Participants included people with experience in clinical care, commissioning research, healthcare financing, developing clinical practice guidelines, and trial methodology and reporting. Twenty-four people participated in 2005 and 42 in 2008, including members of the CONSORT and Practihc groups. After the 2005 meeting, a draft revised checklist for the extension was circulated to a writing group, including some of those invited to the meeting but unable to attend. After several revisions, the writing group produced a draft summary paper. At the 2008 meeting, the draft was discussed and modified. It was circulated to the CONSORT Group for feedback, modified, and submitted for publication.

Evidence of effectiveness of guideline

We are unaware of any evaluations of whether the use of the Practihc extension checklist is associated with an improved quality of trial reporting. One paper has been published suggesting that the PRECIS tool, a sibling to Practihc, but intended for use at the design phase of a randomized trial, was helpful in keeping the design of a trial consistent with the intended purpose [6].

Endorsement and adherence

Thus far, Practihc has not been endorsed by any journal.

Cautions and limitations (including scope)

The Practihc checklist is not intended as an instrument to evaluate the quality of a randomized trial nor it is appropriate to use the checklist to construct a quality score.

The Practihc statement was developed to assist in the reporting of a broad range of intervention trials that aim to evaluate an intervention for use in usual care settings, rather than to test the efficacy of an intervention under idealized conditions.

The flow diagram will need adjustments when reporting cluster trials or other adaptations to the usual two-armed parallel trial.

Creators' preferred bits

Item 2: introduction, background
Scientific background and explanation of rationale

Extension for pragmatic trials: Describe the health or health service problem that the intervention is intended to address and other interventions that may commonly be aimed at this problem.

(a) Describe the health or health service problem, which the intervention is intended to address.

Explanation – Users of pragmatic trial reports seek to solve a health or health service problem in a particular setting. The problem at which the intervention is targeted should thus be described. This enables readers to understand whether the problem confronting them is similar to the problem described in the trial report, and thus whether the study is relevant to them. Ideally, the report should state that the trial is pragmatic in attitude (and why) and explain the purpose of the trial in relationship to the decisions that it is intended to inform and in which settings.

(b) Describe other interventions that may commonly be aimed at this problem.

Explanation – The background of the trial report should mention the intervention under investigation and the usual alternative(s) in relevant settings. To help place the trial in the context of other settings, authors should explain the key features that make the intervention feasible in their trial setting and elsewhere (such as, the widespread availability of the trial drug, the availability of trained staff to deliver the intervention, electronic databases that can identify eligible patients).

Item 3: methods, participants
Eligibility criteria for participants and the settings, and the locations where the data were collected.

Extension for pragmatic trials: Eligibility criteria should be explicitly framed to show the degree to which they include typical participants and, where applicable, typical providers (e.g., nurses), institutions (e.g., hospitals), communities (or localities, e.g., towns), and settings of care (e.g., different healthcare financing systems).

 Explanation – Treatments may perform better when evaluated among selected, highly adherent patients with severe but not intractable disease and few comorbidities. Reports of these restricted trials may be of limited applicability. Excessively stringent inclusion and exclusion criteria reduce the applicability of findings and may result in safety concerns, so the method of recruitment should be completely described. This stringency seems to be reducing over time but remains a problem.

In some trials, the unit of randomization and intervention might be healthcare practitioners, communities, or healthcare institutions such as clinics (i.e., cluster randomized pragmatic trials). In these trials, volunteer institutions may be atypically experienced or well-resourced successful innovators. As the feasibility and success of an intervention may depend on attributes of the healthcare system and setting, reporting this information enables readers to assess the relevance and applicability of the results in their own, possibly different, settings.

Item 4: methods, interventions

Precise details of the interventions intended for each group and how and when they were actually administered.

Extension for pragmatic trials: Describe extra resources added to (or resources removed from) usual settings in order to implement the intervention. Indicate whether efforts were made to standardize the intervention or whether the intervention and its delivery were allowed to vary between participants, practitioners, or study sites. Describe the comparator in similar detail to the intervention.

(a) Describe extra resources added to (or resources removed from) usual settings in order to implement the intervention.

Explanation: If the extra resources to deliver the intervention are not described, readers cannot judge the feasibility of the intervention in their own setting. When relevant, authors should report details (experience, training, etc.) of those who delivered the intervention and its frequency and intensity. If multicomponent interventions are being evaluated, details of the different components should be described.

(b) Indicate whether efforts were made to standardize the intervention or whether the intervention and its delivery were allowed to vary between participants, practitioners, or study sites.

Explanation: In explanatory trials, the intervention is standardized and thus the results may not apply under usual conditions of care where no such standardization is enforced. Pragmatic trials are conducted in typical care settings, and so care may vary between similar participants, by chance, by practitioner preference, or according to institutional policies. For pragmatic trials, efforts that may reduce this natural variation in the intervention and its delivery should be described. However, if reducing variation in a care process or shifting practice patterns is itself the main purpose of the intervention, this should be explicit in the title, abstract, and introduction.

Regardless of the extent to which the intervention was standardized, pragmatic trials should describe the intervention in sufficient detail so that someone could replicate it, or include a reference, or link to a detailed description of the intervention. Unfortunately, this information is often lacking in reports of trials.

(c) Describe the comparator in similar detail to the intervention.

Explanation – In a randomized controlled trial, the effects of the intervention are always related to a comparator. To increase applicability and feasibility, pragmatic trials often compare new interventions to usual care. The chosen comparator should be described in sufficient detail for readers to assess whether the incremental benefits or harms reported are likely to apply in their own setting, where usual care may be more, or less, effective.

Future plans

We plan to update the Practihc extension to match the 2010 CONSORT Statement update.

We plan to undertake systematic reviews of randomized trials to identify the proportion that are explicitly intended to influence decision making, and to evaluate their reporting, using the Practihc CONSORT extension paper as a standard. This will provide a baseline for future assessments of the impact of the Practihc guideline on reporting quality of pragmatic trials.

References

1 Zwarenstein, M., Treweek, S., Gagnier, J. *et al.* (2008) for the CONSORT and Pragmatic Trials in Healthcare (Practihc) groups. Improving the reporting of pragmatic trials: an extension of the CONSORT statement. *BMJ*, **337**, a2390.

2 Moher, D., Schulz, K.F. & Altman, D. (2001) The CONSORT statement: revised recommendations for improving the quality of reports of parallel-group randomized trials. *JAMA*, **285** (15), 1987–1991.

3 Schwartz, D. & Lellouch, J. (1967) Explanatory and pragmatic attitudes in therapeutical trials. *Journal of Chronic Diseases*, **20**, 637–648. (Reprinted in *Journal of Clinical Epidemiology* 2009;62:499–505).

4 Thorpe, K.E., Zwarenstein, M., Oxman, A.D. *et al.* (2009) A pragmatic-explanatory continuum indicator summary (PRECIS): a tool to help trial designers. *Canadian Medical Association Journal*, **180** (10), E47–E57. (Epub 16 April 2009).

5 Treweek, S., McCormack, K., Abalos, E. *et al.* (2006) The Trial Protocol Tool: The PRACTIHC software tool that supported the writing of protocols for pragmatic randomized controlled trials. *Journal of Clinical Epidemiology*, **59** (11), 1127–1133.

6 Riddle, D.L., Johnson, R.E., Jensen, M.P. *et al.* (2010) The Pragmatic-Explanatory Continuum Indicator Summary (PRECIS) instrument was useful for refining a randomized trial design: experiences from an investigative team. *Journal of Clinical Epidemiology*, **63** (11), 1271–1275.

CHAPTER 13

CONSORT for Cluster Randomized Trials

Diana R. Elbourne[1], Marion K. Campbell[2],
Gilda Piaggio[3] and Douglas G. Altman[4]

[1] *London School of Hygiene and Tropical Medicine, London, UK*
[2] *Health Services Research Unit, University of Aberdeen, Aberdeen, UK*
[3] *Statistika Consultoria Ltd, São Paulo, Brazil*
[4] *Centre for Statistics in Medicine, University of Oxford, Oxford, UK*

Timetable

Name of reporting guideline	Notes	Consensus meeting dates	Reporting guideline publication
Extending the CONSORT Statement to cluster randomized trials	Paper for discussion	Workshop Oxford, UK, 1998; Workshop Sheffield, UK, 1999	2001 [1]
CONSORT Statement: extension to cluster randomized trials	Extension of 2001 CONSORT Statement to cluster randomized trials	Montebello, Canada, 2003 Multiple meetings 2000–2004 to finalize paper	2004 [2]
CONSORT Statement 2010: extension to cluster randomized trials	Revision of 2004 paper to extend 2010 CONSORT Statement to cluster randomized trials	Multiple meetings 2009–2012 to finalize paper	2012 [3]

Guidelines for Reporting Health Research: A User's Manual, First Edition. Edited by David Moher, Douglas G. Altman, Kenneth F. Schulz, Iveta Simera and Elizabeth Wager.
© 2014 John Wiley & Sons, Ltd. Published 2014 by John Wiley & Sons, Ltd.

Name of guideline

The Consolidated Standards of Reporting Trials (CONSORT) Statement is a guideline for authors reporting the results of randomized controlled trials (RCTs). The *CONSORT Statement 2010: Extension to Cluster Randomized Trials* [3] is an extension of the 2010 CONSORT Statement [4, 5] for reports of trials in which interventions are randomly allocated to groups (clusters). It aims to elicit clear and complete information on this type of trial. It comprises explanatory text, additions, or amendments to 16 of the 25 items of the CONSORT 2010 checklist, additions to eight items of the CONSORT for Abstracts checklist [6, 7], and design-specific flow diagrams.

History/development

During discussions in 1999 about revising the original 1996 CONSORT Statement [8], it was agreed that this should focus on the simplest and most common trial design (i.e., individually randomized parallel group trials). This revision was published in 2001 [9]. Later in 2001, the CONSORT Group began to consider developing separate papers extending the CONSORT Statement to trials with other designs.

In parallel, two workshops took place in England (Oxford 1998; Sheffield 1999) to discuss cluster randomized controlled trials. One aspect that received attention was how to report this type of trial, and a paper "for discussion" was published in a special issue on cluster RCTs in *Statistics in Medicine* in 2001 [1].

These two trajectories came together in Arlington, Virginia, United States, in May 2002 when a number of CONSORT authors met to consider extensions to the 2001 CONSORT Statement in a range of different designs (including cluster randomized controlled trials). At that meeting, it was decided to write separate guidance statements for different trial designs. The cluster trial extension was the first of these.

A draft manuscript was presented for comments in a CONSORT meeting in Montebello, Canada, in May 2003. Following further discussion, the statement was published in *BMJ* in March 2004 [2].

In preparation for publication of the revised CONSORT Statement for parallel group randomized trials in 2010 [4, 5] and the recommendations for reporting abstracts [6, 7], we began to update the 2004 extension. A number of meetings were held between coauthors in London, Oxford, and Aberdeen in 2009–2010. The updated paper was published in 2012 [3].

When to use this guideline (what types of studies it covers)

The CONSORT cluster extension can be used to guide the reporting of cluster randomized trials. A key aspect of these trials is the extent of similarity within clusters compared to that between clusters, often described in terms of an intraclass correlation coefficient (ICC). The size of the sample required for a trial in which individuals are randomized in clusters is greater than that for a trial in which randomization is based on individuals alone. The extent of this inflation is the design effect, which is a function of both the ICC and the average cluster size.

Although cluster randomized trials are used to evaluate healthcare interventions, they are also used in other fields such as education, crime and justice, and social welfare.

Current version/previous versions

The current version differs from the original CONSORT extension to cluster trials in the following ways:
- The standard CONSORT checklist items and the extension specific to cluster trials are presented separately (Tables 13.1 and 13.2).
- Examples of good reporting practice have been updated.
- A summary of methodological developments published since 2004 is included.
- An augmented checklist for abstracts of cluster RCTs is provided.
- The item on sample size has been expanded to include the possibility of unequal sample sizes.
- A discussion of the item on interim analysis guidelines in the context of cluster RCTs has been included.
- The item on generation of random allocation sequence for participants has been replaced by new items on enrollment of clusters, assignment of clusters to intervention, the methods by which individuals were included in clusters for the purposes of the trial, from whom consent was sought, and whether consent was sought before or after randomization.

Extensions and/or implementations

The extension statement of the 2004 cluster trials has been translated into Spanish [11] and Chinese [12].

Table 13.1 CONSORT 2010 checklist of information to include when reporting a cluster randomized trial.

Section/topic	Item no	Standard checklist item	Extension for cluster designs
Title and abstract			
	1a	Identification as a randomized trial in the title	Identification as a cluster randomized trial in the title
	1b	Structured summary of trial design, methods, results, and conclusions (for specific guidance, see Chapter 8 [6, 7])	See Table 13.2
Introduction			
Background and	2a	Scientific background and explanation of rationale	Rationale for using a cluster design
objectives	2b	Specific objectives or hypotheses	Whether objectives pertain to the cluster level, the individual participant level, or both
Methods			
Trial design	3a	Description of trial design (such as parallel, factorial) including allocation ratio	Definition of cluster and description of how the design features apply to the clusters
	3b	Important changes to methods after trial commencement (such as eligibility criteria), with reasons	
Participants	4a	Eligibility criteria for participants	Eligibility criteria for clusters
	4b	Settings and locations where the data were collected	
Interventions	5	The interventions for each group with sufficient details to allow replication, including how and when they were actually administered	Whether interventions pertain to the cluster level, the individual participant level, or both
Outcomes	6a	Completely defined prespecified primary and secondary outcome measures, including how and when they were assessed	Whether outcome measures pertain to the cluster level, the individual participant level, or both
	6b	Any changes to trial outcomes after the trial commenced, with reasons	
Sample size	7a	How sample size was determined	Method of calculation, number of clusters(s) (and whether equal or unequal cluster sizes are assumed), cluster size, a coefficient of intracluster correlation (ICC or k), and an indication of its uncertainty

(*continued*)

Table 13.1 (*Continued*)

Section/topic	Item no	Standard checklist item	Extension for cluster designs
	7b	When applicable, explanation of any interim analyses and stopping guidelines	
Randomization			
Sequence generation	8a	Method used to generate the random allocation sequence	
	8b	Type of randomization; details of any restriction (such as blocking and block size)	Details of stratification or matching if used
Allocation conceal-ment mechanism	9	Mechanism used to implement the random allocation sequence (such as sequentially numbered containers), describing any steps taken to conceal the sequence until interventions were assigned	Specification that allocation was based on clusters rather than individuals and whether allocation concealment (if any) was at the cluster level, the individual participant level, or both
Implementation	10	Who generated the random allocation sequence, who enrolled participants, and who assigned participants to interventions	Replace by 10a, 10b, and 10c
	10a		Who generated the random allocation sequence, who enrolled clusters, and who assigned clusters to interventions
	10b		Mechanism by which individual participants were included in clusters for the purposes of the trial (such as complete enumeration, random sampling)
	10c		From whom consent was sought (representatives of the cluster, or individual cluster members, or both), and whether consent was sought before or after randomization
Blinding	11a	If done, who was blinded after assignment to interventions (e.g., participants, care providers, those assessing outcomes) and how	
	11b	If relevant, description of the similarity of interventions	

Table 13.1 (*Continued*)

Section/topic	Item no	Standard checklist item	Extension for cluster designs
Statistical methods	12a	Statistical methods used to compare groups for primary and secondary outcomes	How clustering was taken into account
	12b	Methods for additional analyses, such as subgroup analyses and adjusted analyses	
Results			
Participant flow (a diagram is strongly recommended)	13a	For each group, the numbers of participants who were randomly assigned, received intended treatment, and were analyzed for the primary outcome	For each group, the numbers of clusters that were randomly assigned, received intended treatment, and were analyzed for the primary outcome
	13b	For each group, losses and exclusions after randomization, together with reasons	For each group, losses and exclusions for both clusters and individual cluster members
Recruitment	14a	Dates defining the periods of recruitment and follow-up	
	14b	Why the trial ended or was stopped	
Baseline data	15	A table showing baseline demographic and clinical characteristics for each group	Baseline characteristics for the individual and cluster levels as applicable for each group
Numbers analyzed	16	For each group, number of participants (denominator) included in each analysis and whether the analysis was by original assigned groups	For each group, number of clusters included in each analysis
Outcomes and estimation	17a	For each primary and secondary outcome, results for each group, and the estimated effect size and its precision (such as 95% confidence interval)	Results at the individual or cluster level as applicable and a coefficient of intracluster correlation (ICC or k) for each primary outcome
	17b	For binary outcomes, presentation of both absolute and relative effect sizes is recommended	
Ancillary analyses	18	Results of any other analyses performed, including subgroup analyses and adjusted analyses, distinguishing prespecified from exploratory	

(*continued*)

Table 13.1 (*Continued*)

Section/topic	Item no	Standard checklist item	Extension for cluster designs
Harms	19	All important harms or unintended effects in each group (for specific guidance, see CONSORT for harms [10])	
Discussion			
Limitations	20	Trial limitations, addressing sources of potential bias, imprecision, and, if relevant, multiplicity of analyses	
Generalizability	21	Generalizability (external validity, applicability) of the trial findings	Generalizability to clusters and/or individual participants (as relevant)
Interpretation	22	Interpretation consistent with results, balancing benefits and harms, and considering other relevant evidence	
Other information			
Registration	23	Registration number and name of trial registry	
Protocol	24	Where the full trial protocol can be accessed, if available	
Funding	25	Sources of funding and other support (such as supply of drugs), role of funders	

Related activities

In the health field, there is some overlap between the CONSORT extension of cluster trials and that of nonpharmacologic treatments [13] and pragmatic trials [14]. We are not aware of reporting guidelines of particular relevance to cluster trials in the fields of education, crime and justice, or social welfare. However, these issues are relevant to the joint Cochrane Collaboration and Campbell Collaboration Methods.

How best to use the guideline

Chapter 9 explains how best to use the main CONSORT checklist. During the manuscript submission process, editors can ask authors to complete the CONSORT cluster extension checklist and include it as part of the submission process, as well as to reference the published CONSORT cluster

Table 13.2 Extension of CONSORT for Abstracts [6, 7] to reports of cluster randomized trials.

Item	Standard checklist item	Extension to cluster trials
Title	Identification of study as randomized	Identification of study as cluster randomized
Trial design	Description of the trial design (e.g., parallel, cluster, noninferiority)	
Methods		
Participants	Eligibility criteria for participants and the settings where the data were collected	Eligibility criteria for clusters
Interventions	Interventions intended for each group	
Objective	Specific objective or hypothesis	Whether objective or hypothesis pertains to the cluster level, the individual participant level, or both
Outcome	Clearly defined primary outcome for this report	Whether the primary outcome pertains to the cluster level, the individual participant level, or both
Randomization	How participants were allocated to interventions	How clusters were allocated to interventions
Blinding (masking)	Whether participants, care givers, and those assessing the outcomes were blinded to group assignment	
Results		
Numbers randomized	Number of participants randomized to each group	Number of clusters randomized to each group
Recruitment	Trial status[a]	
Numbers analyzed	Number of participants analyzed in each group	Number of clusters analyzed in each group
Outcome	For the primary outcome, a result for each group, and the estimated effect size and its precision	Results at the cluster or individual participant level as applicable for each primary outcome
Harms	Important adverse events or side effects	
Conclusions	General interpretation of the results	
Trial registration	Registration number and name of trial register	
Funding	Source of funding	

[a] Relevant to conference abstracts.

extension. Editors can ask peer reviewers to use the same checklist to guide their assessment.

Although the statement concentrates on reporting (primarily what was done, what was found, and what it means), investigators conducting cluster trials could also consult the CONSORT cluster extension for general information about the design, conduct, and analysis of cluster trials before beginning such a trial.

Although the statement is not a tool for constructing a quality score, readers may find it useful to guide them through the critical appraisal of a published report.

Evidence of effectiveness of guideline

There is some evidence of improvement in the identification of cluster randomized trials in publication titles and abstracts since the 2004 paper [15]. Three recent evaluations of the use of the CONSORT cluster extension checklist and/or flow diagrams in 106 trials in children published in 2004–2010 [16], 300 trials published in 2000–2008 [17], and 15 trials in stroke patients [18] found a slight association with improved quality of reporting of cluster trials, but the fourth review of 50 cancer trials suggested a decline in quality in 2007–2010 [19].

Endorsement and adherence

In supporting the CONSORT Statement, journals are indirectly supporting its extensions. Editors should be aware that the checklist for the cluster extension has additional items specific to these trials, and when endorsing the general CONSORT Statement they are also endorsing the use of this extension guideline.

It is recommended in Chapter 9 that "if a journal supports or endorses CONSORT 2010, it should cite one of the original versions of CONSORT 2010, the Explanation and Elaboration paper, and the CONSORT Website in their 'Instructions to Authors.'" When authors access the CONSORT Website, they will find the cluster extension. We suggest that authors who conduct cluster trials should follow the CONSORT recommendations for reporting their trial and cite the cluster extension.

Cautions and limitations (including scope)

See Chapter 9.

Mistakes and misconceptions

The ICC is very small; therefore, there is no need to adjust for clustering: not true! The relative efficiency of a cluster randomized design with respect to an individually randomized design depends on the design effect, which is a function of both the ICC and the average cluster size. Even if the ICC is very small, a large average cluster size can make the relative efficiency very different from one.

A cluster randomized design always requires a complicated analysis: not true! If the inference is at the cluster level and cluster sizes are similar, a cluster-level analysis using cluster summary measures is satisfactory. A simple analysis using a two-sample *t*-test (in the case of two interventions) is acceptable, perhaps improving power by weighting the summary measures by their inverse variance [20].

A matched-pairs design always provides a gain in efficiency: not always true! It is true that there is a gain in efficiency because of matching that depends on the correlation between the members of a pair. However, this gain might be counterbalanced by the loss of degrees of freedom [21].

The guideline covers clustering that is not by design: not true! Clustering can occur in many types of study not necessarily in the context of a cluster randomized trial or even of a trial. The clustering factor can be included in the model at the analysis stage. However, this type of clustering is outside the scope of this guideline.

The guideline is about cluster analysis: not true! Cluster analysis is a multivariate technique unrelated to cluster randomized trials. It is an exploratory data analysis tool that aims to sort different objects into groups in a way that the degree of association between two objects is maximal if they belong to the same group and minimal otherwise [22].

Creators' preferred bits

Aim of the trial: If the trial is intended to evaluate policy at the hospital level and is not concerned with outcomes on particular subjects, then the hospital is the natural unit of inference and standard methods of sample size estimation, and analysis would apply at the hospital level [20].

Analysis: Application of standard methods for individually randomized trials to cluster randomized trial data, assuming no between-cluster variation, "will tend to bias observed *p*-values downward, thus risking a spurious claim of statistical significance" [20].

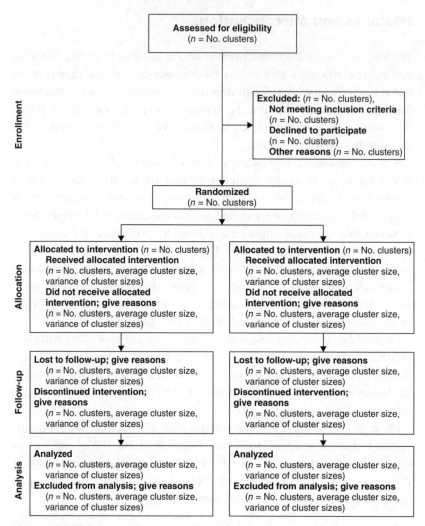

Figure 13.1 Recommended format for flow diagram of the progress of clusters and individuals through the phases of a randomized trial.

Flow diagrams: The addition of bespoke flow diagrams for cluster RCTs has been much appreciated (Figure 13.1).

Future plans

We will update this guidance either because of important new research findings or because of a further update of the CONSORT Statement for individually randomized parallel group trials.

References

1 Elbourne, D.R. & Campbell, M.K. (2001) Extending the CONSORT statement to cluster randomized trials: for discussion. *Statistics in Medicine*, **20**, 489–496.

2 Campbell, M.K., Elbourne, D.R. & Altman, D.G. (2004) CONSORT statement: extension to cluster randomised trials. *BMJ*, **328**, 702–708.

3 Campbell, M.K., Piaggio, G., Elbourne, D.R., Altman, D.G., for the CONSORT group (2012) CONSORT 2010 statement: extension to cluster randomised trials. *BMJ*, **345**, e5661.

4 Schulz, K.F., Altman, D.G. & Moher, D. (2010) CONSORT 2010 statement: updated guidelines for reporting parallel group randomised trials. *BMJ*, **340**, c332.

5 Moher, D. Hopewell, S. Schulz, K.F., *et al.* (2010) CONSORT 2010 Explanation and Elaboration: updated guidelines for reporting parallel group randomised trials. *Journal of Clinical Epidemiology*, **63**, e1–37.

6 Hopewell, S., Clarke, M., Moher, D. *et al.* (2008) CONSORT for reporting randomised trials in journal and conference abstracts. *Lancet*, **371**, 281–283.

7 Hopewell, S., Clarke, M., Moher, D. *et al.* (2008) CONSORT for reporting randomized controlled trials in journal and conference abstracts: explanation and elaboration. *PLoS Medicine*, **5** (1), e20.

8 Begg, C., Cho, M., Eastwood, S. *et al.* (1996) Improving the quality of reporting of randomized controlled trials. The CONSORT statement. *JAMA*, **276** (8), 637–639.

9 Moher, D., Schulz, K.F. & Altman, D. (2001) The CONSORT Statement: revised recommendations for improving the quality of reports of parallel-group randomized trials. *JAMA*, **285** (15), 1987–1991.

10 Ioannidis, J.P., Evans, S.J., Gotzsche, P.C. *et al.* (2004) Better reporting of harms in randomized trials: an extension of the CONSORT statement. *Annals of Internal Medicine*, **141** (10), 781–788.

11 Campbell, M.K., Elbourne, D.R. & Altman, D.G. (2005) The CONSORT statement for cluster randomised trials [Spanish]. *Medicina Clínica (Barcelona)*, **125** (Suppl. 1), 28–31.

12 Campbell, M.J., Elbourne, D., Altman, D.G., for the CONSORT Group (2006) CONSORT statement: extension to cluster randomized trials [Chinese]. *Chinese Journal of Evidence-Based Medicine*, **6** (6), 451–458.

13 Boutron, I., Moher, D., Altman, D.G. *et al.* (2008) Extending the CONSORT statement to randomized trials of nonpharmacologic treatment: explanation and elaboration. *Annals of Internal Medicine*, **148** (4), 295–309.

14 Zwarenstein, M., Treweek, S., Altman, D.G. *et al.* (2008) Improving the reporting of pragmatic trials: an extension of the CONSORT Statement. *BMJ*, **337**, a2390.

15 Taljaard, M., McGowan, J., Grimshaw, J.M. *et al.* (2010) Electronic search strategies to identify reports of cluster randomized trials in MEDLINE: low precision will improve with adherence to reporting standards. *BMC Medical Research Methodology*, **10**, 15.

16 Walleser, S., Hill, S.R. & Bero, L.A. (2011) Characteristics and quality of reporting of cluster randomized trials in children: reporting needs improvement. *Journal of Clinical Epidemiology*, **64**, 1331–1340.

17 Ivers, N.M., Taljaard, M., Dixon, S. *et al.* (2011) Impact of the CONSORT extension for cluster randomised trials on quality of reporting and study methodology: review of a random sample of 300 trials from 2000 to 2008. *BMJ*, **343**, d5886.

18 Sutton, C.J., Watkins, C.L., Dey, P. (2012) Illustrating problems faced by stroke researchers: a review of cluster-randomized controlled trials. *International Journal of Stroke*, **8**, 566–574.

19 Crespi, C.M., Maxwell, A.E. & Wu, S. (2011) Cluster randomized trials of cancer screening interventions: are appropriate statistical methods being used? *Contemporary Clinical Trials*, **32**, 477–484.

20 Donner, A. & Klar, N. (2000) *Design and Analysis of Cluster Randomization Trials in Health Research*. Arnold, London.

21 Hayes, R.J. & Moulton, L.H. (2008) *Cluster Randomised Trials*. Chapman & Hall/CRC.

22 StatSoft, Inc. 2010. *Electronic Statistics Textbook*. StatSoft, Tulsa, OK. Available from http://www.statsoft.com/textbook/.

CHAPTER 14

CONSORT for Noninferiority and Equivalence Trials

Gilda Piaggio[1], Diana Elbourne[2] and Douglas G. Altman[3]

[1] *Statistika Consultoria Ltd, São Paulo, Brazil*
[2] *London School of Hygiene and Tropical Medicine, London, UK*
[3] *Centre for Statistics in Medicine, University of Oxford, Wolfson College, Oxford, UK*

Timetable

Name of reporting guideline	Notes	Consensus meeting date	Reporting guideline publication
Reporting of noninferiority and equivalence randomized trials: an extension of the CONSORT Statement		2003	2006 [1].
Reporting of noninferiority and equivalence randomized trials: extension of the CONSORT 2010 Statement	Revision of 2006 paper to extend 2010 CONSORT Statement to noninferiority and equivalence trials	2010	2012 [2]

Name of guideline

The Consolidated Standards of Reporting Trials (CONSORT) Statement is a guideline for authors reporting randomized controlled trials (RCTs). The *CONSORT Statement 2010: Extension to Noninferiority and Equivalence Trials* [2] is an extension to the CONSORT Statement [3, 4]. Noninferiority trials aim

Guidelines for Reporting Health Research: A User's Manual, First Edition. Edited by David Moher, Douglas G. Altman, Kenneth F. Schulz, Iveta Simera and Elizabeth Wager.
© 2014 John Wiley & Sons, Ltd. Published 2014 by John Wiley & Sons, Ltd.

to show that a new treatment is not worse than a standard active control treatment by a prespecified clinically acceptable difference, the noninferiority margin. Equivalence trials aim to show that a new treatment is equivalent to a standard active control treatment within a prespecified clinically acceptable difference, the margin of equivalence. The new treatment usually has one or more advantages, such as fewer harms, greater ease of administration, lower cost, less invasiveness, or greater convenience in some other respect. This extension guideline aims to elicit clear and complete information on these types of trials [2]. It comprises explanatory text and additions to 12 of the 25 items on the main CONSORT 2010 checklist and additions to five items of the CONSORT for abstracts checklist [5, 6], adapted to noninferiority and equivalence trials [2].

History/development

A revision of the original CONSORT Statement [7], published in 2001 [8], focused on the simplest and most common trial design (i.e., individually randomized parallel group trials). Discussions about extensions of the CONSORT Statement, including applications for equivalence and noninferiority trials, took place in May 2002 in Arlington, Virginia, United States, among some members of the CONSORT Group. At that meeting, it was decided to write separate guidance statements for different trial designs. The equivalence and noninferiority trial extension was one of these. Discussions continued in a CONSORT meeting in Montebello, Canada, in May 2003. Some or all of the authors subsequently met on a number of occasions in London and Geneva and also corresponded by email. A draft manuscript was circulated to members of the CONSORT Group for comments in October 2004. The manuscript was published in *JAMA* in March 2006 [1].

After publication of the revised CONSORT Statement for parallel group randomized trials in 2010, we began to update the 2006 extension. A number of meetings were held in London in 2010. A paper was published in *BMJ* incorporating new advances and adapting the checklist to the CONSORT 2010 checklist [2].

When to use this guideline (what types of studies it covers)

The CONSORT noninferiority and equivalence extension can be used to report noninferiority and equivalence randomized trials (as mentioned earlier).

Noninferiority trials seek to determine whether a new treatment is not worse than an active control by more than an acceptable amount. Because proof of exact equality is impossible, a prestated margin of noninferiority (Δ) is defined for the treatment effect in a primary patient outcome (Figure 14.1). Equivalence trials are very similar, except that equivalence is defined as the treatment effect being between −Δ and +Δ.

The new treatment usually has one or more advantages, such as fewer side effects (harms), greater ease of administration, lower cost, less invasiveness, or greater convenience in some other respect.

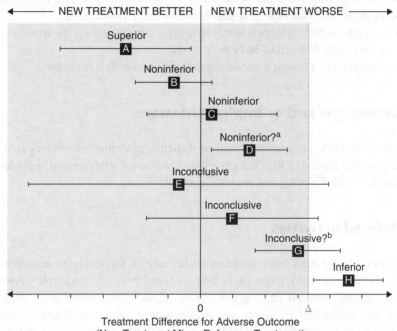

Figure 14.1 (Reproduced with permission from *JAMA*). Error bars indicate 2-sided 95% confidence intervals (CIs). The dashed line at x = Δ indicates the noninferiority margin; the region to the left of x = Δ indicates the zone of noninferiority. A, If the CI lies wholly to the left of zero, the new treatment is superior. B and C, If the CI lies to the left of Δ and includes zero, the new treatment is noninferior but not shown to be superior. D, If the CI lies wholly to the left of Δ and wholly to the right of zero, the new treatment is noninferior in the sense already defined, but it is also inferior in the sense that a null treatment difference is excluded. This puzzling case is rare because it requires a very large sample size. It can also result from having a noninferiority margin that is too wide. E and F, If the CI includes Δ and zero, the difference is nonsignificant but the result regarding noninferiority is inconclusive. G, If the CI includes Δ and is wholly to the right of zero, the difference is statistically significant but the result is inconclusive regarding possible inferiority of magnitude Δ or worse. H, If the CI is wholly above Δ, the new treatment is inferior.

[a]This CI indicates noninferiority in the sense that it does not include Δ, but the new treatment is significantly worse than the standard. Such a result is unlikely because it would require a very large sample size.

[b]This CI is inconclusive in that it is still plausible that the true treatment difference is less than Δ, but the new treatment is significantly worse than the standard.

Current version/previous versions

The current version differs from the original 2006 CONSORT extension to noninferiority and equivalence trials in the following ways:

- The standard CONSORT checklist items and the extension specific to noninferiority trials are presented in separate columns (Tables 14.1 and 14.2).
- An augmented checklist for abstracts of noninferiority RCTs is provided.
- Examples of good reporting practice have been updated.
- Sections on how common noninferiority trials are and on the quality of reporting of these trials have been updated.
- A summary of recent methodological developments is included.

Extensions and/or implementations

The CONSORT noninferiority and equivalence guideline is itself an extension of the general CONSORT guideline. There is no other reporting guideline for noninferiority and equivalence trials.

Related activities

Noninferiority trials have proliferated because of the desire to introduce new drugs that have advantages over standard drugs, for example, fewer side effects, reduced cost, less invasiveness, or more convenience. Regulatory authorities in many countries are developing guidelines for the conduct of noninferiority trials. In particular, the Food and Drug Administration of the United States has recently issued updated guidelines [7].

How best to use the guideline

Chapter 9 explains how best to use the main CONSORT checklist. During the manuscript submission process, editors can ask authors to complete the CONSORT noninferiority and equivalence extension checklist and submit it with their manuscript, as well as to reference the published CONSORT noninferiority and equivalence extension. Editors can ask peer reviewers to use the same checklist to guide their peer review assessment.

Investigators conducting noninferiority or equivalence trials could consult the CONSORT noninferiority and equivalence extension publication for general issues about the design, conduct, and analysis of such trials before beginning a noninferiority or an equivalence trial, in addition to before reporting.

Table 14.1 CONSORT 2010 checklist[a] of information to include when reporting a noninferiority or equivalence trial[b].

Section/topic	Item no	Standard CONSORT 2010 checklist item	Extension for noninferiority trials
Title and abstract			
Title	1a	Identification as a randomized trial in the title	Identification as a noninferiority randomized trial in the title
Abstract	1b	Structured summary of trial design, methods, results, and conclusions (for specific guidance, see Chapter 8 [5, 6]	See Table 14.2
Introduction			
Background and objectives	2a	Scientific background and explanation of rationale	Rationale for using a noninferiority design
	2b	Specific objectives or hypotheses	Hypotheses concerning noninferiority, specifying the noninferiority margin with the rationale for its choice
Methods			
Trial design	3a	Description of trial design (such as parallel, factorial) including allocation ratio	
	3b	Important changes to methods after trial commencement (such as eligibility criteria), with reasons	
Participants	4a	Eligibility criteria for participants	Whether participants in the noninferiority trial are similar to those in any trial(s) that established efficacy of the reference treatment
	4b	Settings and locations where the data were collected	
Interventions	5	The interventions for each group with sufficient details to allow replication, including how and when they were actually administered	Whether the reference treatment in the noninferiority trial is identical (or very similar) to that in any trial(s) that established efficacy
Outcomes	6a	Completely defined prespecified primary and secondary outcome measures, including how and when they were assessed	Specify the noninferiority outcome(s) and whether hypotheses for main and secondary outcome(s) are noninferiority or superiority. Whether the outcomes in the noninferiority trial are identical (or very similar) to those in any trial(s) that established efficacy of the reference treatment

(continued)

Table 14.1 (*Continued*)

Section/topic	Item no	Standard CONSORT 2010 checklist item	Extension for noninferiority trials
	6b	Any changes to trial outcomes after the trial commenced, with reasons	
Sample size	7a	How sample size was determined	Whether the sample size was calculated using a noninferiority criterion and, if so, what the noninferiority margin was
	7b	When applicable, explanation of any interim analyses and stopping guidelines	To which outcome(s) they apply and whether related to a noninferiority hypothesis
Randomization			
Sequence generation	8a	Method used to generate the random allocation sequence	
	8b	Type of randomization; details of any restriction (such as blocking and block size)	
Allocation concealment mechanism	9	Mechanism used to implement the random allocation sequence (such as sequentially numbered containers), describing any steps taken to conceal the sequence until interventions were assigned	
Implementation	10	Who generated the random allocation sequence, who enrolled participants, and who assigned participants to interventions	
Blinding	11a	If done, who was blinded after assignment to interventions (e.g., participants, care providers, those assessing outcomes) and how	
	11b	If relevant, description of the similarity of interventions	
Statistical methods	12a	Statistical methods used to compare groups for primary and secondary outcomes	Whether a one- or two-sided confidence interval approach was used
	12b	Methods for additional analyses, such as subgroup analyses and adjusted analyses	

Table 14.1 (*Continued*)

Section/topic	Item no	Standard CONSORT 2010 checklist item	Extension for noninferiority trials
Results			
Participant flow (a diagram is strongly recommended)	13a	For each group, the number of participants who were randomly assigned, received intended treatment and were analyzed for the primary outcome	
	13b	For each group, losses and exclusions after randomization, together with reasons	
Recruitment	14a	Dates defining the periods of recruitment and follow-up	
	14b	Why the trial ended or was stopped	
Baseline data	15	A table showing baseline demographic and clinical characteristics for each group	
Numbers analyzed	16	For each group, number of participants (denominator) included in each analysis and whether the analysis was by original assigned groups	
Outcomes and estimation	17a	For each primary and secondary outcome, results for each group, the estimated effect size and its precision (such as 95% confidence interval)	For the outcome(s) for which noninferiority was hypothesized, a figure showing confidence intervals and the noninferiority margin may be useful
	17b	For binary outcomes, presentation of both absolute and relative effect sizes is recommended	
Ancillary analyses	18	Results of any other analyses performed, including subgroup analyses and adjusted analyses, distinguishing prespecified from exploratory	
Harms	19	All important harms or unintended effects in each group (for specific guidance, see Chapter 10 [12])	

(*continued*)

Table 14.1 *(Continued)*

Section/topic	Item no	Standard CONSORT 2010 checklist item	Extension for noninferiority trials
Discussion			
Limitations	20	Trial limitations, addressing sources of potential bias, imprecision, and, if relevant, multiplicity of analyses	
Generalizability	21	Generalizability (external validity, applicability) of the trial findings	
Interpretation	22	Interpretation consistent with results, balancing benefits and harms, and considering other relevant evidence	Interpret results in relation to the noninferiority hypothesis. If a superiority conclusion is drawn for outcome(s) for which noninferiority was hypothesized, provide justification for switching
Other information			
Registration	23	Registration number and name of trial registry	
Protocol	24	Where the full trial protocol can be accessed, if available	
Funding	25	Sources of funding and other support (such as supply of drugs), role of funders	

[a] This checklist relates to noninferiority trials, but the same issues apply to equivalence trials.
[b] The CONSORT Group strongly recommends reading this checklist in conjunction with the CONSORT 2010 Explanation and Elaboration [4] for important clarifications on all the items.

Readers may find the guideline useful to guide them through the critical appraisal of published reports of noninferiority and equivalence trials.

Development process

See history/development as mentioned earlier.

Evidence of effectiveness of guideline

We are unaware of any evaluations of whether the use of the CONSORT noninferiority and equivalence extension checklist and/or flow diagram is associated with an improved quality of reporting of noninferiority and equivalence trials.

Table 14.2 Extension of CONSORT for Abstracts to reports of noninferiority trials.

Item	Standard checklist item[a]	Extension for noninferiority trials
Title	Identification of study as randomized	Identification of study as a noninferiority trial
Trial design	Description of the trial design (e.g., parallel, cluster, noninferiority)	
Methods		
Participants	Eligibility criteria for participants and the settings where the data were collected	
Interventions	Interventions intended for each group	
Objective	Specific objective or hypothesis	Specific hypothesis concerning noninferiority including noninferiority margin
Outcome	Clearly defined primary outcome for this report	Clarify for all reported outcomes whether noninferiority or superiority
Randomization	How participants were allocated to interventions	
Blinding (masking)	Whether or not participants, care givers, and those assessing the outcomes were blinded to group assignment	
Results		
Numbers randomized	Number of participants randomized to each group	
Recruitment	Trial status	
Numbers analyzed	Number of participants analyzed in each group	
Outcome	For the primary outcome, a result for each group and the estimated effect size and its precision	For the primary noninferiority outcome, results in relation to noninferiority margin
Harms	Important adverse events or side effects	
Conclusions	General interpretation of the results	Interpretation taking into account the noninferiority hypotheses and any superiority hypotheses
Trial registration	Registration number and name of trial register	
Funding	Source of funding	

[a] Source: From Ref. [6].

Endorsement and adherence

In supporting the CONSORT Statement, journals are indirectly endorsing its extensions. Editors should be aware that the checklist of the noninferiority and equivalence extension has additional items that are specific to these trials.

It is recommended in Chapter 9 that "if a journal supports or endorses CONSORT 2010, it should cite one of the original versions of CONSORT 2010, the E&E, and the CONSORT Website in their 'Instructions to Authors.'" When authors access the CONSORT website, they will find the noninferiority and equivalence extension. We suggest that authors who conduct noninferiority or equivalence trials should cite the noninferiority and equivalence extension [2].

Cautions and limitations (including scope)

All cautions and limitations of the general CONSORT Statement apply to this guideline. As with the general CONSORT Statement, this guideline urges completeness, clarity, and transparency of reporting, which should reflect the actual trial design and conduct. In noninferiority and equivalence trials, flaws in the design, for example, a margin of noninferiority or equivalence that are unreasonably large, could lead to the use of slightly inferior treatments ("biocreep"). Flaws in the conduct of the trial could bias the difference between the new and the standard treatment in either direction, risking the adoption of an inferior treatment or the nonadoption of a noninferior treatment.

Mistakes and misconceptions

Noninferiority and equivalence trials have many features in common but they are not the same: a noninferiority trial seeks to demonstrate that a new treatment is not worse than a standard treatment by more than a small amount (margin of noninferiority). Most therapeutic and prophylactic trials that are not superiority trials address this one-sided question rather than that of equivalence. Two-sided equivalence trials aim to show that two treatments or compounds are similar within specified limits with regard to an outcome; they are more common in the assessment of bioequivalence.

Switching from superiority to noninferiority: a nonsignificant result in a superiority trial does not imply noninferiority or equivalence. Some trials planned as superiority trials report results as if they had been noninferiority or equivalence trials, after failing to demonstrate superiority [11, 12].

Choice of the noninferiority or equivalence margin (Δ): sometimes Δ is too large, which increases the probability of accepting an inferior treatment as noninferior [13], which is of particular concern with major outcomes such as mortality.

Assay sensitivity and constancy assumption: Showing noninferiority of a new treatment with respect to a standard is not a guarantee that the new treatment is effective. The way to ensure assay sensitivity for a noninferiority trial would be to include both a placebo control and an active control (the standard treatment) in the same trial, which is usually not possible for ethical reasons if the standard treatment is known to be effective. A noninferiority trial assumes that the historical difference between the active control and placebo is valid for the present day. With the rapid changes in medical practice and standard of care, this might not be the case [14, 15].

A noninferiority hypothesis does not require calculation of a one-sided confidence interval: even to show noninferiority (one-sided equivalence), the use of two-sided confidence intervals with the appropriate prestated significance level is recommended. This also allows assessment of the superiority of the new treatment if the effect observed is in the opposite direction from the one expected, which cannot be done with one-sided confidence intervals [1, 7, 12].

Creators' preferred bits

Our preferred bits refer to issues related to the aim, analysis, and interpretation of results of noninferiority and equivalence trials that are frequently inadequately stated or reported in the literature:

- *Aim*: Noninferiority trials are intended to show whether a new treatment has at least as much efficacy as the standard *or is worse by an amount less than* Δ.
- *Analysis*: Analyses that exclude patients not taking allocated treatment or otherwise not protocol adherent *could bias the trial in either direction*. The terms intention-to-treat (ITT) (or on-treatment) and per-protocol (PP) analysis are often used but may be inadequately defined [4]. Potentially biased non-ITT analysis is less desirable than ITT in superiority trials but may still provide some insight. In noninferiority and equivalence trials, non-ITT analyses might be desirable as a protection from ITT's increased risk of falsely concluding noninferiority.
- *Interpretation*: It is inappropriate to claim noninferiority *post hoc* from a superiority trial unless clearly related to a predefined margin of noninferiority.
- *Interpretation*: Figure 14.1 showing the possible scenarios of an observed treatment difference for an adverse outcome in a noninferiority trial.

Future plans

We will update this guidance either because of important new research findings or if there is a further update of the CONSORT Statement for individually randomized parallel group trials.

References

1 Piaggio, G., Elbourne, D.R., Altman, D.G. *et al.* (2006) Reporting of noninferiority and equivalence randomized trials: an extension of the CONSORT statement. *JAMA*, **295**, 1152–1160.

2 Piaggio, G., Elbourne, D.R., Pocock, S.J. *et al.* CONSORT Group (2012) Reporting of noninferiority and equivalence randomized trials: extension of the CONSORT 2010 statement. *JAMA*, **308** (24), 2594–2604.

3 Schulz, K.F., Altman, D.G. & Moher, D. (2010) CONSORT 2010 statement: updated guidelines for reporting parallel group randomised trials. *BMJ*, **340**, c332.

4 Moher, D., Hopewell, S., Schulz, K.F. *et al.* (2010) CONSORT 2010 Explanation and Elaboration: updated guidelines for reporting parallel group randomised trials. *BMJ*, **340**, c869.

5 Hopewell, S., Clarke, M., Moher, D. *et al.* (2008) CONSORT for reporting randomised trials in journal and conference abstracts. *Lancet*, **371**, 281–283.

6 Hopewell, S., Clarke, M., Moher, D. *et al.* (2008) CONSORT for reporting randomized controlled trials in journal and conference abstracts: explanation and elaboration. *PLoS Medicine*, **5** (1), e20.

7 Begg, C., Cho, M., Eastwood, S. *et al.* (1996) Improving the quality of reporting of randomized controlled trials. The CONSORT statement. *JAMA*, **276** (8), 637–639.

8 Moher, D., Schulz, K.F. & Altman, D. (2001) The CONSORT Statement: revised recommendations for improving the quality of reports of parallel-group randomized trials. *JAMA*, **285** (15), 1987–1991.

9 FDA (March 2010) *Guidance for Industry. Non-Inferiority Trials.*

10 Ioannidis, J.P., Evans, S.J., Gotzsche, P.C. *et al.* (2004) Better reporting of harms in randomized trials: an extension of the CONSORT statement. *Annals of Internal Medicine*, **141** (10), 781–788.

11 Le Henanff, A., Giraudeau, B., Baron, G. & Ravaud, P. (2006) Quality of reporting of noninferiority and equivalence randomized trials. *JAMA*, **295**, 1147–1151.

12 Boutron, I., Dutton, S., Ravaud, P. & Altman, D.G. (2010) Reporting and interpretation of randomized controlled trials with statistically nonsignificant results for primary outcomes. *JAMA*, **303**, 2058–2064.

13 Gøtzsche, P.C. (2006) Lessons from and cautions about noninferiority and equivalence randomized trials. *JAMA*, **295**, 1172–1174.

14 D'Agostino, R.B. Sr., Massaro, J.M. & Sullivan, L.M. (2003) Non-inferiority trials: design concepts and issues – the encounters of academic consultants in statistics. *Statistics in Medicine*, **22**, 169–186.

15 Kaul, S. & Diamond, G.A. (2006) Good enough: a primer on the analysis and interpretation of noninferiority trials. *Annals of Internal Medicine*, **145**, 62–69.

CHAPTER 15

STRICTA (STandards for Reporting Interventions in Clinical Trials of Acupuncture)

Hugh MacPherson
Department of Health Studies, University of York, York, UK

Name of guideline: STRICTA

The Standards for Reporting Interventions in Clinical Trials of Acupuncture (STRICTA) provides, by means of a six-item checklist, guidance for authors reporting clinical trials involving acupuncture.

When to use STRICTA?

STRICTA is aimed primarily at authors but may also be used by peer and systematic reviewers when they appraise trial designs and reports, in order to make more informed judgments on the quality and style of acupuncture provided within trials.

Although the first version of STRICTA was for controlled trials, the revised version was broadened to be relevant for all clinical trials, that is, whether controlled or not. Therefore, the guideline is applicable for reporting a broad range of clinical evaluation designs, including uncontrolled outcome studies and case reports.

Development process

The impetus for developing the STRICTA reporting guidelines came from a group of acupuncture researchers who met in Exeter University, United Kingdom, in 2001. Our concern at the time was that the reporting of the details of acupuncture interventions in clinical trials was patchy. This limited our confidence in the quality of the acupuncture and potentially

---

Guidelines for Reporting Health Research: A User's Manual, First Edition. Edited by David Moher, Douglas G. Altman, Kenneth F. Schulz, Iveta Simera and Elizabeth Wager.
© 2014 John Wiley & Sons, Ltd. Published 2014 by John Wiley & Sons, Ltd.

compromised the interpretation and appraisal of trial results. The first draft of STRICTA was developed at Exeter and modified by a small group including the editors of the five journals that subsequently published STRICTA. The final version of STRICTA was a checklist with six main items each of which was subdivided, making a total of 20 subitems, along with explanations for each. The six items are the acupuncture rationale, the needling details, the treatment regimen, cointerventions, the practitioner background, and control interventions. The STRICTA website was made available as a resource at www.stricta.info. The five journals published this first version of STRICTA in 2001 and 2002 [1–5]. In their instructions to authors, they included the requirement that the STRICTA guidelines be followed for trials of acupuncture. Translations into Chinese [6, 7], Korean [8], and Japanese [9] were followed.

After six years, it was decided to review how well STRICTA was functioning, whether any impact on quality of reporting could be ascribed to STRICTA, what the experience of authors of trials was when using STRICTA, whether there appeared to be a need for improvements to STRICTA, and what suggestions could be made for improving the content of the guideline itself. To this end, we conducted two studies. In the first study, we surveyed 38 randomly selected authors of clinical trials and 14 authors of Cochrane acupuncture reviews and protocols to determine how useful the STRICTA items were to them [10]. Concurrently with the above review, we conducted a before-and-after systematic review of 90 acupuncture trials to determine whether STRICTA had an impact on the reporting of these trials over time [11]. We summarize the findings of these two studies in the section on the Evidence of Effectiveness of the Guideline. The conclusion from these two reviews was that STRICTA was highly valued and that there was considerable interest in a revision. In particular, we found that most STRICTA items were considered necessary and easy to use although some were seen as poorly reported, ambiguous, or possibly redundant, and a number of suggestions were made for additional items. We now had highly relevant data that would help guide our revision process.

To revise STRICTA, we wanted to involve the wider scientific, research, practitioner, and publishing communities. We also decided that working closely with CONSORT was in the interests of all. This impetus led to a decision to work with the CONSORT Group, as well as the Chinese Cochrane Centre and the Chinese Centre for Evidence-based Medicine, to revise STRICTA as a formal extension to CONSORT. In an initial consultation process in 2008, we surveyed a group of 47 experts drawn from the original STRICTA Group, the CONSORT Group, the World Federation of Acupuncture and Moxibustion Societies, the Acupuncture Trialists' Collaboration [12], the Society for Acupuncture Research [13], and clinical trial authors. These experts came from 15 countries; most had academic positions ($n=41$), were acupuncturists ($n=31$), were involved with journals ($n=18$), were physicians ($n=15$), and had been involved previously in developing reporting guidelines ($n=11$). The survey results were then collated and sent to the participants of a one-day workshop held in Freiburg, Germany, in October 2008. This workshop was attended by 21 individuals from a variety of backgrounds that included experts in epidemiology, trial methodology, statistics, and medical journal editing. Just over half the participants were acupuncturists from a variety of backgrounds, physician and nonphysician. During this workshop, a near-final version of a revised STRICTA was agreed, along with the understanding that STRICTA would be adopted within the CONSORT family as an official extension. Subsequently, a small writing group finalized the guideline, which has now been published [14, 15]. The new version includes not only a revised checklist (see Table 15.1) but also completely rewritten explanations and, in addition, examples of good reporting drawn from the literature. Moreover, the revised STRICTA statement is now shown within the published articles as being embedded within the two-group parallel trial CONSORT checklist [16] and its nonpharmacological treatment extension checklist [17].

There was an agreement at the meeting in Freiburg that STRICTA should continue to function as a stand-alone guideline for reporting acupuncture studies. There was also consensus on a minor change of name, in that the word "controlled" in STRICTA should be replaced by "clinical," as discussed earlier. The group agreed that the rationale behind reporting should be to provide the information needed to allow replication of a study, reduce ambiguity, and enhance transparency. The group recognized that acupuncture trials inevitably differ in the degree of individualization of care that is permitted, and agreed that the reporting guideline should acknowledge this and be applicable across the whole range of designs.

Current version

The current version of STRICTA comprises a checklist with 6 items broken out into 17 subitems (Table 15.1). Each of the six items and their subitems have explanations of the need for the item/subitem to be reported well. Also provided are examples of good reporting from the published literature.

The first of the six items relates to the reporting of the acupuncture rationale within a clinical trial, which includes the style of acupuncture, the reasoning for treatment provided, and the extent to which the treatment varied. The last of these is highly relevant for acupuncture trials in

Table 15.1 STRICTA 2010 checklist of information to include when reporting interventions in a clinical trial of acupuncture.

Item	Detail	
1. Acupuncture rationale	1a)	Style of acupuncture (e.g., Traditional Chinese Medicine, Japanese, Korean, Western medical, Five Element, ear acupuncture)
	1b)	Reasoning for treatment provided, based on historical context, literature sources, and/or consensus methods, with references where appropriate
	1c)	Extent to which treatment was varied
2. Details of needling	2a)	Number of needle insertions per subject per session (mean and range where relevant)
	2b)	Names (or location if no standard name) of points used (uni/bilateral)
	2c)	Depth of insertion based on a specified unit of measurement or on a particular tissue level
	2d)	Response sought (e.g., *de qi* or muscle twitch response)
	2e)	Needle stimulation (e.g., manual, electrical)
	2f)	Needle retention time
	2g)	Needle type (diameter, length, and manufacturer or material)
3. Treatment regimen	3a)	Number of treatment sessions
	3b)	Frequency and duration of treatment sessions
4. Other components of treatment	4a)	Details of other interventions administered to the acupuncture group (e.g., moxibustion, cupping, herbs, exercises, lifestyle advice)
	4b)	Setting and context of treatment, including instructions to practitioners, and information and explanations to patients
5. Practitioner background	5)	Description of participating acupuncturists (qualification or professional affiliation, years in acupuncture practice, other relevant experience)
6. Control or comparator interventions	6a)	Rationale for the control or comparator in the context of the research question, with sources that justify this choice
	6b)	Precise description of the control or comparator. If sham acupuncture or any other type of acupuncture-like control is used, provide details as for Items 1 to 3 mentioned earlier.

Note: This checklist, which should be read in conjunction with the explanations of the STRICTA items provided in the main text, is designed to replace CONSORT 2010's item 5 when reporting an acupuncture trial.

that traditional acupuncture treatments are customized for each patient, and, commonly, treatments are varied for the same patient at different treatment sessions.

The second item relates to the reporting of acupuncture needling details. These include the number of needles inserted, the names of the acupuncture points, the depth of needle insertion, the responses elicited from the patients from the needle(s) itself, the methods of needle stimulation, the needle retention time, and the needle type.

The third item focuses on reporting of the treatment regimen, including the number of sessions provided and the frequency and duration of the treatment sessions.

The fourth item is related to the reporting of other components of treatment administered to patients alongside acupuncture. Within the practice of Chinese medicine, acupuncture is often provided in conjunction with moxibustion, cupping, herbal medicine, and lifestyle advice, and depending on the research question, these components may (or may not) be thought of as specific to the intervention and whether the decision to add the components is driven by acupuncture theory and presumed to influence outcome.

The fifth item recommends reporting of the practitioner background, for example, qualifications and professional affiliation, years in practice, and other relevant experience.

The sixth and last item focuses on reporting of the control or comparator interventions. The rationale for the control should be explained, and a precise description of the control or comparator intervention(s) should be reported. Sham acupuncture is sometimes used as a control, and in this case the needling details and treatment regimen should also be reported at the level of detail as set out in the second and third items discussed earlier.

Evidence of effectiveness of guideline

We conducted two studies that addressed the question of the effectiveness of STRICTA. In the first study, we asked acupuncture trial authors and systematic reviewers about their experiences of using the STRICTA guideline and their opinion on its utility. We randomly selected a group of 38 trial authors from the reports of clinical trials published in 2004 and 2005, and to them added authors of 14 Cochrane acupuncture systematic reviews or protocols. To these 52 individuals, we sent a questionnaire asking them to rank the utility of STRICTA items and also elicited qualitative responses about their experience of using the guideline. Of these, 54% (28/52) responded. Fifty-seven percent (11/19) of trial authors used STRICTA to help guide their writing. However, over half of these reported that the editing process had removed some or all of the STRICTA-specific items. Overall, the respondents tended to rank the utility of STRICTA highly. Five items in particular were less highly valued, three of which were related to the details on the practitioner's background. In conclusion, we found that respondents considered STRICTA to be a useful framework for improving the reporting of acupuncture interventions. Authors also highlighted the difficulties of reporting pragmatic trials where the design allows practitioners to follow normal practice. Journals that had not adopted STRICTA were found by some authors to be requesting editing changes, usually reductions in word length, which resulted in their not being able to report all the STRICTA items. Respondents also reported on aspects of the items, or their wording, that were unclear or needed clarification. We also noted that very few acupuncture studies were published in the five STRICTA-adopting journals.

In the second study, we aimed to measure whether any improvement in the quality of reporting for randomized controlled trials of acupuncture had occurred since the publication of the STRICTA and CONSORT statements [11]. To do this, we selected at random 90 peer-reviewed journal articles reporting the results of acupuncture trials. We selected three distinct time periods: 1994–1995 (before the publication of the original CONSORT [18]), 1999–2000 (before the publication of the revised version of CONSORT [19] and before the publication of the original STRICTA), and 2004–2005 (for sufficient time to pass). We assessed published papers within these periods using the CONSORT and STRICTA checklists. We detected a statistically significant improvement in the reporting of CONSORT items over time for these acupuncture trials. With regard to STRICTA items, we did not find a difference between the number of items reported in journal articles published before and three to four years following the publication of STRICTA. We concluded that general standards of reporting for acupuncture trials have improved significantly since the introduction of the CONSORT statement in 1996. However, we noted that the quality in reporting details specific to acupuncture interventions had not changed following the publication of the first version of STRICTA. These studies provided a platform for the latest revision of STRICTA.

Endorsement

When STRICTA was first published, it was endorsed by five journals: *Acupuncture in Medicine, Complementary Therapies in Medicine, Journal of Alternative and Complementary Medicine, Medical Acupuncture*, and *Clinical Acupuncture and Oriental Medicine* (now ceased publication). The revised version of STRICTA is currently being copublished by six journals: *Acupuncture in Medicine* [14], *Australian Journal of Acupuncture and Chinese Medicine, Journal of Alternative and Complementary Medicine, Journal of Evidence-Based Medicine, Medical Acupuncture*, and *PLoS Medicine* [15]. It is hoped that all these journals will continue, or start, to endorse STRICTA and will include the requirement to follow the reporting of STRICTA items in their instructions to authors.

Misconceptions

The STRICTA guideline has a focus only on the reporting of the intervention in acupuncture trials. It is not designed to improve the design or quality of acupuncture trials.

Creator's preferred bits

The item within STRICTA that initially sets the scene for understanding and interpreting an acupuncture trial is the item on the rationale for the style of acupuncture. Acupuncture has an unusually long history over 2000 years and has been practised in many cultures and countries over that period of time. For this reason, acupuncture can be characterized as having a broad diversity of styles and approaches in both East Asia and the West [20]. Therefore, authors of trials of acupuncture should have a clear rationale for their choice of acupuncture and provide sufficient context for those reading such reports to be able to understand what style of acupuncture is being delivered.

Probably the most important item within the STRICTA guidelines is the item related to the number of treatment sessions. This item recommends that both the number of sessions and the frequency of treatment be clearly documented. If there was only one item reported, then this should be it. There is some evidence that for chronic conditions, for which acupuncture is most widely used, six or more sessions have been observed to be associated with increased effectiveness [21].

The third item that is of great value relates to the other components of treatment administered to the acupuncture group. Additional components of treatment refer to the auxiliary techniques, prescribed self-treatment, and lifestyle advice provided by the practitioner. This includes the setting and context of treatment, which might comprise instructions to practitioners and information and explanations to patients. We know that the setting and context of treatment can provide additional therapeutic benefits [22]. The context here might include instructions to practitioners to modify their normal practice, for example, prescribing or proscribing explanations to patients about their diagnosis. For patients, the context includes the information they have been given about the trial that might be expected to modify outcomes.

Future plans

The revised STRICTA statement has only recently been published (mid-2010). The primary focus in the short term is to complete the publication program of the revised STRICTA guideline. The second step is to ensure accurate translations and their publication in China, Japan, and Korea. Third, the journals that have published STRICTA will be encouraged to endorse STRICTA and add a requirement to follow the guideline. We do not plan to update STRICTA for at least five years. However, an update of the studies on the impact of STRICTA on reporting will be useful after more time has elapsed since its publication.

References

1 MacPherson, H., White, A., Cummings, M. *et al.* (2001) Standards for reporting interventions in controlled trials of acupuncture: the STRICTA recommendations. *Complementary Therapies in Medicine*, **9** (4), 246–249.

2 MacPherson, H., White, A., Cummings, M. *et al.* (March 2002) Standards for reporting interventions in controlled trials of acupuncture: the STRICTA statement. *Acupuncture in Medicine*, **20** (1), 22–25.

3 MacPherson, H., White, A., Cumming, M. *et al.* (2002) Standards for reporting interventions in controlled trials of acupuncture: the STRICTA statement. *Clinical Acupuncture & Oriental Medicine*, **3** (1), 6–9.

4 MacPherson, H., White, A., Cumming, M. *et al.* (2002) Standards for reporting interventions in controlled trials of acupuncture: the STRICTA statement. *Medical Acupuncture*, **13** (3), 9–11.

5 MacPherson, H., White, A., Cummings, M. *et al.* (2002) Standards for reporting interventions in controlled trials of acupuncture: the STRICTA recommendations. *Journal of Alternative and Complementary Medicine*, **8** (1), 85–89.

6 Xuemei, L., Mingming, Z. & Huilin, L. (2003) Improving the quality of reports in controlled trials of acupuncture by using CONSORT and STRICTA. *Zhongguo Zhenjiu Chinese Acupuncture and Moxibustion*, **23** (12), 699–701.

7 Jianping, L. (2005) Standards for reporting interventions in controlled trials of acupuncture: the STRICTA recommendations. *Chinese Journal of Integrated Traditional and Western Medicine*, **25** (6), 556–558.

8 Lee, H., Park, J., Seo, J. *et al.* (2002) Standards for reporting interventions in controlled trials of acupuncture: the STRICTA Recommendations. *Journal of Korean Society for Acupuncture & Moxibustion*, **19** (6), 134–154.

9 Yamashita, H. Japanese translation of the revised STRICTA. http://www.stricta.info/uploads/1/7/1/5/17150358/revised_stricta2010_japanese_version_in_jjsam_2013.pdf (Accessed 16th Feb 2014)

10 Prady, S.L. & MacPherson, H. (November 2007) Assessing the utility of the standards for reporting trials of acupuncture (STRICTA): a survey of authors. *Journal of Alternative and Complementary Medicine*, **13** (9), 939–943.

11 Prady, S.L., Richmond, S.J., Morton, V.M. & MacPherson, H. (2008) A systematic evaluation of the impact of STRICTA and CONSORT recommendations on quality of reporting for acupuncture trials. *PLoS ONE*, **3** (2), e1577.

12 Acupuncture Trialists Collaboration. http://www.mskcc.org/cancer-care/integrative-medicine/acupuncture-trialists-collaboration (Accessed 16 Feb 2014).

13 Society for Acupuncture Research. http://www.acupunctureresearch.org/ (Accessed 16 Feb 2014).

14 MacPherson, H., Altman, D.G., Hammerschlag, R. *et al.* (June 2010) Revised STandards for Reporting Interventions in Clinical Trials of Acupuncture (STRICTA): extending the CONSORT statement. *Acupuncture in Medicine*, **28** (2), 83–93.

15 MacPherson, H., Altman, D.G., Hammerschlag, R. *et al.* (2010) Revised STandards for Reporting Interventions in Clinical Trials of Acupuncture (STRICTA): extending the CONSORT statement. *PLoS Medicine*, **7** (6), e1000261.

16 Schulz, K.F., Altman, D.G., Moher, D., for the CONSORT Group (2010) CONSORT 2010 Statement: updated guidelines for reporting parallel group randomised trials. *BMJ*, **340**, c332.

17 Boutron, I., Moher, D., Altman, D.G. *et al.* (2008) Extending the CONSORT statement to randomized trials of nonpharmacologic treatment: explanation and elaboration. *Annals of Internal Medicine*, **148** (4), 295–309.

18 Begg, C., Cho, M., Eastwood, S. *et al.* (1996) Improving the quality of reporting of randomized controlled trials. The CONSORT statement. *JAMA*, **276** (8), 637–639.

19 Moher, D., Schulz, K.F. & Altman, D. (2001) The CONSORT statement: revised recommendations for improving the quality of reports of parallel-group randomized trials. *JAMA*, **285** (15), 1987–1991.

20 Birch, S. & Felt, R. (1999) *Understanding Acupuncture*. Churchill Livingstone, Edinburgh.

21 Ezzo, J., Berman, B., Hadhazy, V.A. *et al.* (2000) Is acupuncture effective for the treatment of chronic pain? A systematic review. *Pain*, **86** (3), 217–225.

22 Di Blasi, Z., Harkness, E., Ernst, E. *et al.* (2001) Influence of context effects on health outcomes: a systematic review. *Lancet*, **357** (9258), 757–762.

CHAPTER 16

TREND (Transparent Reporting of Evaluations with Nonrandomized Designs)

Don C. Des Jarlais

Baron Edmond de Rothschild Chemical Dependency Institute, Beth Israel Medical Center, New York, NY, USA

Timetable

Name of reporting guideline initiative	Consensus meeting date	Reporting guideline publication
TREND Transparent Reporting of Evaluations with Nonrandomized Designs	March 2003	April 2004

Name of guideline

TREND – Transparent Reporting of Evaluations with Nonrandomized Designs

History/development

The TREND statement grew out of the meta-analysis work on HIV prevention interventions being conducted by the Centers for Disease Control Prevention Research Synthesis (PRS) project in the late 1990s and early 2000s [1]. It is worth revisiting some of the original concerns that led to the development of the TREND statement because many of these are still relevant today. Indeed, many are now of increased importance.

Ethical issues in HIV research: In almost all of the early HIV prevention studies, it was considered ethically necessary to provide some services to the "control/comparison" group. Given that AIDS was a fatal disease and

Guidelines for Reporting Health Research: A User's Manual, First Edition. Edited by David Moher, Douglas G. Altman, Kenneth F. Schulz, Iveta Simera and Elizabeth Wager.
© 2014 John Wiley & Sons, Ltd. Published 2014 by John Wiley & Sons, Ltd.

that there was a great misunderstanding of how the virus was and was not transmitted, providing accurate information about HIV and AIDS was usually considered a minimum service to be provided to people in the control/comparison condition. HIV counseling and testing were also typically provided to the control/comparison group, both as a valued service and because determining HIV seroprevalence among the target population was an important part of the research.

The data from these early studies were often very difficult to interpret. Most of the studies used randomization into experimental and comparison groups, and there were usually no differences in the outcome measures between these groups, but there were large pre- versus post-differences (reductions in HIV risk behavior) for both the experimental and comparison groups. When analyzed as randomized clinical trials (RCTs), most of these studies indicated that the interventions were not successful. However, when analyzed as non-RCTs, the interventions (for both the experimental and comparison groups) showed large effects. The study reports, however, usually provided very little detail about the actual content of the services received by the comparison group.

Conceptual issues: A second aspect of the lack of detail was the common failure to utilize an identified theoretical framework for developing the experimental intervention. Within a rigorous RCT design, it is usually possible to determine if an intervention "works" without having much of an understanding of the mechanism. However, in a non-RCT design, having a theoretical framework for interpreting the evaluation data can be critical for assessing whether the observed outcomes are likely to be because of the intervention or other factors.

The combination of lack of detail about services provided to comparison groups and lack of theory meant that it is usually not possible to make even preliminary inferences about what might have been the "active ingredients" in evaluations that did show positive outcomes.

Research synthesis and meta-analysis: By the late 1990s, quantitative research synthesis and meta-analysis [2] had become the standard method for assessing the effectiveness of interventions. The sheer number of intervention studies in most fields had made the limitations of qualitative research syntheses apparent, and a variety of developments, from computerized literature databases and new statistical techniques [2], had greatly increased the ability to conduct quantitative systematic reviews and meta-analyses.

The situation in the late 1990s faced by the PRS project was that the reduction in HIV change/risk behavior was occurring both inside and outside of structured evaluation studies, and that much of the relevant data was being collected and reported, but that the reporting was so incomplete that it was not possible to synthesize the data. This led the

PRS team to organize the 2003 meeting of journal editors that led to the TREND statement, which was published in the *American Journal of Public Health* in 2004. The TREND website was created by the CDC at the time of publication.

When to use this guideline (what types of studies it covers)

The objective of the TREND statement was to improve the completeness and reporting of evaluations with nonrandomized designs. It was viewed as parallel to the CONSORT statement. Thus, the TREND statement would be applicable for the same types of evaluation research as CONSORT, except that the research design did not include randomization. It was expected that greater completeness and transparency would permit more evaluations to be included in meta-analyses for topics where it is difficult (for practical or ethical reasons) to conduct randomized trials.

The TREND statement emphasizes reporting the theoretical bases of interventions. Clear statement of the theories underlying the interventions, with measurement of the intervening processes, can serve to provide a conceptual basis for assessing the likelihood that the intervention did "cause" the outcome even in the absence of a truly randomized trial.

Current versions

The statement and checklist have not required updating so far.

Previous versions

None.

Extensions to be aware of

There are no extensions to the TREND checklist.

Related activities

The PRS group and the journal editors who participated in the development of the TREND statement were not the only people who were dissatisfied with the over-reliance on RCTs for generating evidence for the effectiveness of different interventions in public health. Victora *et al.* published an influential article on the importance of using nonrandomized evaluation designs in the same issue of the *American Journal of Public Health* in which the TREND statement was published. Victora *et al.* noted that many public health interventions have relatively long and complex causal pathways between the initial intervention and the desired outcomes [2]. They cite an example of child nutrition where there needs to be a high coverage of public health workers for the target population in which the public health workers are trained in nutritional counseling and these workers counsel a large number of mothers; the mothers then improve the child-feeding behaviors; and then the children improve dietary intake and, finally, have an improved nutritional status. There clearly are many opportunities for such an intervention to fail. There are also some opportunities for the intervention to exceed expectations, for example, counseled mothers may counsel other mothers who were not reached by public health workers, new social norms might emerge to support improved feeding behaviors. A randomized controlled trial that produces a *p*-value for the difference in nutritional status of the experimental group versus the control group does not provide much useful information for evaluating an intervention with a long, complex (and possibly branching) causal pathway.

Victora *et al.* argue for using both "plausibility" designs and "adequacy" designs to supplement and/or to replace RCT designs. "Plausibility" designs include comparison of the experimental condition with some other condition – though this may be only a simple pre- versus post-comparison – and also measure and assess the variables on the causal pathway. "Adequacy" designs focus on whether the effect size reaches an epidemiological level and on modifiers of the effect size.

Victora *et al.*'s call for using designs other than randomized trials is fully consistent with the rationale for the TREND statement. If other than randomized trial designs are to be used, then using the TREND statement becomes increasingly important so that the individual nonrandomized evaluations can be incorporated into systematic reviews [2].

Glasgow *et al.* developed the RE-AIM framework to improve the translation of experimental behavioral interventions into public health practice [3]. Behavioral interventions were assessed in terms of the components of RE-AIM: Reach (the size of the target population for an intervention), Effectiveness (the extent to which an intervention produced the desired effects in field settings), Adoption (the extent to which the intervention was used in field settings), Implementation (the quality and fidelity with which the intervention was applied in field settings) and Maintenance (the extent to which the intervention was sustained in field settings). The RE-AIM framework is useful for identifying barriers to successful utilization of behavioral interventions and studying diffusion and implementation processes.

The TREND statement is focused on improving the reporting of non-randomized evaluations of interventions, whereas RE-AIM is focused on the actual implementation and performance of interventions in the field. There are, however, several areas of overlap between TREND and RE-AIM. Both are concerned with assessing the effectiveness of interventions and both are concerned with assessments in settings other than the highly controlled settings in which RCTs are typically conducted.

The Cochrane Collaboration (http://www.cochrane.org) and the Campbell Collaboration (http://www.campbellcollaboration.org) are also addressing the issues involved in utilizing nonrandomized trials in systematic reviews. In particular, the Cochrane Nonrandomized Study Methods Group (Reeves, B., University of Bristol) and the Cochrane Risk of Bias Group (Mayhew, A., University of Ottawa) have been working on these issues.

How best to use the guideline

The TREND statement should be used in the reporting of evaluations of interventions when designs other than the "standard" RCT design were used. In particular, the TREND statement should be helpful in reporting designs that might be considered to have a substantial methodological rigor, such as interrupted time series, controlled before-and-after studies, and studies using statistical techniques such as propensity matching. The TREND statement was developed in order to include more non-RCT evaluations into systematic review, so that use of the TREND statement should increase the likelihood that a specific non-RCT evaluation will be included in systematic reviews and meta-analyses.

We would encourage authors, reviewers, and editors to bear in mind that much of the value of an evaluation study may be lost if the study is not reported transparently (so that it can be included in systematic reviews/meta-analyses).

Development process

The CDC PRS project convened a two-day meeting of journal editors in 2003. The meeting produced a list of recommended items for a checklist for the reporting of evaluations with nonrandomized designs. Following this meeting, the three primary authors of the TREND statement paper (Des Jarlais, D.C., Lyles, C., and Crepaz, N.) drafted the checklist and the paper containing the TREND statement. The draft was circulated to the editors who had attended the initial meeting for comment and revision. These editors were then included as coauthors (as members of the TREND group) in the publication of the paper in 2004.

Evidence of effectiveness of guideline

There have been no formal evaluations of the effectiveness of the TREND statement. However, to our knowledge, more nonrandomized evaluation studies are being included in meta-analyses of public health interventions than earlier, which suggests that the TREND statement has had an impact on the reporting of such studies. But the continuing interest in the issue of assessing nonrandomized designs [4] suggests that the issues related to optimal use and optimal reporting of nonrandomized designs have not been satisfactorily resolved.

Endorsement and adherence

Publication of the TREND statement was accompanied by several editorials, with statements of endorsement from editors and incorporation of the statement into the "instructions for authors" of journals. The journals that have adopted the TREND statement are listed on the web site (see http://www.cdc.gov/trendstatement/supporters.html).

Cautions and limitations (including scope)
Mistakes and/or misconceptions

The TREND statement should not be seen as an assessment of the "quality" of a non-RCT study. The report of a non-RCT study may be transparent (follow the TREND checklist), and the study may still contain inappropriate use of theoretical concepts, biased/erroneous data, misinterpretation of the data, and so on. However, if the report of a non-RCT evaluation does utilize the TREND statement, it generally will be easier for readers of the report to assess the quality of the evaluation.

Creators' preferred bits

There are many situations in which it is important to evaluate an intervention but practical and/or ethical concerns prevent the use of a randomized controlled design. A number of statistical techniques, such as propensity scoring, have been developed to compensate for the lack of true randomization and produce useful data about the effectiveness of an intervention.

The difficulties in conducting randomized trials are particularly applicable for evaluations of public health/population-level interventions in which the local community may be the unit of analysis. By changing the environment in which health and disease are generated, such structural interventions may have important advantages over interventions that focus on individuals and are thus amenable to randomized trials.

The value of nonrandomized evaluations, however, can be severely compromised by a lack of transparency in their reporting. Lack of transparency can make it impossible to abstract the information needed to use quantitative research synthesis methods to compare such evaluations and to compare nonrandomized evaluations with randomized evaluations.

Finally, the primary strength of randomized evaluations is that, by isolating a single independent variable and then studying the relationship of that independent variable on specified outcome variables, one can be relatively certain that variation in the independent variable is the "cause" of change in the outcomes, even if one does not understand the causal processes. Drawing causal inferences from nonrandomized evaluations is typically considerably more difficult. The TREND statement directly confronts this problem by asking researchers to specify the theories/causal pathways that link the independent variables, through moderator and mediator variables, to the outcome variables. Progress in developing effective interventions depends not only on amassing large amounts of empirical data but also on developing sophisticated theoretical understanding of how an intervention works, for whom it works, and under what conditions it works. By explicitly requiring specification of the theory utilized in intervention studies with nonrandomized designs, the TREND statement has the potential to advance the development of theory underlying different types of interventions.

Future plans

When the TREND statement was first published, it was expected that there would be continuous development of the statement. Unfortunately, lack of resources and competing priorities have limited the amount of further development that has occurred so far. A moderately large number of journals support TREND (see http://www.cdc.gov/trendstatement/ supporters.html) through requiring authors to use the statement when submitting papers that report nonrandomized evaluations. However, it is appropriate to make a few statements here about current and future use of the TREND statement.

First, the rationale for using TREND is as strong or stronger now as it was when the statement was first published. Evaluations using nonrandomized designs are at least as important and the need to incorporate data from such evaluations into systematic reviews and meta-analyses is also as important as before.

Second, the TREND checklist, if somewhat long, is relatively straightforward. There should not be any great difficulties in using the checklist.

There are two areas in which the checklist might be elaborated. As noted above, there has been additional work on developing and classifying non-randomized designs, such as the West *et al.*'s paper [4]. Incorporating such work into the checklist would undoubtedly be helpful.

The need for utilizing identified theories for designing and reporting evaluations has become more important. Having a checklist item for specifying the underlying theory in an intervention was an important aspect of the TREND statement. The number of evaluation studies continues to grow in most fields of public health, and theories have become even more useful for conceptually organizing the studies. The checklist would be strengthened by asking authors to specify the theoretical concepts in the interventions and to state how those concepts were operationalized. In particular, it would be helpful to specify how mediating variables were operationalized and whether statistical testing was performed to test the functions of the mediating variables.

Finally, the TREND statement could also be strengthened by requiring more complete reporting of primary and secondary outcomes. In many evaluation studies, it is not clear how primary and secondary outcomes were decided, with the suspicion that statistical significance levels were used in the decision. There is also an important question – both for theory and for practice – of how the different potential outcome measures are or are not related to each other. One of the primary goals of the TREND statement is to advance understanding of the theories underlying interventions, and the relationships among different outcome measures can provide important insights for refining theories.

References

1 Des Jarlais, D.C., Lyles, C., Crepaz, N. *et al.* (2004) Improving the reporting quality of non-randomized evaluations of behavioral and public health interventions: the TREND Statement. *American Journal of Public Health*, **94** (3), 361–366.
2 Victora, C., Habicht, J.-P. & Bryce, J. (2004) Evidence-based public health: moving beyond randomized trials. *American Journal of Public Health*, **94** (3), 400–405.
3 Glasgow, R.E., Askew, S., Percell, P. *et al.* (2013). Use of RE-AIM to address health inequities: application in a low-income community health center based weight loss and hypertension self-management program. *Translation Behavioral Medicine*, **3** (2), 200–210.
4 West, S., Duan, N., Peqiegmat, W. *et al.* (2008) Alternatives to the randomized controlled trial. *American Journal of Public Health*, **98** (8), 1359–1366.

Trend statement checklist

Paper Section/ Topic	Item No	Descriptor	Reported? ✓	Pg #
Title and Abstract				
Title and Abstract	1	• Information on how unit were allocated to interventions • Structured abstract recommended • Information on target population or study sample		
Introduction				
Background	2	• Scientific background and explanation of rationale • Theories used in designing behavioral interventions		
Methods				
Participants	3	• Eligibility criteria for participants, including criteria at different levels in recruitment/sampling plan (e.g., cities, clinics, subjects) • Method of recruitment (e.g., referral, self-selection), including the sampling method if a systematic sampling plan was implemented • Recruitment setting • Settings and locations where the data were collected		

Interventions	4	• Details of the interventions intended for each study condition and how and when they were actually administered, specifically including:
		  ○ Content: what was given?
		  ○ Delivery method: how was the content given?
		  ○ Unit of delivery: how were the subjects grouped during delivery?
		  ○ Deliverer: who delivered the intervention?
		  ○ Setting: where was the intervention delivered?
		  ○ Exposure quantity and duration: how many sessions or episodes or events were intended to be delivered? How long were they intended to last?
		  ○ Time span: how long was it intended to take to deliver the intervention to each unit?
		  ○ Activities to increase compliance or adherence (e.g., incentives)		

Paper Section/ Topic	Item No	Descriptor	Reported? ✓	Pg #
Objectives	5	• Specific objectives and hypotheses		
Outcomes	6	• Clearly defined primary and secondary outcome measures • Methods used to collect data and any methods used to enhance the quality of measurements • Information on validated instruments such as psychometric and biometric properties		
Sample Size	7	• How sample size was determined and, when applicable, explanation of any interim analyses and stopping rules		
Assignment Method	8	• Unit of assignment (the unit being assigned to study condition, e.g., individual, group, community) • Method used to assign units to study conditions, including details of any restriction (e.g., blocking, stratification, minimization) • Inclusion of aspects employed to help minimize potential bias induced due to non-randomization (e.g., matching)		
Blinding (masking)	9	• Whether or not participants, those administering the interventions, and those assessing the outcomes were blinded to study condition assignment; if so, statement regarding how the blinding was accomplished and how it was assessed.		
Unit of Analysis	10	• Description of the smallest unit that is being analyzed to assess intervention effects (e.g., individual, group, or community) • If the unit of analysis differs from the unit of assignment, the analytical method used to account for this (e.g., adjusting the standard error estimates by the design effect or using multilevel analysis)		
Statistical Methods	11	• Statistical methods used to compare study groups for primary methods outcome(s), including complex methods of correlated data • Statistical methods used for additional analyses, such as a subgroup analyses and adjusted analysis • Methods for imputing missing data, if used • Statistical software or programs used		

(continued)

Paper Section/ Topic	Item No	Descriptor	Reported? ✓	Pg #
Results				

Participant flow	12	• Flow of participants through each stage of the study: enrollment, assignment, allocation, and intervention exposure, follow-up, analysis (a diagram is strongly recommended)
		  ∘ Enrollment: the numbers of participants screened for eligibility, found to be eligible or not eligible, declined to be enrolled, and enrolled in the study
		  ∘ Assignment: the numbers of participants assigned to a study condition
		  ∘ Allocation and intervention exposure: the number of participants assigned to each study condition and the number of participants who received each intervention
		  ∘ Follow-up: the number of participants who completed the follow-up or did not complete the follow-up (i.e., lost to follow-up), by study condition
		  ∘ Analysis: the number of participants included in or excluded from the main analysis, by study condition
		• Description of protocol deviations from study as planned, along with reasons		

Recruitment	13	• Dates defining the periods of recruitment and follow-up		
Baseline Data	14	• Baseline demographic and clinical characteristics of participants in each study condition • Baseline characteristics for each study condition relevant to specific disease prevention research • Baseline comparisons of those lost to follow-up and those retained, overall and by study condition • Comparison between study population at baseline and target population of interest		
Baseline equivalence	15	• Data on study group equivalence at baseline and statistical methods used to control for baseline differences		

Paper Section/ Topic	Item No	Descriptor	Reported?	
			✓	Pg #
Numbers analyzed	16	• Number of participants (denominator) included in each analysis for each study condition, particularly when the denominators change for different outcomes; statement of the results in absolute numbers when feasible • Indication of whether the analysis strategy was "intention to treat" or, if not, description of how non-compliers were treated in the analyses		
Outcomes and estimation	17	• For each primary and secondary outcome, a summary of results for each estimation study condition, and the estimated effect size and a confidence interval to indicate the precision • Inclusion of null and negative findings • Inclusion of results from testing pre-specified causal pathways through which the intervention was intended to operate, if any		
Ancillary analyses	18	• Summary of other analyses performed, including subgroup or restricted analyses, indicating which are pre-specified or exploratory		
Adverse events	19	• Summary of all important adverse events or unintended effects in each study condition (including summary measures, effect size estimates, and confidence intervals)		
DISCUSSION				
Interpretation	20	• Interpretation of the results, taking into account study hypotheses, sources of potential bias, imprecision of measures, multiplicative analyses, and other limitations or weaknesses of the study • Discussion of results taking into account the mechanism by which the intervention was intended to work (causal pathways) or alternative mechanisms or explanations • Discussion of the success of and barriers to implementing the intervention, fidelity of implementation • Discussion of research, programmatic, or policy implications		

(continued)

Paper Section/ Topic	Item No	Descriptor	Reported? ✓	Pg #
Generalizability	21	• Generalizability (external validity) of the trial findings, taking into account the study population, the characteristics of the intervention, length of follow-up, incentives, compliance rates, specific sites/settings involved in the study, and other contextual issues		
Overall Evidence	22	• General interpretation of the results in the context of current evidence and current theory		

From: Des Jarlais, D. C., Lyles, C., Crepaz, N., & the Trend Group (2004). Improving the reporting quality of nonrandomized evaluations of behavioral and public health interventions: The TREND statement. *American Journal of Public Health*, 94, 361–366. For more information, visit: http://www.cdc.gov/trendstatement/

CHAPTER 17

STROBE (STrengthening the Reporting of Observational studies in Epidemiology)

Myriam Cevallos[1] and Matthias Egger[2]

[1]*CTU Bern and Insititute of Social and Preventative Medicine, University of Bern, Bern, Switzerland*
[2]*Institute of Social and Preventive Medicine (ISPM), University of Bern, Bern, Switzerland*

Timetable

Meeting/event date	Objective
March 2001	Idea first discussed
November 2001	Small exploratory meeting at University of Bristol, United Kingdom
April 2003	Planning meeting at University of Bristol, United Kingdom
August 2003	Need for reporting guidelines discussed at World Epidemiology Conference in Montreal, Canada
September 2004	Large workshop at University of Bristol, funded by European Science Foundation
May 2005	First draft checklist posted on STROBE website
October 2007	Publication of checklist and Explanation and Elaboration document in several journals
August 2010	Revision meeting at University of Bern, Switzerland

STROBE Statement

The STrengthening the Reporting of OBservational Studies in Epidemiology (STROBE) statement is a set of recommendations to improve the reporting of observational studies. STROBE addresses the three main types of observational studies: cohort, case–control, and cross-sectional studies. The statement consists of a checklist of 22 items that relate to the title, abstract, introduction, methods, results, and discussion sections of articles.

Guidelines for Reporting Health Research: A User's Manual, First Edition. Edited by David Moher, Douglas G. Altman, Kenneth F. Schulz, Iveta Simera and Elizabeth Wager.
© 2014 John Wiley & Sons, Ltd. Published 2014 by John Wiley & Sons, Ltd.

A diagram showing the number of individuals at each stage of the study, from assessment of eligibility to inclusion in the analysis, may also be considered.

The STROBE checklist, the accompanying comprehensive Explanation and Elaboration (E&E) document, and the website, offer guidance to authors on how to prepare reports on observational research, enhance the completeness and transparency of reporting, and facilitate the critical appraisal and interpretation of studies by reviewers, journal editors, and readers.

History/development

The STROBE statement is the result of an international collaborative effort by epidemiologists, methodologists, statisticians, and journal editors. The idea of a reporting guideline for observational studies was first discussed by a small group of epidemiologists working in the United Kingdom in 2001 and further developed in several meetings. The STROBE initiative was formally established in 2004 in Bristol, United Kingdom, during a two-day workshop funded by the European Science Foundation. In the same year, the STROBE website (www.strobe-statement.org) was launched. Prior to the workshop, the group conducted an extensive literature search of textbooks, bibliographic databases, previous recommendations, etc., to collect all relevant information related to observational research. The group decided early on to restrict the scope of the STROBE statement to three study designs.

The workshop was attended by 23 epidemiologists, methodologists, statisticians, journal editors, and practitioners from Europe and North America and was used to write the first draft of the checklist. The draft was subsequently revised during several meetings of the coordination group and in email discussions with the wider group. Subsequently three revisions were published on the website, two summaries of received comments were prepared, and any changes were documented. During this process, the coordinating group met on eight occasions and held several telephone conferences to revise the checklist and to prepare the article reporting the STROBE statement as well as the E&E document. The STROBE statement and the E&E paper were finally simultaneously published in several journals, with open access to both articles.

When to use this guideline
(what types of studies it covers)

The STROBE recommendations are designed to inform the reporting of observational epidemiological studies. STROBE covers descriptive studies of, for example, the prevalence or incidence of a disease, as well as analytical studies that investigate associations between exposures and health outcomes. STROBE is limited to the three main observational study designs: cohort, case–control, and cross-sectional studies.

The cohort design refers to studies where the investigators follow people over time. They obtain information about people and their exposures at baseline, let time pass, and then assess the occurrence of outcomes. Investigators often compare people who are exposed to a factor of interest (e.g., particle matter in the air) with people who are not exposed or exposed to a lesser degree, and assess exposure and outcome variables at multiple points during follow-up. Incidence rates, rate ratios, and relative risks may then be calculated.

In case–control studies, investigators compare exposures between people with a particular disease outcome (cases) with people without that outcome (controls). All cases or a large fraction of cases diagnosed during a period are typically included in the study. The sample of controls represents the cohort or population of people from which the cases arose. Depending on the sampling strategy for cases and controls and the nature of the population studied, the odds ratio obtained in a case–control study is interpreted as the risk ratio, rate ratio, or (prevalence) odds ratio [1].

In cross-sectional studies, investigators assess all individuals in a sample at the same point in time, often to examine the prevalence of exposures, risk factors, or disease.

Other designs such as genetic linkage studies, infectious disease modeling or case reports and case series are *not* covered by STROBE. However, as many of the key elements in STROBE also apply to these designs, authors who report such studies may nevertheless find the recommendations useful. The STROBE statement was not developed to assess the methodological quality of epidemiological studies and should not be used for this purpose.

Current versions

The STROBE statement includes a checklist of 22 items that relate to the title, abstract, introduction, methods, results, and discussion sections of articles. Eighteen items are common to cohort studies, case–control studies, and cross-sectional studies and four items are specific to each of the three study designs. For some items, information should be given separately for cases and controls in case–control studies or exposed and unexposed groups in cohort and cross-sectional studies. Separate checklists for each of the three study designs are available on the STROBE website.

The E&E paper offers detailed explanations of each checklist item, gives methodological background, and provides published examples of what the STROBE group considered transparent reporting.

The STROBE recommendations have so far been published in eight journals, including the *BMJ*, *Annals of Internal Medicine*, *PLoS Medicine*, and *The Lancet* [2–9]. The E&E article was published in *PLoS Medicine*, *Annals of Internal Medicine*, and *Epidemiology* [10–12].

Previous versions

No major changes to the original version have been published.

Extensions to be aware of

The STrengthening the REporting of Genetic Association (STREGA) recommendations were published in 2009 and are the first extension of STROBE [13]. STREGA provides additions to 12 of the 22 original items of the STROBE checklist to facilitate the reporting of genetic association studies. An extension in the field of molecular epidemiology has been published [27] and one on neuro-epidemiology is in preparation.

Translations

The STROBE recommendations have been translated into Chinese, Spanish, German, Italian, Japanese, Portuguese, Greek, and Persian. Translations to French, Korean, and Bahasa Indonesian are under way. The E&E document is available in Spanish, Japanese, and a Korean version will become available soon.

Related activities

An idea that was discussed during the 2010 workshop was to bring STROBE and PRISMA together and extend the PRISMA guidelines [14] for systematic reviews and meta-analyses of clinical trials to observational studies. In the first step, conceptual issues specific to observational studies were identified and the first impression was gained of the PRISMA items that would need to be changed and the new items that may need to be added.

How best to use the guideline

We strongly recommend authors to use the checklist alongside the STROBE E&E document when writing reports of observational studies, to make sure that they understand what is meant (and what is not) by a given item. Many authors will also find the examples of good reporting useful. The STROBE website may also be useful to identify additional information and background. The STROBE checklist can also support editors and reviewers when assessing submitted articles for completeness of reporting of important methodological details.

The recommendations are only intended to provide guidance on how to report observational research in a transparent and complete manner. They are not prescriptions for designing or conducting studies or an instrument to assess the quality of published articles.

Development process

The STROBE statement and other reporting guidelines should be considered as evolving documents that require periodic changes and updates in light of experience and new evidence [15]. Indeed, two distinguished commentators argued that STROBE should come with an "expiration date," and should be updated in 2010 [16]. This was the aim of the workshop held in Bern, Switzerland, in August 2010.

During this workshop the group discussed the impact of STROBE and its endorsement by journals, and the uses (and misuses) of STROBE. The group revisited the checklist to identify items in need of revision and discussed the addition of new items, based on recent developments in study methodology and new empirical evidence on the reporting of cohort, case–control, and cross-sectional studies. The group identified only minor revisions and additions, and it was felt that these did not justify a new version of the checklist. A draft of a revised checklist with the suggestions for modifications proposed during the meeting will serve as the basis for further discussions at the next meeting.

Evidence of effectiveness of guideline

The possible contribution of the STROBE statement in improving the quality of reporting of observational studies has been a matter for discussion and criticism in more than 30 commentaries and editorials [17]. The fact that the STROBE website receives about 3000 hits per month gives further indication of its impact.

Several recent bibliographic studies have used the STROBE statement to assess the quality of reporting of observational studies in defined medical fields [18–24]. We are, however, not aware of any systematic study comparing the quality of reporting before and after the publication of the STROBE guidelines.

Endorsement and adherence

The STROBE recommendations have been cited over 600 times and have been endorsed by over 100 journals and the International Committee of Medical Journal Editors (see website for complete list of endorsing journals) [17]. The type of endorsement and instructions to authors on the use of STROBE, however, vary widely between journals.

Cautions and limitations (including scope)

The STROBE developers stress that their recommendations are about reporting and should not be seen as prescriptions for designing or conducting studies. Moreover, the checklist should not be used as an instrument to evaluate the quality of observational research. In a recent bibliographic study [25] we looked at a sample of 100 randomly selected articles and examined where, when, and why STROBE was cited. We found that in most observational study reports, STROBE was used as a reporting guideline, whereas half of systematic reviews used STROBE inappropriately as a tool to assess the methodological quality of studies. The absence of reliable tools to assess the quality of observational studies [26] may explain why authors sometimes use reporting guidelines for this purpose.

The STROBE recommendations are limited to three common observational study designs but do not cover many other designs and variations that exist in epidemiological research. The group welcomes extensions that adapt the checklist to other study designs.

Creators' preferred bits

The creators of STROBE do not have preferred items as such, but generally feel that the items closely linked to the prevention of bias in a given observational study are those where transparent and complete reporting is most likely to make a difference. These items will vary between the different study designs and within designs from study to study.

Future plans

The STROBE group will meet again in one or two years to review the need for a revision of the statement. The group is in the process of developing a short checklist for journal and conference abstracts of observational studies based on the STROBE statement. Last but not least and also resulting from our first revision meeting in 2010, we plan to explore an extension of the PRISMA recommendations for systematic reviews and meta-analyses of observational studies.

References

1 Knol, M.J. (2008) What do case-control studies estimate? Survey of methods and assumptions in published case-control research. *American Journal of Epidemiology*, **168** (9), 1073–1081.
2 von Elm, E., Altman, D.G., Egger, M. *et al.* (2007) The Strengthening the Reporting of Observational Studies in Epidemiology (STROBE) statement: guidelines for reporting observational studies. *Lancet*, **370** (9596), 1453–1457.
3 von Elm, E. *et al.* (2007) The Strengthening the Reporting of Observational Studies in Epidemiology (STROBE) statement: guidelines for reporting observational studies. *Epidemiology*, **18** (6), 800–804.
4 von Elm, E. *et al.* (2007) The Strengthening the Reporting of Observational Studies in Epidemiology (STROBE) statement: guidelines for reporting observational studies. *Bulletin of the World Health Organization*, **85** (11), 867–872.
5 von Elm, E. *et al.* (2007) The Strengthening the Reporting of Observational Studies in Epidemiology (STROBE) statement: guidelines for reporting observational studies. *Preventive Medicine*, **45** (4), 247–251.
6 von Elm, E. *et al.* (2007) Strengthening the Reporting of Observational Studies in Epidemiology (STROBE) statement: guidelines for reporting observational studies. *BMJ*, **335** (7624), 806–808.
7 von Elm, E. *et al.* (2007) The Strengthening the Reporting of Observational Studies in Epidemiology (STROBE) statement: guidelines for reporting observational studies. *PLoS Medicine*, **4** (10), e296.
8 von Elm, E. *et al.* (2007) The Strengthening the Reporting of Observational Studies in Epidemiology (STROBE) statement: guidelines for reporting observational studies. *Annals of Internal Medicine*, **147** (8), 573–577.
9 von Elm, E. *et al.* (2008) The Strengthening the Reporting of Observational Studies in Epidemiology (STROBE) statement: guidelines for reporting observational studies. *Journal of Clinical Epidemiology*, **61** (4), 344–349.
10 Vandenbroucke, J.P. *et al.* (2007) Strengthening the Reporting of Observational Studies in Epidemiology (STROBE): explanation and elaboration. *Epidemiology*, **18** (6), 805–835.
11 Vandenbroucke, J.P. *et al.* (2007) Strengthening the Reporting of Observational Studies in Epidemiology (STROBE): explanation and elaboration. *PLoS Medicine*, **4** (10), e297.
12 Vandenbroucke, J.P. *et al.* (2007) Strengthening the Reporting of Observational Studies in Epidemiology (STROBE): explanation and elaboration. *Annals of Internal Medicine*, **147** (8), W163–W194.
13 Little, J. *et al.* (2009) STrengthening the REporting of Genetic Association Studies (STREGA): an extension of the STROBE statement. *PLoS Medicine*, **6** (2), e22.
14 Liberati, A. *et al.* (2009) The PRISMA statement for reporting systematic reviews and meta-analyses of studies that evaluate health care interventions: explanation and elaboration. *PLoS Medicine*, **6** (7), e1000100.

15 Moher, D. *et al.* (2010) Guidance for developers of health research reporting guidelines. *PLoS Medicine*, **7** (2), e1000217.

16 Rothman, K.J. & Poole, C. (2007) Some guidelines on guidelines: they should come with expiration dates. *Epidemiology*, **18** (6), 794–796.

17 STROBE statement. Strengthening the reporting of observational studies in epidemiology. Available from http://www.strobe-statement.org/.

18 Langan, S. *et al.* (2010) The reporting of observational research studies in dermatology journals: a literature-based study. *Archives of Dermatology*, **146** (5), 534–541.

19 Brand, R.A. (2009) Standards of reporting: the CONSORT, QUORUM, and STROBE guidelines. *Clinical Orthopaedics and Related Research*, **467** (6), 1393–1394.

20 Fung, A.E. *et al.* (2009) Applying the CONSORT and STROBE statements to evaluate the reporting quality of neovascular age-related macular degeneration studies. *Ophthalmology*, **116** (2), 286–296.

21 Lystad, R.P., Pollard, H. & Graham, P.L. (2009) Epidemiology of injuries in competition taekwondo: a meta-analysis of observational studies. *Journal of Science and Medicine in Sport*, **12** (6), 614–621.

22 Papathanasiou, A.A. & Zintzaras, E. (2010) Assessing the quality of reporting of observational studies in cancer. *Annals of Epidemiology*, **20** (1), 67–73.

23 Theobald, K. *et al.* (2009) Quality assurance in non-interventional studies. *German Medical Science*, **7**, Doc29.

24 Yoon, U. & Knobloch, K. (2010) Quality of reporting in sports injury prevention abstracts according to the CONSORT and STROBE criteria: an analysis of the World Congress of Sports Injury Prevention in 2005 and 2008. *British Journal of Sports Medicine*, **46** (3), 202–206.

25 Da Costa, B., Cevallos, M., Altman, D.G. *et al.* (2011) Uses and misuses of the STROBE statement: bibliographic study. *BMJ Open*; 1:e000048.

26 Sanderson, S., Tatt, I.D. & Higgins, J.P. (2007) Tools for assessing quality and susceptibility to bias in observational studies in epidemiology: a systematic review and annotated bibliography. *International Journal of Epidemiology*, **36** (3), 666–676.

27 Gallo, V., Egger, M., McCormack, V. *et al.* (2011) STrengthening the Reporting of OBservational studies in Epidemiology – Molecular Epidemiology (STROBE-ME): an extension of the STROBE Statement. *PLoS Med.*; 8:e1001117.

STROBE statement – checklist of items that should be included in reports of observational studies

	Item No	Recommendation
Title and abstract	1	(a) Indicate the study's design with a commonly used term in the title or the abstract
		(b) Provide in the abstract an informative and balanced summary of what was done and what was found
Introduction		
Background/rationale	2	Explain the scientific background and rationale for the investigation being reported
Objectives	3	State specific objectives, including any prespecified hypotheses
Methods		
Study design	4	Present key elements of study design early in the paper
Setting	5	Describe the setting, locations, and relevant dates, including periods of recruitment, exposure, follow-up, and data collection
Participants	6	(a) *Cohort study* – Give the eligibility criteria, and the sources and methods of selection of participants. Describe methods of follow-up
		Case-control study – Give the eligibility criteria, and the sources and methods of case ascertainment and control selection. Give the rationale for the choice of cases and controls
		Cross-sectional study – Give the eligibility criteria, and the sources and methods of selection of participants
		(b) *Cohort study* – For matched studies, give matching criteria and number of exposed and unexposed
		Case-control study – For matched studies, give matching criteria and the number of controls per case
Variables	7	Clearly define all outcomes, exposures, predictors, potential confounders, and effect modifiers. Give diagnostic criteria, if applicable
Data sources/ measurement	8*	For each variable of interest, give sources of data and details of methods of assessment (measurement). Describe comparability of assessment methods if there is more than one group
Bias	9	Describe any efforts to address potential sources of bias
Study size	10	Explain how the study size was arrived at

(*continued*)

	Item No	Recommendation
Quantitative variables	11	Explain how quantitative variables were handled in the analyses. If applicable, describe which groupings were chosen and why
Statistical methods	12	(a) Describe all statistical methods, including those used to control for confounding
		(b) Describe any methods used to examine subgroups and interactions
		(c) Explain how missing data were addressed
		(d) *Cohort study* – If applicable, explain how loss to follow-up was addressed *Case-control study* – If applicable, explain how matching of cases and controls was addressed *Cross-sectional study* – If applicable, describe analytical methods taking account of sampling strategy
		(e) Describe any sensitivity analyses
Results		
Participants	13*	(a) Report numbers of individuals at each stage of study – eg numbers potentially eligible, examined for eligibility, confirmed eligible, included in the study, completing follow-up, and analysed
		(b) Give reasons for non-participation at each stage
		(c) Consider use of a flow diagram
Descriptive data	14*	(a) Give characteristics of study participants (eg demographic, clinical, social) and information on exposures and potential confounders
		(b) Indicate number of participants with missing data for each variable of interest
		(c) *Cohort study* – Summarise follow-up time (eg, average and total amount)
Outcome data	15*	*Cohort study* – Report numbers of outcome events or summary measures over time
		Case-control study – Report numbers in each exposure category, or summary measures of exposure
		Cross-sectional study – Report numbers of outcome events or summary measures
Main results	16	(a) Give unadjusted estimates and, if applicable, confounder-adjusted estimates and their precision (eg, 95% confidence interval). Make clear which confounders were adjusted for and why they were included
		(b) Report category boundaries when continuous variables were categorized
		(c) If relevant, consider translating estimates of relative risk into absolute risk for a meaningful time period

	Item No	Recommendation
Other analyses	17	Report other analyses done – eg analyses of subgroups and interactions, and sensitivity analyses
Discussion		
Key results	18	Summarise key results with reference to study objectives
Limitations	19	Discuss limitations of the study, taking into account sources of potential bias or imprecision. Discuss both direction and magnitude of any potential bias
Interpretation	20	Give a cautious overall interpretation of results considering objectives, limitations, multiplicity of analyses, results from similar studies, and other relevant evidence
Generalisability	21	Discuss the generalisability (external validity) of the study results
Other information		
Funding	22	Give the source of funding and the role of the funders for the present study and, if applicable, for the original study on which the present article is based

*Give information separately for cases and controls in case-control studies and, if applicable, for exposed and unexposed groups in cohort and cross-sectional studies.

Note: An Explanation and Elaboration article discusses each checklist item and gives methodological background and published examples of transparent reporting. The STROBE checklist is best used in conjunction with this article (freely available on the Web sites of PLoS Medicine at http://www.plosmedicine.org/, Annals of Internal Medicine at http://www.annals.org/, and Epidemiology at http://www.epidem.com/). Information on the STROBE Initiative is available at www.strobe-statement.org.

CHAPTER 18

STREGA (Strengthening the Reporting of Genetic Associations)

Julian Little

Department of Epidemiology and Community Medicine, Canada Research Chair in Human Genome Epidemiology, University of Ottawa, Ottawa, ON, Canada

STREGA timetable

Reporting guideline	Notes	Meeting date	Publication date
STREGA	For case–control, cross-sectional, and cohort studies of genetic associations – brought together group of epidemiologists, geneticists, statisticians, journal editors, and graduate students	June 2006	2009

Strengthening the Reporting of Genetic Associations

The Strengthening the Reporting of Genetic Association Health Studies (STREGA) statement is a guideline for authors reporting genetic association studies. There has been a tremendous increase in the reporting of associations between genes and diseases; more than 50,000 articles have now been published, and the annual number has tripled between 2001 and 2009 [1, 2]. However, the evidence base on gene disease associations is fraught with methodological problems [3–5]. Inadequate reporting of results, even from well-conducted studies, hampers assessment of a study's strengths and weaknesses, and hence the integration of evidence [6]. Some studies have noted inadequate reporting of genetic association studies [7, 8] (and in developing the guidelines, we also noted that some methodological features of studies were very poorly reported).

Guidelines for Reporting Health Research: A User's Manual, First Edition. Edited by David Moher, Douglas G. Altman, Kenneth F. Schulz, Iveta Simera and Elizabeth Wager.
© 2014 John Wiley & Sons, Ltd. Published 2014 by John Wiley & Sons, Ltd.

The STREGA guideline was developed to address this problem. The guideline does not describe or dictate how a genetic association study should be designed but seeks to enhance the transparency of its reporting, regardless of choices made during design, conduct, or analysis. It builds on the STROBE statement, providing additions to 12 of the 22 items on the STROBE checklist. The additions concern population stratification, genotyping errors, modeling haplotype variation, Hardy–Weinberg equilibrium (HWE), replication, selection of participants, rationale for choice of genes and variants, treatment effects in studying quantitative traits, statistical methods, relatedness, reporting of descriptive and outcome data, and the volume of data issues that are important to consider in genetic association studies.

When to use STREGA

As is the case for the STROBE statement to which STREGA is an extension, the STREGA guideline can be used to report case–control, cross-sectional, and cohort studies of genetic associations.

The case–control study is the most commonly used design in studies of genetic associations. In case–control studies, investigators compare exposures or genotypes between people with a particular disease outcome (cases) and people without that outcome (controls) [9]. Investigators aim to collect cases and controls who are representatives of an underlying cohort or a cross section of a population. The case sample may be all or a large fraction of available cases, whereas the control sample is usually only a small fraction of people in the cohort or the population that does not have the outcome of interest. Thus, controls represent the cohort or population of people from which the cases arose. The design has been applied to the investigation of candidate genes, that is, where there is an *a priori* hypothesis about associations with variants of genes thought to be important in influencing the outcome of interest [10, 11], and to genome-wide association studies in which there is an "agnostic" assessment of associations between the outcome of interest and many thousands of genetic variants [12–14].

In cross-sectional studies, all individuals in a sample are assessed at the same point in time. These assessments often address the prevalence of exposures, risk factors, or disease [9]. Examples of cross-sectional studies of genetic associations include investigations in the National Health and Nutrition Examination Survey in the United States of variants of the gene encoding apolipoprotein E and chronic kidney disease [15] and candidate genetic variation in quantitative traits related to heart disease [16, 17].

In cohort studies, people are followed over time [9]. Information is obtained about people and their exposures at a baseline, and after time has passed, the occurrence of disease or an outcome is assessed. Groups within the cohort may be compared, or the whole cohort may be compared with an external comparison cohort. In the context of genetic association studies, comparison is made between individuals with one or more gene variants of interest and those who have one or more of the common variants of those genes. Investigators may assess several different outcomes within a single cohort study, and may assess exposure and outcome variables at multiple points during follow-up. Examples of cohort studies of genetic associations include investigations of *APOE* and late-onset dementia [18–20] and the gene encoding the adipokine resistin (*RETN*) and diabetes-related traits in the Framingham offspring cohort [21].

Articles that present and synthesize data from several studies in a single report are becoming increasingly common. In particular, many genome-wide association analyses include several different study populations, sometimes with different study designs and genotyping platforms, and in various stages of discovery and replication [12–14]. The STREGA guideline addresses this development by recommending that when data from several studies are presented in a single report, each of the constituent studies and the composite result should be fully described.

Current version

The STREGA statement was published in eight journals in 2009 [22] and in one book chapter [23]. It comprises explanatory text, a 22-item set of recommendations that make clear where additions have been made to the STROBE checklist and a table providing complementary information on the areas and rationale for the additional STREGA recommendations. In addition, the STREGA recommendations are available at www.strega-statement.org.

Extensions

A statement on "Strengthening the reporting of genetic risk prediction studies (GRIPS)" was published in 10 journals in 2011 [24], with further exploration and elaboration in 4 articles [25].

Genetic-risk prediction studies typically concern the development and/or the evaluation of models for the prediction of a specific health outcome. There is considerable variation in the design, conduct, and analysis of these studies, and many publications do not provide sufficient details to judge methodological or analytical aspects. As the number of discovered genetic markers that could be used in future genetic-risk prediction studies continues to increase, it is crucial to enhance the quality of the reporting of these studies, since valid interpretation could be compromised by the lack of reporting of key information.

The GRIPS statement addresses this need. It was developed by a multidisciplinary panel of 25 risk-prediction researchers, epidemiologists, geneticists, methodologists, statisticians, and journal editors, 7 of whom were also part of the STREGA initiative. This panel attended a two-day meeting in which they discussed a draft version of a checklist that was developed from STREGA because of its focus on observational study designs and genetic factors, REMARK [26] because of its focus on prediction models, and STARD [27, 28] because of its focus on test evaluation. The initial recommendations were revised both during the meeting and in extensive electronic correspondence after the meeting.

The strategy followed in developing the GRIPS guidelines was consistent with recommendations proposed on how to develop health research reporting guidelines [29], which was published after the workshop. In formulating the GRIPS statement, methodological advances in the design and assessment of genetic-risk prediction models, which are still developing, were anticipated. Thus, similar to STREGA, the GRIPS statement focuses on recommending how a study should be reported and not how a study should be designed, conducted, or analyzed.

Related activities

Improving the reporting of genetic association studies will facilitate the synthesis of evidence. Guidelines for the systematic review and meta-analysis of genetic association studies have been published in the form of a handbook [30] and commentary [31]. Systematic reviews and meta-analyses typically deal with one or a few variants of one or a few genes. However, there is considerable value in pulling together evidence about the overall effects of genetic variation on disease or other outcomes, and also in looking at the effects of gene variants on a range of disease outcomes. To meet this need, interim guidelines on the assessment of cumulative evidence on genetic associations have been developed [32, 33]. Examples of the operationalization of these include field synopses relating to Alzheimer's disease [34] and colorectal cancer [35]. In addition, a workshop was held to develop guidelines for the assessment of cumulative evidence on gene environment interaction, which have been published [36].

How best to use the guideline
Authors

The STREGA guideline is intended to maximize the transparency, quality, and completeness of reporting of what was done and found in a particular study. The recommendations are not intended to support or oppose the choice of any particular study design or method. When authors use STREGA, we suggest that the format of the article should conform with the journal style, editorial directions, and, where possible, author preferences. It has been suggested that reporting guidelines are most helpful if authors keep the general content of the guideline items in mind when they write their initial drafts, and then refer to the details of individual items as they critically appraise what they have written during the revision process [37]. Adherence to recommendations may make some manuscripts longer and this may be seen as a drawback when there is limited space in a print journal. However, the ability to post information on the Web should alleviate this concern, and the place in which supplementary information is presented can be decided by authors and editors of individual journals. The availability of supplementary information raises possible concerns including the care with which the supplemental material was evaluated in the review process and the continuation of availability of supplementary information. Some journals have started to address these issues [38, 39].

Peer reviewers and editors

The STREGA Reporting Guidelines should not be used to assess submitted manuscripts to determine the quality or validity of the study being reported, but the checklist can be a useful guide to peer reviewers and editors in being an aide memoire for aspects of the review process and for making a decision about a manuscript. If editors include the STREGA checklist as part of their guidance for reviewers, this should encourage a thorough review process. Guidance for reviewers is particularly important given the multidisciplinary nature of research on genetic association, gene–environment, and gene–gene interactions. In addition, if authors, peer reviewers, and editors use the same checklist, this should facilitate communication about the transparency of reporting of genetic association studies. In particular, transparent reporting of study design and methods can advance understanding of whether specific methodological aspects can influence the direction or the magnitude of the association observed.

Development process

A multidisciplinary group developed the STREGA statement by using literature review, workshop presentations and discussion, and iterative electronic correspondence after the workshop. Thirty-three of 74 invitees participated in the STREGA workshop in Ottawa, Ontario, Canada, in June 2006. Participants included epidemiologists, geneticists, statisticians, journal editors, and graduate students.

Before the workshop, an electronic search was performed to identify reporting guidance for genetic association studies. Workshop participants were also asked to identify any existing guidance. They prepared brief presentations on existing reporting guidelines, empirical evidence on reporting of genetic association studies, the development of the STROBE statement, and several key areas for discussion that were identified on the basis of consultations before the workshop. These areas included the selection and participation of study participants; rationale for choice of genes and variants investigated; genotyping errors; methods for inferring haplotypes; population stratification; assessment of HWE; multiple testing; reporting of quantitative (continuous) outcomes; selectively reporting study results; joint effects; and inference of causation in single studies. Additional resources to inform workshop participants were the HuGENet handbook [30, 31], examples of data extraction forms from systematic reviews or meta-analyses, articles on guideline development [40, 41], and the checklists developed for STROBE. To harmonize our recommendations for genetic association studies with those for observational epidemiologic studies, we communicated with the STROBE group during the development process and sought their comments on the STREGA draft documents. We also provided comments on the developing STROBE statement and its associated explanation and elaboration document [9].

Evidence of effectiveness of guideline

We are unaware of any evaluations as to whether the use of the STREGA recommendations is associated with an improved quality of reporting of genetic association studies. As part of completing such an assessment, we reviewed the reporting of a random sample of genetic association studies published in 2007 [8], which follows an earlier assessment made for studies published in 2001–2003 [7].

Endorsement and adherence

Fifteen journals have explicitly supported STREGA either by publishing the statement, or a commentary on it, or referring to it in their instructions to authors. In addition, the statement is included on the EQUATOR, CONSORT, and US National Library of Medicine websites. We are unaware of any data on journal adherence to STREGA.

Cautions and limitations

The STREGA checklist is not intended as an instrument to evaluate the quality of a genetic association study, and it is not appropriate to use the checklist to construct a quality score.

We have already mentioned the increased frequency of articles that present and synthesize data from several studies in a single publication. We have observed that publication of additional information on the study online is a common practice in this situation. STREGA recommends that the methods and results be described in sufficient detail to enable assessment of the strengths and weaknesses of the evidence provided. However, we have noted considerable variation in practice and we plan to address this in the future.

Because it was based on STROBE, the study designs included were limited to cross-sectional studies, cohort studies, and case–control studies. The STREGA statement does not provide explicit guidance for designs that are specific to genetic epidemiology studies, such as case-only studies or case–parent–trio studies, although the latter can be considered as a special type of case–control study. Explicit guidance on the reporting of gene–environment and gene–gene joint effects is not provided. With regard to gene–environment joint effects, in particular, concerns about ensuring adequate statistical power [42] have stimulated efforts to enable the pooling of data, including promoting the harmonization of exposure assessment across studies [43, 44]. It will be crucial to have reporting sufficiently transparent not only to specify what variables and measures have been harmonized, but also what procedures were used to collect these [45]. In addition, because of the development of novel methods for analyses of both gene–gene [46] and gene–environment [47] joint effects, we would underline the recommendations made in both STROBE and STREGA about transparency of reporting analysis of subgroups and joint effects.

Creators' preferred bits

First, the recommendation to state whether the study is the first report of a genetic association, a replication effort, or both, has become particularly important in an era of genome-wide association analyses. Moreover, this is likely to continue to be very important with the continued development of new genotyping technologies such as assessment of copy number variation [48] and full genomic sequencing [49]. Second, there is an ongoing debate about the methods to address the possible effects of population stratification [22, 50–52]. Population stratification occurs when there exist subgroups within a population between which both allele (or genotype or haplotype) frequencies and disease risks differ. When the population groups compared differ in the proportions of the subgroups, an association between a genotype and the disease being investigated may reflect the genotype of an indicator gene identifying the subgroup rather than a disease-related causal variant. In this situation, population subgroup is a confounder because it is associated with both genotype frequency and disease risk. Third, at the STREGA workshop, there were differing views about whether testing for departure from HWE is a useful method to detect errors or peculiarities in the data set and also the method of testing [22, 53]. Transparent reporting of whether such testing was done, and if so the method used, is important for allowing the empirical evidence to accrue.

Future plans

We plan to work further to disseminate the STREGA guideline and evaluate whether the dissemination activities are associated with improvements in the reporting of genetic association studies. As part of this evaluation, we have analyzed reporting from 2002 to 2003 [7] and 2007 [8]. In addition, we have completed an assessment of the reporting of genome-wide association studies [54].

References

1 Lin, B.K., Clyne, M., Walsh, M. *et al.* (2006) Tracking the epidemiology of human genes in the literature: the HuGE Published Literature Database. *American Journal of Epidemiology*, **164**, 1–4.

2 Yu, Y., Yesupriya, A., Clyne, M. *et al.* HuGE Literature Finder. HuGE Navigator. Available from http://www.hugenavigator.net/HuGENavigator/startPagePubLit.do [accessed on 26 October 2010].

3 Little, J., Khoury, M.J., Bradley, L. *et al.* (2003) The human genome project is complete. How do we develop a handle for the pump? *American Journal of Epidemiology*, **157**, 667–673.

4 Ioannidis, J.P., Bernstein, J., Boffetta, P. *et al.* (2005) A network of investigator networks in human genome epidemiology. *American Journal of Epidemiology*, **162**, 302–304.

5 Ioannidis, J.P., Gwinn, M., Little, J. *et al.* (2006) A road map for efficient and reliable human genome epidemiology. *Nature Genetics*, **38**, 3–5.

6 von Elm, E. & Egger, M. (2004) The scandal of poor epidemiological research. *BMJ*, **329**, 868–869.

7 Yesupriya, A., Evangelou, E., Kavvoura, F.K., *et al.* (2008) Reporting of human genome epidemiology (HuGE) association studies: an empirical assessment. *BMC Medical Research Methodology*, **8**, 31.

8 Aljasir, B., Ioannidis, J.P., Yurkiewich, A. *et al.* (2013) Assessment of systematic effects of methodological characteristics on candidate genetic associations. *Human Genetics*, **132**, 167–178.

9 Vandenbroucke, J.P., von Elm, E., Altman, D.G. *et al.* (2007) Strengthening the Reporting of Observational Studies in Epidemiology (STROBE): explanation and elaboration. *Annals of Internal Medicine*, **147**, W163–W194.

10 Daly, A.K. (2003) Candidate gene case-control studies. *Pharmacogenomics*, **4**, 127–139.

11 Siontis, K.C., Patsopoulos, N.A. & Ioannidis, J.P. (2010) Replication of past candidate loci for common diseases and phenotypes in 100 genome-wide association studies. *European Journal of Human Genetics*, **18**, 832–837.

12 McCarthy, M.I., Abecasis, G.R., Cardon, L.R. *et al.* (2008) Genome-wide association studies for complex traits: consensus, uncertainty and challenges. *Nature Reviews Genetics*, **9**, 356–369.

13 Pearson, T.A. & Manolio, T.A. (2008) How to interpret a genome-wide association study. *JAMA*, **299**, 1335–1344.

14 Hindorff, L.A., Junkins, H.A., Hall, P.N. *et al.* A catalog of published genome-wide association studies. Available from www.genome.gov/gwastudies [accessed on 20 October 2010].

15 Chu, A.Y., Parekh, R.S., Astor, B.C. *et al.* (2009) Association of APOE polymorphism with chronic kidney disease in a nationally representative sample: a Third National Health and Nutrition Examination Survey (NHANES III) Genetic Study. *BMC Medical Genetics*, **10**, 108.

16 Crawford, D.C., Sanders, C.L., Qin, X. *et al.* (2006) Genetic variation is associated with C-reactive protein levels in the Third National Health and Nutrition Examination Survey. *Circulation*, **114**, 2458–2465.

17 Keebler, M.E., Sanders, C.L., Surti, A. *et al.* (2009) Association of blood lipids with common DNA sequence variants at 19 genetic loci in the multiethnic United States National Health and Nutrition Examination Survey III. *Circulation Cardiovascular Genetics*, **2**, 238–243.

18 Myers, R.H., Schaefer, E.J., Wilson, P.W. *et al.* (1996) Apolipoprotein E epsilon4 association with dementia in a population-based study: The Framingham study. *Neurology*, **46**, 673–677.

19 Slooter, A.J., Cruts, M., Kalmijn, S. *et al.* (1998) Risk estimates of dementia by apolipoprotein E genotypes from a population-based incidence study: the Rotterdam Study. *Archives of Neurology*, **55**, 964–968.

20 Tang, M.X., Stern, Y., Marder, K. *et al.* (1998) The APOE-epsilon4 allele and the risk of Alzheimer disease among African Americans, whites, and Hispanics. *JAMA*, **279**, 751–755.

21 Hivert, M.F., Manning, A.K., McAteer, J.B. *et al.* (2009) Association of variants in RETN with plasma resistin levels and diabetes-related traits in the Framingham Offspring Study. *Diabetes*, **58**, 750–756.

22 Little, J., Higgins, J.P., Ioannidis, J.P. *et al.* (2009) STrengthening the REporting of Genetic Association Studies (STREGA): an extension of the STROBE statement. *PLoS Medicine*, **6**, e22.

23 Little, J., Higgins, J.P., Ioannidis, J.P. *et al.* (2010) STrengthening the REporting of Genetic Association studies (STREGA) – an extension of the STROBE statement. In: Khoury, M.J., Bedrosian, S.R., Gwinn, M., *et al.* (eds), *Human Genome Epidemiology. Building the Evidence for Using Genetic Information to Improve Health and Prevent Disease*, 2nd. edn., pp. 188–214, Oxford University Press, New York.

24 Janssens, A.C., Ioannidis, J.P., van Duijn, C.M. *et al.* (2011) Strengthening the reporting of genetic risk prediction studies: the GRIPS statement. *BMJ*, **342**, d631.

25 Janssens, A.C., Ioannidis, J.P., Bedrosian, S. *et al.* (2011) Strengthening the reporting of Genetic RIsk Prediction Studies (GRIPS): explanation and elaboration. *Journal of Clinical Epidemiology*, **64**, e1–e22.

26 McShane, L.M., Altman, D.G., Sauerbrei, W. *et al.* (2005) Reporting recommendations for tumor marker prognostic studies (REMARK). *Journal of the National Cancer Institute*, **97**, 1180–1184.

27 Bossuyt, P.M., Reitsma, J.B., Bruns, D.E. *et al.* (2003) Towards complete and accurate reporting of studies of diagnostic accuracy: the STARD Initiative. *Annals of Internal Medicine*, **138**, 40–44.

28 Bossuyt, P.M., Reitsma, J.B., Bruns, D.E. *et al.* (2003) The STARD statement for reporting studies of diagnostic accuracy: explanation and elaboration. *Annals of Internal Medicine*, **138**, W1–W12.

29 Moher, D., Schulz, K.F., Simera, I. & Altman, D.G. (2010) Guidance for developers of health research reporting guidelines. *PLoS Medicine*, **7**, e1000217. [PMID: 20169112].

30 Little, J., & Higgins, J.P.T. The HuGENet™ HuGE Review Handbook, version 1.0. Available from http://www.med.uottawa.ca/public-health-genomics/web/assets/documents/HuGE_Review_Handbook_V1_0.pdf [accessed on 20 July 2011].

31 Higgins, J.P., Little, J., Ioannidis, J.P. *et al.* (2007) Turning the pump handle: evolving methods for integrating the evidence on gene-disease association. *American Journal of Epidemiology*, **166**, 863–866.

32 Ioannidis, J.P., Boffetta, P., Little, J. *et al.* (2008) Assessment of cumulative evidence on genetic associations: interim guidelines. *International Journal of Epidemiology*, **37**, 120–132.

33 Khoury, M.J., Bertram, L., Boffetta, P. *et al.* (2009) Genome-wide association studies, field synopses, and the development of the knowledge base on genetic variation and human diseases. *American Journal of Epidemiology*, **170**, 269–279.

34 Bertram, L., McQueen, M.B., Mullin, K. *et al.* (2007) Systematic meta-analyses of Alzheimer disease genetic association studies: the AlzGene database. *Nature Genetics*, **39**, 17–23.

35 Theodoratou, E., Montazeri, Z., Hawken, S. *et al.* (2012) Systematic meta-analyses and field synopsis of genetic association studies in colorectal cancer. *Journal of the National Cancer Institute*, **104**, 1433–1457.

36 Boffetta, P., Winn, D.M., Ioannidis, J.P. *et al.* (2012) Recommendations and proposed guidelines for assessing the cumulative evidence on joint effects of genes and environments on cancer occurrence in humans. *International Journal of Epidemiology*, **41**, 686–704.

37 Davidoff, F., Batalden, P., Stevens, D. *et al.* (2008) Publication guidelines for improvement studies in health care: evolution of the SQUIRE Project. *Annals of Internal Medicine*, **149**, 670–676.

38 Marcus, E. (2009) Taming supplemental material. *Cell*, **139**, 11.

39 Marcus, E. (2010) 2010: a Publishing Odyssey. *Cell*, **140**, 9.

40 Altman, D.G., Schulz, K.F., Moher, D. *et al.* (2001) The revised CONSORT statement for reporting randomized trials: explanation and elaboration. *Annals of Internal Medicine*, **134**, 663–694.

41 Moher, D., Schultz, K.F. & Altman, D. (2001) The CONSORT statement: revised recommendations for improving the quality of reports of parallel-group randomized trials. *JAMA*, **285**, 1987–1991.

42 Burton, P.R., Hansell, A.L., Fortier, I. *et al.* (2009) Size matters: just how big is BIG?: Quantifying realistic sample size requirements for human genome epidemiology. *International Journal of Epidemiology*, **38**, 263–273.

43 Knoppers, B.M., Fortier, I., Legault, D. & Burton, P. (2008) The Public Population Project in Genomics (P3G): a proof of concept? *European Journal of Human Genetics*, **16**, 664–665.

44 Stover, P.J., Harlan, W.R., Hammond, J.A. *et al.* (2010) PhenX: a toolkit for interdisciplinary genetics research. *Current Opinion in Lipidology*, **21**, 136–140.

45 Fortier, I., Burton, P.R., Robson, P.J. *et al.* (2010) Quality, quantity and harmony: the DataSHaPER approach to integrating data across bioclinical studies. *International Journal of Epidemiology*. **39**, 1383–1393.

46 Cordell, H.J. (2009) Detecting gene-gene interactions that underlie human diseases. *Nature Reviews Genetics*, **10**, 392–404.

47 Thomas, D. (2010) Methods for investigating gene-environment interactions in candidate pathway and genome-wide association studies. *Annual Review of Public Health*, **31**, 21–36.

48 Wain, L.V., Armour, J.A. & Tobin, M.D. (2009) Genomic copy number variation, human health, and disease. *Lancet*, **374**, 340–350.

49 Tucker, T., Marra, M. & Friedman, J.M. (2009) Massively parallel sequencing: the next big thing in genetic medicine. *American Journal of Human Genetics*, **85**, 142–154.

50 Astle, W. & Balding, D.J. (2009) Population structure and cryptic relatedness in genetic association studies. *Statistical Science*, **24**, 451–471.

51 Dadd, T., Weale, M.E. & Lewis, C.M. (2009) A critical evaluation of genomic control methods for genetic association studies. *Genetic Epidemiology*, **33**, 290–298.

52 Price, A.L., Zaitlen, N.A., Reich, D. & Patterson, N. (2010) New approaches to population stratification in genome-wide association studies. *Nature Reviews Genetics*, **11**, 459–463.

53 Minelli, C., Thompson, J.R., Abrams, K.R. *et al.* (2008) How should we use information about HWE in the meta-analyses of genetic association studies? *International Journal of Epidemiology*, **37**, 136–146.

54 Yurkiewich, A.J., (2011) An analysis of genome-wide association studies to produce evidence useful in guiding their reporting and synthesis. MSc thesis, University of Ottawa, Ottawa, ON, Canada, 1–181.

STREGA reporting recommendations, extended from STROBE statement

Item	Item number	STROBE Guideline	Extension for Genetic Association Studies (STREGA)
Title and Abstract	1	(a) Indicate the study's design with a commonly used term in the title or the abstract. (b) Provide in the abstract an informative and balanced summary of what was done and what was found.	
Introduction			
Background rationale	2	Explain the scientific background and rationale for the investigation being reported.	
Objectives	3	State specific objectives, including any pre-specified hypotheses.	*State if the study is the first report of a genetic association, a replication effort, or both.*
Methods			
Study design	4	Present key elements of study design early in the paper.	
Setting	5	Describe the setting, locations and relevant dates, including periods of recruitment, exposure, follow-up, and data collection.	
Participants	6	(a) **Cohort study** – Give the eligibility criteria, and the sources and methods of selection of participants. Describe methods of follow-up. **Case-control study** – Give the eligibility criteria, and the sources and methods of case ascertainment and control selection. Give the rationale for the choice of cases and controls. **Cross-sectional study** – Give the eligibility criteria, and the sources and methods of selection of participants	*Give information on the criteria and methods for selection of subsets of participants from a larger study, when relevant.*

(*continued*)

Item	Item number	STROBE Guideline	Extension for Genetic Association Studies (STREGA)
		(b) **Cohort study** – For matched studies, give matching criteria and number of exposed and unexposed. **Case-control study** – For matched studies, give matching criteria and the number of controls per case.	
Variables	7	(a) Clearly define all outcomes, exposures, predictors, potential confounders, and effect modifiers. Give diagnostic criteria, if applicable.	*(b) Clearly define genetic exposures (genetic variants) using a widely-used nomenclature system. Identify variables likely to be associated with population stratification (confounding by ethnic origin).*
Data sources measurement	8*	(a) For each variable of interest, give sources of data and details of methods of assessment (measurement). Describe comparability of assessment methods if there is more than one group.	*(b) Describe laboratory methods, including source and storage of DNA, genotyping methods and platforms (including the allele calling algorithm used, and its version), error rates and call rates. State the laboratory/centre where genotyping was done. Describe comparability of laboratory methods if there is more than one group. Specify whether genotypes were assigned using all of the data from the study simultaneously or in smaller batches.*
Bias	9	(a) Describe any efforts to address potential sources of bias.	*(b) For quantitative outcome variables, specify if any investigation of potential bias resulting from pharmacotherapy was undertaken. If relevant, describe the nature and magnitude of the potential bias, and explain what approach was used to deal with this.*

Item	Item number	STROBE Guideline	Extension for Genetic Association Studies (STREGA)
Study size	10	Explain how the study size was arrived at.	
Quantitative variables	11	Explain how quantitative variables were handled in the analyses. If applicable, describe which groupings were chosen, and why.	*If applicable, describe how effects of treatment were dealt with.*
Statistical methods	12	(a) Describe all statistical methods, including those used to control for confounding.	*State software version used and options (or settings) chosen.*
		(b) Describe any methods used to examine subgroups and interactions.	
		(c) Explain how missing data were addressed.	
		(d) **Cohort study** – If applicable, explain how loss to follow-up was addressed. **Case-control study** – If applicable, explain how matching of cases and controls was addressed. **Cross-sectional study** – If applicable, describe analytical methods taking account of sampling strategy	
		(e) Describe any sensitivity analyses	
			(f) State whether Hardy-Weinberg equilibrium was considered and, if so, how.
			(g) Describe any methods used for inferring genotypes or haplotypes.
			(h) Describe any methods used to assess or address population stratification.
			(i) Describe any methods used to address multiple comparisons or to control risk of false positive findings.
			(j) Describe any methods used to address and correct for relatedness among subjects

(continued)

Item	Item number	STROBE Guideline	Extension for Genetic Association Studies (STREGA)
Results			
Participants	13*	(a) Report the numbers of individuals at each stage of the study – e.g., numbers potentially eligible, examined for eligibility, confirmed eligible, included in the study, completing follow-up, and analysed. (b) Give reasons for non-participation at each stage. (c) Consider use of a flow diagram.	*Report numbers of individuals in whom genotyping was attempted and numbers of individuals in whom genotyping was successful.*
Descriptive data	14*	(a) Give characteristics of study participants (e.g., demographic, clinical, social) and information on exposures and potential confounders. (b) Indicate the number of participants with missing data for each variable of interest. (c) **Cohort study** – Summarize follow-up time, e.g. average and total amount.	*Consider giving information by genotype.*
Outcome data	15*	**Cohort study**-Report numbers of outcome events or summary measures over time. **Case-control study** – Report numbers in each exposure category, or summary measures of exposure. **Cross-sectional study** – Report numbers of outcome events or summary measures.	*Report outcomes (phenotypes) for each genotype category over time* *Report numbers in each genotype category* *Report outcomes (phenotypes) for each genotype category*
Main results	16	(a) Give unadjusted estimates and, if applicable, confounder-adjusted estimates and their precision (e.g., 95% confidence intervals). Make clear which confounders were adjusted for and why they were included. (b) Report category boundaries when continuous variables were categorized.	

Item	Item number	STROBE Guideline	Extension for Genetic Association Studies (STREGA)
		(c) If relevant, consider translating estimates of relative risk into absolute risk for a meaningful time period.	
			(d) Report results of any adjustments for multiple comparisons.
Other analyses	17	(a) Report other analyses done – e.g., analyses of subgroups and interactions, and sensitivity analyses.	
			(b) If numerous genetic exposures (genetic variants) were examined, summarize results from all analyses undertaken. *(c) If detailed results are available elsewhere, state how they can be accessed.*

Discussion

Key results	18	Summarize key results with reference to study objectives.	
Limitations	19	Discuss limitations of the study, taking into account sources of potential bias or imprecision. Discuss both direction and magnitude of any potential bias.	
Interpretation	20	Give a cautious overall interpretation of results considering objectives, limitations, multiplicity of analyses, results from similar studies, and other relevant evidence.	
Generalizability	21	Discuss the generalizability (external validity) of the study results.	

Other Information

Funding	22	Give the source of funding and the role of the funders for the present study and, if applicable, for the original study on which the present article is based.	

STREGA = STrengthening the REporting of Genetic Association studies; STROBE = STrengthening the Reporting of Observational Studies in Epidemiology.
*Give information separately for cases and controls in case-control studies and, if applicable, for exposed and unexposed groups in cohort and cross-sectional studies.

CHAPTER 19

STARD (STAndards for Reporting of Diagnostic Accuracy Studies)

Patrick M.M. Bossuyt

Department of Clinical Epidemiology & Biostatistics, Academic Medical Center, University of Amsterdam, Amsterdam, the Netherlands

Timetable

Name of reporting guideline initiative	Consensus meeting date	Reporting guideline publication
STARD Standards for Reporting of Diagnostic Accuracy Studies	16–17 September 2000	January 2003

History/development

Like all other interventions in healthcare, medical tests should be carefully evaluated before they are introduced into practice and whenever doubts exist about their value. In general, the methods for evaluating tests in medicine are not as well developed as those for evaluating drugs or other forms of treatment [1, 2]. One of the crucial steps in the evaluation of a diagnostic test is an assessment of its accuracy: the test's ability to distinguish between individuals with and without disease, or more, generally, between individuals with and without the target condition [3]. For a long time, the sensitivity and specificity of a test were regarded as stable test properties. Over the years, evidence has accumulated showing that sensitivity and specificity vary across subgroups, defined by history, sex, and previous test results [4, 5]. In addition, our understanding of sources of bias in test accuracy studies has grown considerably in the past decades [6–8].

As test accuracy may vary across populations, readers of reports of diagnostic accuracy studies have to be able to identify the inclusion and exclusion criteria of the study and the process for identifying eligible patients.

Guidelines for Reporting Health Research: A User's Manual, First Edition. Edited by David Moher, Douglas G. Altman, Kenneth F. Schulz, Iveta Simera and Elizabeth Wager.
© 2014 John Wiley & Sons, Ltd. Published 2014 by John Wiley & Sons, Ltd.

Because deficiencies in study design and execution of diagnostic accuracy studies can introduce bias, readers should be well informed about the actual design of the study, and the way it was conducted.

At the 1999 Cochrane Colloquium meeting in Rome, the Diagnostic and Screening Test Methods Working Group of the Cochrane Collaboration discussed the low methodological quality and substandard reporting of accuracy studies. Inspired by the undeniably successful CONSORT initiative to improve the quality of reporting of randomized trials, the group set out to develop something similar for diagnostic accuracy studies: developing Standards for the Reporting of Diagnostic Accuracy studies (STARD).

A STARD steering committee led the initiative and started with an extensive literature search. They extracted a list of 75 potential items that could be included in the checklist. Subsequently, the STARD steering committee convened a consensus meeting in September 2000 in Amsterdam, for invited researchers, editors, methodologists, and professional organizations. During this meeting, the participants eliminated and consolidated items, to form a final 25-item checklist (see Table 19.1). In addition, the STARD group put considerable effort into the development of a flow diagram prototype for test accuracy studies (see Figure 19.1). The flow diagram provides information about the method of participant recruitment, the order of test execution, the number of participants undergoing the test under evaluation and the reference test, the number of participants with positive and negative test results and the number with indeterminate test results. Such a flow diagram has the potential to communicate vital information about the design of a study and the flow of participants in a transparent manner.

Potential users field-tested the first version of the checklist and flow diagram. The checklist was placed on the CONSORT web site with a call for comments. It was also circulated by email to various groups. The STARD steering committee then assembled the final, single page checklist which was made public in January 2003. The STARD Statement was accompanied by a separate explanatory document, explaining the meaning and rationale of each item and briefly summarizing the available evidence [9, 10].

When to use this guideline (what types of studies it covers)

The objective of the STARD initiative is to improve the accuracy and completeness of reporting of studies of diagnostic accuracy, to allow readers to assess the potential for bias in the study and to evaluate its generalizability.

The diagnostic accuracy of a test refers to its ability to distinguish between individuals with and without disease, or more generally, between individuals with and without the target condition [3]. Diagnostic accuracy

Table 19.1 STARD checklist for reporting of studies of diagnostic accuracy.

Section and Topic	Item #		On page #
TITLE/ABSTRACT/ KEYWORDS	1	Identify the article as a study of diagnostic accuracy (recommend MeSH heading 'sensitivity and specificity').	
INTRODUCTION	2	State the research questions or study aims, such as estimating diagnostic accuracy or comparing accuracy between tests or across participant groups.	
METHODS			
Participants	3	The study population: The inclusion and exclusion criteria, setting and locations where data were collected.	
	4	Participant recruitment: Was recruitment based on presenting symptoms, results from previous tests, or the fact that the participants had received the index tests or the reference standard?	
	5	Participant sampling: Was the study population a consecutive series of participants defined by the selection criteria in item 3 and 4? If not, specify how participants were further selected.	
	6	Data collection: Was data collection planned before the index test and reference standard were performed (prospective study) or after (retrospective study)?	
Test methods	7	The reference standard and its rationale.	
	8	Technical specifications of material and methods involved including how and when measurements were taken, and/or cite references for index tests and reference standard.	
	9	Definition of and rationale for the units, cut-offs and/or categories of the results of the index tests and the reference standard.	
	10	The number, training, and expertise of the persons executing and reading the index tests and the reference standard.	
	11	Whether or not the readers of the index tests and reference standard were blind (masked) to the results of the other test and describe any other clinical information available to the readers.	
Statistical methods	12	Methods for calculating or comparing measures of diagnostic accuracy, and the statistical methods used to quantify uncertainty (eg 95% confidence intervals).	
	13	Methods for calculating test reproducibility, if done.	

(*continued*)

Table 19.1 (*Continued*)

Section and Topic	Item #		On page #
RESULTS			
Participants	14	When study was performed, including beginning and end dates of recruitment.	
	15	Clinical and demographic characteristics of the study population (at least information on age, gender, spectrum of presenting symptoms).	
	16	The number of participants satisfying the criteria for inclusion who did or did not undergo the index tests and/or the reference standard; describe why participants failed to undergo either test (a flow diagram is strongly recommended).	
Test results	17	Time-interval between the index tests and the reference standard, and any treatment administered in between.	
	18	Distribution of severity of disease (define criteria) in those with the target condition; other diagnoses in participants without the target condition.	
	19	A cross tabulation of the results of the index tests (including indeterminate and missing results) by the results of the reference standard; for continuous results, the distribution of the test results by the results of the reference standard.	
	20	Any adverse events from performing the index tests or the reference standard.	
Estimates	21	Estimates of diagnostic accuracy and measures of statistical uncertainty (eg 95% confidence intervals).	
	22	How indeterminate results, missing data, and outliers of the index tests were handled.	
	23	Estimates of variability of diagnostic accuracy between subgroups of participants, readers or centers, if done.	
	24	Estimates of test reproducibility, if done.	
DISCUSSION	25	Discuss the clinical applicability of the study findings.	

is often expressed as the test's sensitivity and specificity: the proportion of the diseased correctly classified as such by the test, and the proportion of participants without the target condition correctly classified as such, respectively. Alternative expressions of accuracy exist, such as the positive and negative predictive value, likelihood ratios, the diagnostic odds ratio, or – when multiple positivity cutoffs are possible – the area under the ROC curve [3].

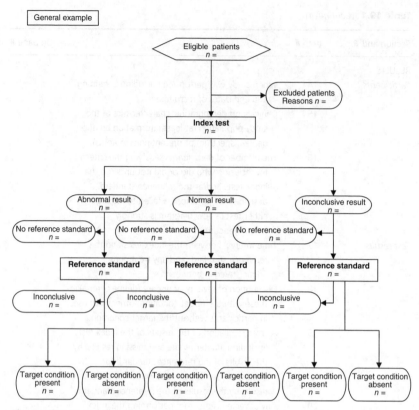

Figure 19.1 Template flow diagram for a diagnostic accuracy study.

In a typical diagnostic accuracy study, a consecutive series of participants, sampled from a well-defined study population, are subjected to the index test – the test under evaluation – and then to the clinical reference standard – the best available procedure for establishing the presence or absence of the target condition. If the clinical reference standard is error-free, it is usually referred to as the gold standard.

Current versions

The STARD Statement was published in the first issues in 2003 of seven leading general and specialty journals, including *Annals of Internal Medicine, Radiology, BMJ*, and *Clinical Chemistry* and, subsequently, in several other journals [11–24]. The documents are also available on several web sites, including that of *Clinical Chemistry*, the CONSORT web site, and on the STARD web site itself (see www.stard-statement.org).

The checklist has not required updating so far.

Previous versions

None.

Extensions be aware of

There are no extensions to the STARD checklist.

The STARD group believes that one general checklist for studies of diagnostic accuracy, rather than different checklists for each field, will be more widely disseminated and more easily accepted by authors, peer reviewers, and journal editors.

A number of publications have discussed the application of the STARD criteria to specific type of diagnostic tests, such as to history and physical examination [25].

Related activities

Medical tests and biomarkers are used for many purposes, not just for making a diagnosis. It is to be expected that more checklists will be developed, once our understanding about the sources of bias and variability for treatment selection markers, monitoring tests, screening tests, and other types of tests develops. A checklist has been developed for prognostic tumor markers [26].

How best to use the guideline

The checklist can be used by authors to evaluate the completeness and transparency of a report of a diagnostic accuracy study. The checklist can also be used by editors for the same purposes. Several journals, such as *Clinical Chemistry*, require submission of the checklist before processing of a submitted manuscript. Reviewers also use the checklist and the explanatory document to highlight incomplete or unclear sections in manuscripts, with suggestions for improving the clarity of the paper. The checklist is also being used to evaluate the completeness of grant proposals and protocols for diagnostic accuracy studies.

Evidence of effectiveness of guideline

An early evaluation of 265 diagnostic accuracy studies published in high-impact journals in 2000 (prior to the publication of STARD) and in 2004 (post-STARD) revealed that the quality of reporting in articles on diagnostic accuracy had slightly but significantly improved after the publication of the STARD statement. Papers published in 2004 reported on average 14 of the 25 essential STARD items [27].

Other evaluations of STARD have also shown that there is still room for improvement. Fontela *et al.* studied 90 diagnostic accuracy studies of commercial tests for TB, malaria, and HIV published between 2004 and 2006 [28]. They concluded that the studies were of moderate to low quality and were poorly reported. None referred to STARD. Wilczynski evaluated 240 diagnostic accuracy studies published between 2001 and 2005 using a subset of the STARD items and detected no meaningful changes over the years [29]. Coppus *et al.* examined 24 studies reporting on test accuracy in reproductive medicine in 1999 and 27 studies in 2004 [30]. Overall, less than half of the studies reported adequately on 50% or more of the STARD items.

A possible reason for the slow uptake could be the way the STARD statement is used within the editorial process. Smidt *et al.* identified the top 50 journals that frequently publish studies on diagnostic accuracy, and examined the instructions for authors on each journal's web site, extracting all text mentioning STARD or other text regarding the reporting of diagnostic accuracy studies. They found variable language in journals that had adopted the STARD statement. Most adopting journals refer to the STARD statement, without describing their expectations regarding the exact use of the STARD statement [31].

Endorsement and adherence

Publication of the STARD documents was accompanied by several editorials, with statements of endorsement from editors and their boards [32–38]. By now, more than two dozen journals have published the statement and about 120 journals have officially endorsed the STARD reporting guidelines and encourage their authors and reviewers to use these reporting guidelines. (A full list of endorsing journals is available on the STARD web site www.stard-statement.org).

Cautions and limitations (including scope)
Mistakes and/or misconceptions

The STARD statement was originally developed for diagnostic tests. Diagnosis is the most readily recognized purpose of medical testing – often referred to as simply "diagnostics" – but there are many other purposes of testing, such as the selection and monitoring of treatment. Many of the principles behind STARD, and a large part of the items in the STARD checklist, probably apply equally well to these other forms of testing, but STARD does not cover all these other purposes fully. Specific sources of bias, accompanying other types of study design, should be added for test evaluations that are targeted at other forms of testing.

Creators' preferred bits

Contrary to what is written in many textbooks, the accuracy of a medical test that is used for diagnostic purposes is not a fixed test property: it described the behavior of the test in specific circumstances. For that reason it is critically important that estimates of the sensitivity and specificity of a test, or other expressions of diagnostic accuracy, are accompanied by a clear and unambiguous description of how and where eligible participants were identified, and what prior testing they had undergone.

The most serious sources of bias in diagnostic accuracy studies have to do with the flow of study participants: Did all included participants receive the clinical reference standard? Was only a single reference standard used? It is absolutely desirable to use a flow diagram to inform readers about the flow of participants.

Estimates of test accuracy not only vary across patient groups and settings, or from risk of bias: they are also affected by chance variability. Most studies of test accuracy are small in number, and provide pairs of estimates: sensitivity and specificity, or positive and negative predictive values, or likelihood ratios. These estimates should be accompanied by expressions of the statistical uncertainty, such as confidence intervals.

Future plans

The STARD group plans the development of a richer web environment, to reflect the dissemination of ideas and notions that led to the development of the STARD statement. The web site will have short tutorials, lectures, and other teaching material that can be used to teach students and professionals in different fields about test accuracy studies.

The new web environment will also have tools for reviewers and editors, such as boilerplate text for journal instructions and templates to point study authors to incomplete reporting and to offer ways of improving the transparency and completeness of manuscripts.

References

1 Straus, S.E. (2006) Bridging the gaps in evidence based diagnosis. *BMJ*, **333** (7565), 405–406.

2 Knottnerus, J.A., van, W.C. & Muris, J.W. (2002) Evaluation of diagnostic procedures. *BMJ*, **324** (7335), 477–480.

3 Bossuyt, P.M. (2008) Interpreting diagnostic test accuracy studies. *Seminars in Hematology*, **45** (3), 189–195.

4 Moons, K.G. *et al.* (1997) Limitations of sensitivity, specificity, likelihood ratio, and Bayes' theorem in assessing diagnostic probabilities: a clinical example. *Epidemiology*, **8** (1), 12–17.

5 Hlatky, M.A. *et al.* (1984) Factors affecting sensitivity and specificity of exercise electrocardiography. Multivariable analysis. *American Journal of Medicine*, **77** (1), 64–71.

6 Whiting, P. *et al.* (2004) Sources of variation and bias in studies of diagnostic accuracy: a systematic review. *Annals of Internal Medicine*, **140** (3), 189–202.

7 Lijmer, J.G. *et al.* (1999) Empirical evidence of design-related bias in studies of diagnostic tests. *JAMA*, **282** (11), 1061–1066.

8 Rutjes, A.W., *et al.* (2006) Evidence of bias and variation in diagnostic accuracy studies. *Canadian Medical Association Journal*, **174** (**4**), 469–476.

9 Bossuyt, P.M. *et al.* (2003) The STARD statement for reporting studies of diagnostic accuracy: explanation and elaboration. *Annals of Internal Medicine*, **138** (1), W1–W12.

10 Bossuyt, P.M. *et al.* (2003) The STARD statement for reporting studies of diagnostic accuracy: explanation and elaboration. *Clinical Chemistry*, **49** (1), 7–18.

11 Bossuyt, P.M. & Reitsma, J.B. (2003) The STARD initiative. *Lancet*, **361** (9351), 71.

12 Bossuyt, P.M. *et al.* (2003) Towards complete and accurate reporting of studies of diagnostic accuracy: the STARD initiative. The Standards for Reporting of Diagnostic Accuracy Group. *Croatian Medical Journal*, **44** (5), 635–638.

13 Bossuyt, P.M. *et al.* (2003) Towards complete and accurate reporting of studies of diagnostic accuracy: the STARD initiative. *Clinical Radiology*, **58** (8), 575–580.

14 Bossuyt, P.M. *et al.* (2003) Towards complete and accurate reporting of studies of diagnostic accuracy: the STARD initiative. *Annals of Clinical Biochemistry*, **40** (Pt 4), 357–363.

15 Bossuyt, P.M. *et al.* (2003) Towards complete and accurate reporting of studies of diagnostic accuracy: the STARD initiative. *American Journal of Roentgenology*, **181** (1), 51–55.

16 Bossuyt, P.M. *et al.* (2003) Toward complete and accurate reporting of studies of diagnostic accuracy: the STARD initiative. *Academic Radiology*, **10** (6), 664–669.

17 Bossuyt, P.M. *et al.* (2003) Reporting studies of diagnostic accuracy according to a standard method; the Standards for Reporting of Diagnostic Accuracy (STARD). *Nederlands tijdschrift voor geneeskunde*, **147** (8), 336–340.

18 Bossuyt, P.M. *et al.* (2003) Towards complete and accurate reporting of studies of diagnostic accuracy: the STARD initiative. *Clinical Chemistry and Laboratory Medicine*, **41** (1), 68–73.

19 Bossuyt, P.M. *et al.* (2003) Towards complete and accurate reporting of studies of diagnostic accuracy: the STARD initiative. *Clinical Biochemistry*, **36** (1), 2–7.

20 Bossuyt, P.M. *et al.* (2003) Toward complete and accurate reporting of studies of diagnostic accuracy. The STARD initiative. *American Journal of Clinical Pathology*, **119** (1), 18–22.

21 Bossuyt, P.M. *et al.* (2003) Towards complete and accurate reporting of studies of diagnostic accuracy: the STARD Initiative. *Annals of Internal Medicine*, **138** (1), 40–44.

22 Bossuyt, P.M. *et al.* (2003) Towards complete and accurate reporting of studies of diagnostic accuracy: the STARD Initiative. *Radiology*, **226** (1), 24–28.

23 Bossuyt, P.M. *et al.* (2003) Towards complete and accurate reporting of studies of diagnostic accuracy: the STARD initiative. *BMJ*, **326** (7379), 41–44.

24 Bossuyt, P.M. *et al.* (2003) Towards complete and accurate reporting of studies of diagnostic accuracy: the STARD initiative. Standards for Reporting of Diagnostic Accuracy. *Clinical Chemistry*, **49** (1), 1–6.

25 Simel, D.L., Rennie, D. & Bossuyt, P.M. (2008) The STARD statement for reporting diagnostic accuracy studies: application to the history and physical examination. *Journal of General Internal Medicine*, **23** (6), 768–774.

26 McShane, L.M. *et al.* (2005) Reporting recommendations for tumor marker prognostic studies (REMARK). *Journal of the National Cancer Institute*, **97** (16), 1180–1184.

27 Smidt, N. *et al.* (2006) The quality of diagnostic accuracy studies since the STARD statement: has it improved? *Neurology*, **67** (5), 792–797.

28 Fontela, P.S. *et al.* (2009) Quality and reporting of diagnostic accuracy studies in TB, HIV and malaria: evaluation using QUADAS and STARD standards. *PLoS ONE*, **4** (11), e7753.

29 Wilczynski, N.L. (2008) Quality of reporting of diagnostic accuracy studies: no change since STARD statement publication – before-and-after study. *Radiology*, **248** (3), 817–823.

30 Coppus, S.F. *et al.* (2006) Quality of reporting of test accuracy studies in reproductive medicine: impact of the Standards for Reporting of Diagnostic Accuracy (STARD) initiative. *Fertility and Sterility*, **86** (5), 1321–1329.

31 Smidt, N. *et al.* (2007) Endorsement of the STARD Statement by biomedical journals: survey of instructions for authors. *Clinical Chemistry*, **53** (11), 1983–1985.

32 Gatsonis, C. (2003) Do we need a checklist for reporting the results of diagnostic test evaluations? The STARD proposal. *Academic Radiology*, **10** (6), 599–600.

33 Hansell, D.M. & Wells, A.U. (2003) Towards complete and accurate reporting of studies of diagnostic accuracy: the STARD initiative. *Clinical Radiology*, **58** (8), 573–574.

34 McQueen, M. (2003) Evidence-based laboratory medicine: addressing bias, generalisability and applicability in studies on diagnostic accuracy. The STARD initiative. *Clinical Chemistry and Laboratory Medicine*, **41** (1), 1.

35 McQueen, M.J. (2003) The STARD initiative: a possible link to diagnostic accuracy and reduction in medical error. *Annals of Clinical Biochemistry*, **40** (Pt 4), 307–308.

36 Meyer, G.J. (2003) Guidelines for reporting information in studies of diagnostic test accuracy: the STARD initiative. *Journal of Personality Assessment*, **81** (3), 191–193.

37 Price, C.P. (2003) Improving the quality of peer reviewed literature on diagnostic tests: the STARD initiative. *Clinica Chimica Acta*, **334** (1–2), 1–3.

38 Rennie, D. (2003) Improving reports of studies of diagnostic tests: the STARD initiative. *JAMA*, **289** (1), 89–90.

CHAPTER 20

SURGE (The SUrvey Reporting GuidelinE)

Jeremy Grimshaw
Ottawa Hospital Research Institute and University of Ottawa, Ottawa, ON, Canada

Timetable

Name of reporting guideline initiative	Notes	Consensus meeting date	Reporting guideline publication
SURGE	Under development	Pending	Background development paper published [22]

Name of proposed guideline

The SUrvey Reporting GuidelinE (SURGE) is primarily intended to provide guidance to authors reporting information that has been collected via self-administered, postal surveys.

History/overview

Surveys are often used in health and health services research to gather quantitative and qualitative information from a target group. A substantial body of literature exists to show that the methods used in conducting survey research can significantly affect the validity, reliability, and generalizability of the findings [1, 2].

Although standards exist for the development and administration of surveys used in research (Dillman's Tailored Design Method being among the best known) [3], validated standards for the reporting of survey research have not been identified to date [4, 5]. Without consistency in how and/or what is reported, it may be difficult or impossible to distinguish between high-quality and low-quality surveys.

Guidelines for Reporting Health Research: A User's Manual, First Edition. Edited by David Moher, Douglas G. Altman, Kenneth F. Schulz, Iveta Simera and Elizabeth Wager.
© 2014 John Wiley & Sons, Ltd. Published 2014 by John Wiley & Sons, Ltd.

With this in mind, we conducted the foundational work necessary to develop a reporting guideline for survey research; here we describe the three phases of this work. First, we conducted a systematic review of the literature designed to identify any existing guidelines or quality criteria relevant to the reporting of survey research, and any research evaluating the quality of reporting for survey research; results from this phase indicated that while some criteria have been identified to inform the reporting of survey research, no validated reporting guidelines exist. Second, results from this review informed the development and pilot-testing of a 33-item assessment tool designed to identify the most important criteria to be reported. Third, we applied this tool to a representative sample of published papers reporting the results of surveys from the health and health services literature.

When to use this guideline (what types of studies it will cover)

The planned SURGE document is intended for use when reporting the results of survey research for health and health services. SURGE may be useful to a variety of groups, such as authors, peer reviewers, and editors, reviewing submissions involving survey research and readers assessing the validity of the findings in survey reports. By extension, the guideline may also be suitable for informing reports of survey research in other areas where surveys are commonly used, such as psychology and sociology.

Development process

The proposal for developing SURGE was conceived by researchers at the Ottawa Hospital Research Institute. The executive SURGE research group was assembled and a series of planning meetings were followed.

Existing guidance for developing reporting guidelines suggests carrying out a series of preparatory activities, which include identification of participants for the development group, identification of any existing guidelines, a comprehensive literature review for relevant evidence on the quality of reporting in the area of interest, and generation of a list of items for consideration [6]. In accordance with these recommendations, we settled on a three-phase approach:

1 searching the literature on existing guidelines, criteria and/or empirical research examining survey reporting are as follows:
  (a) a systematic search of the published, peer-reviewed literature,
  (b) a search of journals' instructions to authors,

2 developing and piloting a set of quality assessment criteria for survey research reports, and
3 applying the quality assessment criteria to a representative sample of survey research papers.

We limited our work to self-administered postal surveys in the health sciences literature and defined survey as a research method where information is gathered by asking people questions on a specific topic, and where the data collection procedure is standardized and well defined; the information is gathered from a subset of the population of interest with the intent of generating summary statistics that are generalizable to the larger population [7, 8]. Although we recognize that this approach excludes in-person, telephone, web-based, and other survey methods, we hope the resulting guideline will form the basis for developing guidelines for other types of survey research.

1a. Systematic review of available guidelines for reporting surveys and empirical research on the quality of reporting surveys

We conducted a systematic review to identify: (i) existing validated guidelines and/or any items deemed critical to reporting survey research, (ii) empirical research that had already evaluated the quality of reporting of survey research.

Table 20.1 describes the results of the first search that yielded four independent but unvalidated checklists [9–12], which included 38 distinct reporting items. We categorized these items into eight broad themes: background, methods, sample selection, research tool, results, response rates, interpretation and discussion, and ethics and disclosure.

We identified eight relevant empirical studies evaluating the quality of reporting for survey research. Five of these [13–17] examined the reporting of response rates; three [14–18] evaluated the reporting of nonresponse analyses in survey research; and two [19, 20] assessed the degree to which authors make their survey instrument available to readers. Overall, all eight papers indicated that there was suboptimal reporting of these domains.

1b. Search of journals' instructions to authors

We examined the websites of medical journals of high-impact factor to determine whether any provided guidance for authors of survey research. Our sampling strategy was adapted from Altman [21] and identified the top five journals from 33 medical specialties and the top 15 journals from general and internal medicine producing a total of 165 titles. We found most journals (90%) contained no mention of, or guidance for, reporting of survey research. (This proportion was essentially unchanged (88%) when we focused on the 137 journals that had actually published survey research articles.)

Table 20.1 Items present in four checklists providing guidance for reporting of survey research.

Reporting item	Number of checklists including the item
Background	
Justification of research method	3
Background literature review	2
Explicit research question	3
Clear study objectives	3
Methods	
Description of methods used for data analysis	3
Method of questionnaire administration	3
Location of data collection	3
Dates of data collection	1
Number and types of contact	3
Methods sufficiently described for replication	2
Evidence of reliability	1
Evidence of validity	1
Methods for verifying data entry	1
Use of a codebook	2
Sample selection	
Sample size calculation	3
Representativeness	4
Method of sample selection	3
Description of population and sample frame	1
Research tool	
Description of the research tool	4
Description of the development of the research tool	2
Instrument pretesting	2
Instrument reliability and validity	3
Scoring methods	2
Results	
Results of research presented	2
Results address objectives	2
Clear description of which results based on part of the sample	2
Generalizability	2
Response rates	
Response rate stated	4
How response rate was calculated	2
Discussion of nonresponse bias	1
All respondents accounted for	2
Interpretation and discussion	
Interpret and discuss findings	3
Conclusions and recommendations	2
Limitations	2
Ethics and disclosure	
Consent	2
Sponsorship	2
Research ethics approval	1
Evidence of ethical treatment of human subjects	1

Only 17/165 journals (10%) included one or more of the terms: "survey," "questionnaire," "response rate," or "nonresponder." Of these, six included the word "survey" in their instructions, but provided no guidance for reporting survey research (i.e., the term was used to state whether surveys were an acceptable study design for submission to the journal or not). Eight provided only one brief phrase or statement addressing survey research: that is, they stated that survey papers should report response rates ($n = 6$), provided references that address methodological issues around the conduct of survey research ($n = 1$) or included a statement that authors should "consider" response rates and nonresponder bias ($n = 1$). The remaining three instructions provided more than one directive or statement (two of which contained precisely the same text). However, both of these contained limited guidance (comprising only 110 or 133 words) with no additional or novel items that were not already represented in the 38 items produced by our literature search (Table 20.1).

2. Developing and piloting a set of quality assessment criteria for survey research reports

Having failed to locate any existing validated guidelines for survey research, we proceeded to develop a set of quality criteria for reporting survey research and apply it to a representative sample of survey research reports.

Using the 38 items identified in the first step of our process (Table 20.1), 32 items were selected as most critical to the reporting of survey research because of the frequency with which they appeared in the literature and the consensus of the executive group. These 32 items were compiled and categorized into a draft evaluation tool that was reviewed and revised iteratively by the executive group. The resulting draft instrument was piloted by two researchers on a convenience sample of survey research articles identified by the authors. Items were added, edited, and removed following group discussion and consensus. The revised final draft was approved by the executive group and comprised 33 items (Table 20.2).

3. Applying the quality assessment criteria to a representative sample of survey research papers

We aimed to identify a minimum of 100 survey reports by searching the top 15 journals (by impact factor) from four broad areas of health research (health science, public health, general/internal medicine, and medical informatics) chosen primarily for their propensity to publish survey research in the period January 2008–February 2009.

We identified 117 papers eligible for inclusion and found considerable variation in the degree to which the items were reported. Most notably, a significant proportion of the studies (34%) lacked any description of the

Table 20.2 Data abstraction quality criteria

Category	Item
Title and abstract	Is the design of the study stated in the title and/or abstract?
Introduction	Is there an explanation of why the research is necessary, placing the study in context of previous work in relevant fields?
	Is the purpose or aim of the paper explained?
Methods	
Research tool	Is the questionnaire described?
	If an existing tool was used, are its psychometric properties presented?
	If an existing tool was used, are references to the original work provided?
	If a new tool was used, are the procedures used to develop and pre-test provided?
	If a new tool was used, have its reliability and validity been reported?
	Is a description of the scoring procedures provided?
Sample selection	Is there a description of the survey population and the sample frame used to identify this population?
	Do the authors provide a description of how representative the sample is of the underlying population?
	Is a sample size calculation or rationale/justification for the sample size presented?
Survey administration	Mode of administration?
	Do the authors provide information on the type of contact and how many attempts were made to contact subjects (i.e., prenotification by letter or telephone, reminder postcard, duplicate questionnaire with reminder)?
	Do the authors report whether incentives were provided (financial or other)?
	Is there a description of who approached potential participants (e.g., identification of who signed the covering letter)?
Analysis	Is the method of data analysis described?
	Do the authors provide methods for analysis of nonresponse error?
	Is the method for calculating response rate provided?
	Are definitions provided for complete versus partial completions?
	Are the methods for handling item missing data provided?
Results	Is the response rate reported?
	Are all respondents accounted for?
	Is information given on how nonrespondents differ from respondents?
	Are the results clearly presented?
	Do the results address the objective(s)?
Discussion	Are the results summarized with reference to the study objectives?
	Are the strengths of the study stated?
	Are the limitations of the study (taking into account potential sources of bias or imprecision) stated?
	Is there explicit discussion of the generalizability (external validity) of the results?
Ethical quality indicators	Study funding reported?
	Research Ethics Board (REB) review reported?
	Reporting of subject consent procedures?

survey instrument, 75% did not provide the survey questions in the article or an accessible document, 75% did not report validity or reliability of the survey instrument, and 54% failed to describe scoring procedures for the survey instrument used in the study. Most (89%) did not provide a description of how representative the sample was of the underlying population. Several studies (35%) did not provide information on the type of contact nor the number of contact attempts made; and a number of studies (20%) did not explicitly state the mode of survey administration (which was determined from descriptions of other methods in the paper). Methods for handling missing data were rarely (11%) reported, and response rates were infrequently defined (25%).

Future plans/next steps

We have determined that no validated guideline for reporting survey research exists, and that the quality of reporting of published, self-administered postal surveys is suboptimal. Critical methodological details often go unreported in survey research papers or are not reported in sufficient detail. A reporting guideline specific to survey research may aid in improving the quality of reporting in this important area of health and health services research.

We therefore plan to move forward with the development of SURGE based on our findings. We plan to hold a consensus meeting, including a broad group of stakeholders, and to follow this by iterative development, validation, publication, and evaluation of the guideline and its impact.

Evidence of effectiveness of guideline

In the long term, we plan to determine whether the use of SURGE is associated with an improved quality of reporting of survey research.

References

1 McColl, E., Jacoby, A., Thomas, L. *et al.* (2001) Design and use of questionnaires: a review of best practice applicable to surveys of health service staff and patients. *Health Technology Assessment (Winchester, England)*, **5**, 1–256.

2 Edwards, P. (2010) Questionnaires in clinical trials: guidelines for optimal design and administration. *Trials*, **11**, 2.

3 Dillman, D.A. (2007) *Mail and Internet Surveys: The Tailored Design Method*. John Wiley & Sons, Inc., Hoboken.

4 EQUATOR Network Website. http://www.equator-network.org [accessed on October 2009].

5 Bennett, C., Khangura, S., Brehaut, J. *et al*. Reporting Guidelines for Surveys: Limited Guidance and Little Adherence. Sixth International Congress on Peer Review and Biomedical Publication 2009.

6 Moher, D., Schulz, K., Simera, I., Altman, D. (2010) Guidance for Developers of Health Research Reporting Guidelines. *PLos Medicine*, **7** (2), e10000217. doi:10.1371/journal.pmed.10000217.

7 Groves, R.M., Fowler, F.J., Couper, M.P. *et al*. (2004) *An Introduction to Survey Methodology*. John Wiley & Sons, Inc., Hoboken.

8 Aday, L.A. & Cornelius, L.J. (2006) *Designing and Conducting Health Surveys: A Comprehensive Guide*. Jossey-Bass, San Francisco.

9 Kelley, K., Clark, B., Brown, V. & Sitzia, J. (2003) Good practice in the conduct and reporting of survey research. *International Journal for Quality in Health Care*, **15**, 261–266.

10 Draugalis, J.R., Coons, S.J. & Plaza, C.M. (2008) Best Practices for survey research reports: a synopsis for authors and reviewers. *American Journal of Pharmaceutical Education*, **72**, 11.

11 Huston, P. (1996) Reporting on surveys: information for authors and peer reviewers. *Canadian Medical Association Journal*, **154**, 1695–1704.

12 AAPOR. American Association of Public Opinion Research (AAPOR). Available from www.aapor.org.

13 Badger, F. & Werrett, J. (2005) Room for improvement? Reporting response rates and recruitment in nursing research in the past decade. *Journal of Advanced Nursing*, **51**, 502–510.

14 Asch, D.A., Jedrziewski, M.K. & Christakis, N.A. (1997) Response rates to mail surveys published in medical journals. *Journal of Clinical Epidemiology*, **50**, 1129–1136.

15 Cummings, S.M., Savitz, L.A. & Konrad, T.R. (2001) Reported response rates to mailed physician questionnaires. *Health Services Research*, **35**, 1347–1355.

16 Johnson, T. & Owens, L. (2003) Survey Response Rate Reporting in the Professional Literature. American Association for Public Opinion Research – Section on Survey Research Methods.

17 Smith, T.W. (2002) Reporting survey nonresponse in academic journals. *International Journal of Public Opinion Research*, **14**, 469–474.

18 Werner, S., Praxedes, M. & Kim, H. (2007) The reporting of nonresponse analyses in survey research. *Organizational Research Methods*, **10**, 287–295.

19 Schilling, L.M., Kozak, K., Lundahl, K. & Dellavalle, R.P. (2006) Inaccessible novel questionnaires in published medical research: hidden methods, hidden costs. *American Journal of Epidemiology*, **164**, 1141–1144.

20 Rosen, T. & Olsen, J. (2006) Invited commentary: the art of making questionnaires better. *American Journal of Epidemiology*, **164**, 1145–1149.

21 Altman, D.G. (2005) Endorsement of the CONSORT statement by high impact medical journals: survey of instructions for authors. *BMJ*, **330**, 1056–1057.

22 Bennett, C., Khangura, S., Brehaut, J.C. *et al*. (2011) Reporting guidelines for survey research: an analysis of published guidance and reporting practices. *PLoS Med* 8:e1001069.

CHAPTER 21

COREQ (Consolidated Criteria for Reporting Qualitative Studies)

Andrew Booth[1], Karin Hannes[1], Angela Harden[1], Jane Noyes[2], Janet Harris[1] and Allison Tong[3]

[1] *Cochrane Collaboration Qualitative Research Methods Group*
[2] *Centre for Health-Related Research, School for Healthcare Sciences, College of Health & Behavioural Sciences, Bangor University, Bangor, UK*
[3] *Sydney School of Public Health, University of Sydney, Sydney, Australia*

Timetable

Name of reporting guideline initiative	Notes	Consensus meeting date	Reporting guideline publication
COREQ	–	NA	2007

Name of guideline

The Consolidated Criteria for Reporting Qualitative Studies (COREQ) covers the reporting of studies using interviews and focus groups [1]. It is the only reporting guidance for qualitative research to have received other than isolated endorsement although it applies to only a few of the many qualitative methods in use. It comprises a 32-item checklist that was developed by reviewing and identifying items from other tools and checklists for qualitative studies. Despite its narrow focus, COREQ can be used by peer reviewers and editors reviewing many qualitative research submissions. COREQ can also be used by readers wishing to gauge the validity of the results of a published report of qualitative research and by researchers preparing systematic reviews of qualitative research.

Guidelines for Reporting Health Research: A User's Manual, First Edition. Edited by David Moher, Douglas G. Altman, Kenneth F. Schulz, Iveta Simera and Elizabeth Wager.
© 2014 John Wiley & Sons, Ltd. Published 2014 by John Wiley & Sons, Ltd.

History/development

The qualitative research community has been slow in developing and adopting reporting standards for both ideological and practical reasons. First, the plethora of research methodologies, each with considerable variation in data collection methods, makes development of a single reporting standard problematic. Second, researchers may perceive a prescriptive, overarching framework as limiting their ability to capture rich and important contextual data [2]. Third, descriptions of methods and presentation of narrative and graphical data (which may include field notes, documents, transcriptions of interviews and interactions, and artifacts) vary considerably between articles with different underlying purposes.

Recent years have, however, seen wider recognition that the systematic and careful documentation of all procedures – an "account of practice" – is located securely within the tradition of qualitative inquiry [4]. Description and the corresponding documentation of the procedure are acknowledged as critical in driving forward methodological innovation and in advocating the value of a published research study.

When to use this guideline (what types of studies it covers)

The COREQ checklist was developed to promote explicit and comprehensive reporting of interviews and focus groups [2]. These two methods are widely used for eliciting patient and consumer opinions, priorities, barriers, expectations, and needs to improve the quality of health care [6]. In-depth interviews are often used to study the experiences and meanings of disease and to explore personal and sensitive themes. Focus groups employ semistructured discussions between groups of 4–12 participants to explore a specific set of issues [7].

At the time of its publication, the developers of COREQ reported that only the *BMJ* of the mainstream biomedical journals had criteria for reviewing qualitative research [2]. However, this checklist was not used as the basis for COREQ as the developers concluded that the *BMJ* checklist was not comprehensive and did not provide specific guidance for the key aspects of study reporting. The *Journal of Advanced Nursing* has both a reporting framework to structure a paper and a supplementary guidance on appropriate use of methods.

Current version

The COREQ checklist consists of 32 criteria, with a descriptor to supplement each item. It is organized into three domains (Table 21.1).

Table 21.1 Domains and items covered by the COREQ checklist.

Domain	Total number of items	Details of items
Domain 1: research team and reflexivity	8 items	Personal characteristics [5 items] • Interviewer; credentials; occupation; gender; experience; and training Relationship with participants [3 items] • Prior relationship; participant knowledge of interviewer; interviewer characteristics
Domain 2: study design	15 items	Theoretical framework [1 item] Participant selection [4 items] Sampling; method of approach; sample size; and non-participation Setting [3 items] Setting of data collection; presence of nonparticipants; description of sample Data collection [7 items] Interview guide; repeat interviews; audio/visual recording; field notes; duration; data saturation; transcripts returned
Domain 3: analysis and findings	9 items	Data analysis [5 items] Number of data coders; description of coding tree; derivation of themes; software; participant checking Reporting [4 items] Quotations presented; data and findings consistent; clarity of major themes; clarity of minor themes

The COREQ statement with full explanation and supporting detail is only published in full in one journal article [2]. Several editorials have reproduced abbreviated variants such as the COREQ checklist [11].

Extensions and/or implementations

No extensions or implementations of COREQ have been published to date. One potential reason is a lack of international consensus on reporting criteria for qualitative research. The COREQ statement differs from such statements as CONSORT and STROBE (see Chapters 8 and 18) as it does not result from extensive exploration or sharing of opinions from experts in the field. It is primarily the result of individual academic effort with supporting literature searches. Delphi studies or consensus meetings might optimize the COREQ statement increasing uptake among key stakeholders.

Related activities

The Robert Wood Johnson Foundation has sponsored the Qualitative Research Guidelines Project to develop a website for people developing, evaluating, and engaging in qualitative research projects in healthcare settings (http://www.qualres.org/index.html). Entitled *Using Qualitative Methods in Healthcare Research*: *A Comprehensive Guide for Designing, Writing, Reviewing and Reporting Qualitative Research*, the project has identified two sets of guidelines for publishing qualitative research, those by Malterud [17] and those created by Miller & Crabtree [18] for the *Journal of Family Practice*.

In addition to the COREQ statement and the publication by Malterud [17], the EQUATOR Network documents three further sources of guidance for reporting qualitative research. Those by Blignault & Ritchie [19] and Clark [20] are generic, the latter known as "the RATS guidelines" are specifically intended for the purpose of peer review. Earlier guidelines by Elliott [21] are specific to qualitative research studies in psychology and its related fields.

How best to use the guideline

Authors
Authors should follow the COREQ checklist if they are reporting findings from interviews or focus groups. However, the checklist may need to be supplemented with reference to critical features of the methodology used (e.g., ethnography, grounded theory) and by looking at a good published example of that methodology, preferably from the target journal. The checklist can be adapted if authors use methods other than interviews and focus groups.

Peer reviewers
Peer reviewers will likely find the COREQ checklist helpful as a series of general prompts rather than a prescriptive structure. Journal editors could encourage reviewers to use the checklist to encourage completeness of reporting within the overall framework required by each journal's Instructions to Authors.

Editors
Editors can encourage authors to complete the checklist before submission. If the completed checklist is included with the submitted manuscript, it can

function as an additional quality assurance mechanism before peer review. Alternatively editors can draw the contents of the checklist to the attention of peer reviewers while emphasizing that the guideline is designed to ensure completeness of reporting rather than standardization of the format. In this way, the COREQ checklist will contribute to the clarity, accuracy, and transparency of reporting without any loss of the richness of content and context that occur with standardized formats.

Development process

Search strategy. The developers of COREQ performed a comprehensive search for published checklists used to assess or review qualitative studies, and guidelines for reporting qualitative studies. Sources included Medline and CINAHL from the respective start dates of each database (1966 and 1982) to April 2006, Cochrane and Campbell protocols, systematic reviews of qualitative studies, author or reviewer guidelines of major medical journals, and reference lists of relevant publications [2]. They used citation pearl growing (i.e., index terms from relevant articles were used to conduct a broad search). The electronic databases were searched using terms and text words for research (standards), health services research (standards), and qualitative studies (evaluation). Duplicate checklists and instructions focusing on the conduct and analysis of qualitative research, rather than the reporting, of qualitative studies were excluded.

  Data extraction. From each included publication, the COREQ developers extracted all criteria for assessing or reporting qualitative studies. They compiled 76 items from 22 checklists into a comprehensive list [2]. They recorded the frequency of each item across all the publications. Items most frequently included in the checklists related to sampling method, setting for data collection, method of data collection, respondent validation of findings, method of recording data, description of the derivation of themes, and inclusion of supporting quotations. They grouped all items into three domains: (i) research team and reflexivity, (ii) study design, and (iii) data analysis and reporting.

  Duplicate items and those that were ambiguous, too broadly defined, not specific to qualitative research, or impractical to assess were removed. Where necessary, the remaining items were rephrased for clarity. Based on consensus among the authors, two new items that were considered relevant for reporting qualitative research using interviews or focus groups were added. The two new items were as follows:

1 identifying those who conducted the interview or focus group, and
2 reporting the presence of nonparticipants during the interview or focus group.

Evidence of the effectiveness of guideline

In introducing COREQ, its developers acknowledged that "there is no empiric basis that shows that the introduction of COREQ will improve the quality of reporting of qualitative research" [2].

Endorsement and adherence

Thus far, COREQ is endorsed by the *Croatian Medical Journal; Headache; International Journal of Nursing Studies; Journal of Pediatric Psychiatry; Journal of Sexual Medicine; Palliative Care; Physiotherapy; Radiographer; Scandinavian Journal of Work, Environment & Health.*

Cautions and limitations (including scope)

The COREQ checklist tool is appropriate for studies that use focus groups and interviews. Its value is more limited when applied to studies that use different data collection methods, and it may be more or less appropriate for different qualitative methodologies. Additional considerations may also apply when researching particular populations such as children or those in other vulnerable groups.

In this context, debates regarding reporting standards mirror issues related to the use of checklists for assessment of qualitative research. Some researchers prefer to use quality criteria as prompts rather than prescriptive guidelines [23, 24]. Quality in qualitative research may be viewed as holistic in nature and not constructed over a scaffold of individual criteria. Unlike a randomized controlled trial where problems with internal validity can completely compromise the results, a limited qualitative study can still yield useful insights [23]. However, none of the above is an argument for poor reporting of the research.

Key features

Appropriateness of sample

The appropriateness of the sample is critical when appraising qualitative research, and therefore researchers should report sufficient detail on the sampling methods and approach to allow reviewers to assess the sample.

The *sample size* of a qualitative study is not judged in strictly quantitative terms but readers should be able to assess the diversity of included perspectives. Details of how participants were approached to take part, any reasons for refusal to participate or for dropping out, and characteristics of the included sample are also helpful in this respect.

Clarity of data collection

One way in which readers can understand the focus of the research and judge the adequacy of data collection methods is to ensure that a report provides sufficient details of questions and prompts, or in the case of children and young people description of any age-appropriate methods and activities used to develop engagement. This enables readers to assess whether participants were encouraged to openly convey their viewpoints, or in the case of children and young people that individual communication and developmental needs were taken into consideration. With the relationship between researcher and participants being central (requiring reflexivity, i.e., consideration of its likely effect on collection, analysis, and interpretation) [28], the reader needs to know whether repeat interviews were conducted, possibly influencing rapport and affecting the richness of data obtained. This is also true of recording the participants' words, as audio recording and transcription more accurately capture the participants' views than contemporaneous researcher notes. A further provision may be for participants to check their own transcript for accuracy (respondent validation), although the value of this is not universally agreed and the approach may not be useful or practical with some populations such as children [28]. Participants are typically able to validate their own perceptions, not the researcher's interpretations of them. If audio recording was not provided, reasons should be given. Field notes can be used to record contextual details and nonverbal expressions for data analysis and interpretation [29]. With children and young people, interviews and focus groups may involve production of drawings, use of stickers and symbols to attribute opinions, and smaller staged activities within an overall framework. Collection of data may involve filming; collection of material produced; photographing; or keeping drawings, models, flipcharts, and so on. Duration of the interview or focus group may affect the amount of data obtained. A specific consideration is whether participants were recruited until no new relevant knowledge was obtained from new participants (known as data saturation) [30].

Clarity of data analysis and findings

It is important that researchers provide sufficient detail on their methods of data analysis and the relationship between the analysis and the findings in the research report so that reviewers can assess the rigor of the analysis and the credibility of the findings. Strategies for increasing rigor in data analysis may include use of multiple coders or methods of researcher triangulation and searching for negative cases that contradict initial researcher analysis and interpretations of the data [28]. The credibility of the findings can be assessed from whether the process of coding (selecting significant sections from participant statements) and how themes are derived and identified is made explicit. Systematic use of coding and memoing increases confidence in how the researchers developed their understanding of the data and hence the credibility of the findings [29]. If children or young people are involved, then a range of data types may be collected, depending on the age and communication abilities of the participants. Reporting should describe how various types of data were organized, synthesized, and analyzed in age-appropriate ways. Obtaining feedback from participants on the research findings, if consistent with the research approach, may help to ensure that the participants' own meanings and perspectives have been faithfully interpreted and not distorted by the researchers' own beliefs, assumptions, prior agenda, or knowledge [28].

Other considerations related to reporting include whether researchers have included quotations from different participants so that reviewers can assess the extent to which all participants' data have contributed to the analysis and the diversity of perspectives represented [31]. In the case of children and young people, it may be important to report findings by age and context and consider other variables such as gender, family structure, and socioeconomic circumstances.

Thickness of detail

Although not explicitly covered in the COREQ guidelines, the concept of "thickness" relates to both the details of the methods and details of the findings [30]. The context in which data were collected, for example, in the participants' homes, will illuminate why they responded in a particular way. If nonparticipants, for example, parents or formal or informal caregivers, were present during either interviews or focus groups, this can affect the freeness of expression for participants. In common with quantitative studies, participant characteristics, including demographic data, should be reported so that readers can consider the relevance of interpretations to their own situation. Readers should be able to assess whether perspectives from different affected parties have been explored, such as patients and healthcare providers (fair dealing) [28].

Future plans

The developers of the COREQ checklist acknowledge that their initiative is a first step and they invite readers to comment to improve the checklist. This is particularly important given the intended limited scope of the checklist and its immaturity compared with other more established checklists. The Centre for Methodology of Educational Research from

Katholieke Universiteit Leuven, Belgium, is currently considering a further investigation of the COREQ checklist's wider applicability. The Cochrane Collaboration's Qualitative Research Methods Group is keen that momentum from steps taken to improve the quality of primary research material will further extend to producing Standards for Reporting Qualitative Evidence Syntheses.

It remains to be seen whether COREQ sees increased uptake, expansion to other types of qualitative research, or is superseded by a more generic statement. Engagement with experts in the field in evaluating and improving the COREQ statement could be an important step to increase its use.

References

1 Tong, A., Sainsbury, P. & Craig, J. (2007) Consolidated criteria for reporting qualitative research (COREQ): a 32-item checklist for interviews and focus groups. *International Journal for Quality in Health Care*, **19** (6), 349–357.

2 Barbour, R. (2001) Checklists for improving rigour in qualitative research: a case of the tail wagging the dog? *BMJ*, **322**, 1115–1117.

3 Freeman, M., deMarrais, K.D., Preissle, J. *et al.* (2007) Standards of evidence in qualitative research: an incitement to discourse. *Educational Researcher*, **36** (1), 25–32.

4 Atkins, S., Lewin, S., Smith, H. *et al.* (2008) Conducting a meta-ethnography of qualitative literature: lessons learnt. *BMC Medical Research Methodology*, **8**, 21.

5 Sofaer, S. (2002) Qualitative research methods. *International Journal for Quality in Health Care*, **14**, 329–336.

6 Kitzinger, J. (2006) Focus groups. In: Pope, C. & Mays, N. (eds), *Qualitative Research in Health Care*, 3rd edn. Blackwell Publishing, Oxford.

7 Mills, E., Jadad, A.R., Ross, C. & Wilson, K. (2005) Systematic review of qualitative studies exploring parental beliefs and attitudes toward childhood vaccination identified common barriers to vaccination. *Journal of Clinical Epidemiology*, **58**, 1081–1088.

8 Sandelowski, M. & Barroso, J. (2003) Classifying the findings in qualitative studies. *Qualitative Health Research*, **13** (7), 905–923.

9 Sandelowski, M. (1998) Writing a good read: strategies for re-presenting qualitative data. *Research in Nursing & Health*, **21**, 375–382.

10 Agustin, C. (2009) How can reporting guidelines help you write your research findings? *The Radiographer*, **56** (1), 5–9.

11 Dixon-Woods, M., Booth, A. & Sutton, A.J. (2007) Synthesising qualitative research: a review of published reports. *Qualitative Research*, **7**, 375–422.

12 Hannes, K. & Macaitis, K. (2010). A move to more systematic and transparent approaches in qualitative evidence synthesis: update on a review of published papers. *Qualitative Research*, **12**, 402–442.

13 Booth, A. (2006) "Brimful of STARLITE": toward standards for reporting literature searches. *Journal of the Medical Library Association*, **94** (4), 421–429.

14 Des Jarlais, D.C., Lyles, C. & Crepaz, N. (2004) Improving the reporting quality of nonrandomized evaluations of behavioral and public health interventions: the TREND Statement. *American Journal of Public Health*, **94** (3), 361–366.

15 Gilpatrick, E. (1999) *Quality Improvement Projects in Health Care*. Sage Publications, London.

16 Robson, C. (2002) *Real World Research*. Blackwell Publishing, Oxford.

17 Malterud, K. (2001) Qualitative research: standards, challenges, guidelines. *Lancet*, **358**, 483–488.

18 Frankel, R.M. (1999) Standards of Qualitative Research. In: Crabtree, B.F. & Miller, W.L. (eds), *Doing Qualitative Research*, 2nd edn., pp. 341, Sage Publications, Thousand Oaks.

19 Blignault, I. & Ritchie, J. (2009) Revealing the wood and the trees: reporting qualitative research. *Health Promotion Journal of Australia*, **20** (2), 140–145.

20 Clark, J.P. (2003) How to peer review a qualitative manuscript. In: Godlee, F. & Jefferson, T. (eds), *Peer Review in Health Sciences*, 2nd edn., pp. 219–235, BMJ Books, London.

21 Elliott, R. (1999) Evolving guidelines for publication of qualitative research studies in psychology and related fields. *British Journal of Clinical Psychology*, **38** (3), 215–229.

22 Dixon-Woods, M., Shaw, R.L., Agarwal, S. & Smith, J.A. (2004) The problem of appraising qualitative research. *Quality & Safety in Health Care*, **13** (3), 223–225.

23 Hannes, K. (2009). Chapter 6. Critical Appraisal of Qualitative Research. Draft Cochrane Guidance. Cochrane Collaboration Qualitative Research Methods Group, Adelaide. Available from http://www.joannabriggs.edu.au/cqrmg/documents/Cochrane_Guidance/Chapter6_Guidance_Critical_Appraisal.pdf. [accessed on 30 September 2010].

24 Elder, N.C. & William, L. (1995) Reading and evaluating qualitative research studies. *Journal of Family Practice*, **41**, 279–285.

25 Altheide, D. & Johnson, J. (1994) Criteria for assessing interpretive validity in qualitative research. In: Denzin, N. & Lincoln, Y. (eds), *Handbook of Qualitative Research*. Sage Publications, Thousand Oaks, CA.

26 Giacomini, M.K. & Cook, D.J. (2000) Users' guides to the medical literature XXIII. Qualitative research in health care. A. Are the results of the study valid? *JAMA*, **284**, 357–362.

27 Mays, N. & Pope, C. (2000) Assessing quality in qualitative research. *BMJ*, **320** (7226), 50–52.

28 Pope, C. & Mays, N. (2006) Observational methods. In: Pope, C. & Mays, N. (eds), *Qualitative Research in Health Care*, 3rd edn., pp. 32–42, Blackwell, UK.

29 Popay, J., Rogers, A. & Williams, G. (1998) Rationale and standards for the systematic review of qualitative literature in health services research. *Qualitative Health Research*, **8**, 341–351.

30 Mays, N. & Pope, C. (2006) Quality in qualitative health research. In: Pope, C. & Mays, N. (eds), *Qualitative Research in Health Care*, 3rd edn., pp. 82–101, Blackwell, UK.

Consolidated criteria for reporting qualitative studies (COREQ): 32-item checklist

Developed from:

Tong A, Sainsbury P, Craig J. Consolidated criteria for reporting qualitative research (COREQ): a 32-item checklist for interviews and focus groups. *International Journal for Quality in Health Care*. 2007. Volume 19, Number 6: pp. 349 – 357.

YOU MUST PROVIDE A RESPONSE FOR ALL ITEMS. ENTER N/A IF NOT APPLICABLE

No. Item	Guide questions/description	Reported on Page #
Domain 1: Research team and reflexivity		
Personal Characteristics		
1. Inter viewer/facilitator	Which author/s conducted the inter view or focus group?	Results
2. Credentials	What were the researcher's credentials? E.g. PhD, MD	Methods
3. Occupation	What was their occupation at the time of the study?	Methods
4. Gender	Was the researcher male or female?	N/A
5. Experience and training	What experience or training did the researcher have?	Methods
Relationship with participants		
6. Relationship established	Was a relationship established prior to study commencement?	N/A
7. Participant knowledge of the interviewer	What did the participants know about the researcher? e.g. personal goals, reasons for doing the research	N/A
8. Interviewer characteristics	What characteristics were reported about the inter viewer/facilitator? e.g. Bias, assumptions, reasons and interests in the research topic	Methods
Domain 2: study design		
Theoretical framework		
9. Methodological orientation and Theory	What methodological orientation was stated to underpin the study? e.g. grounded theory, discourse analysis, ethnography, phenomenology, content analysis	Methods

No. Item	Guide questions/description	Reported on Page #
Participant selection		
10. Sampling	How were participants selected? e.g. purposive, convenience, consecutive, snowball	Methods
11. Method of approach	How were participants approached? e.g. face-to-face, telephone, mail, email	Methods
12. Sample size	How many participants were in the study?	Results
13. Non-participation	How many people refused to participate or dropped out? Reasons?	Methods
Setting		
14. Setting of data collection	Where was the data collected? e.g. home, clinic, workplace	Methods
15. Presence of non-participants	Was anyone else present besides the participants and researchers?	Results
16. Description of sample	What are the important characteristics of the sample? e.g. demographic data, date	Results
Data collection		
17. Interview guide	Were questions, prompts, guides provided by the authors? Was it pilot tested?	Methods
18. Repeat interviews	Were repeat inter views carried out? If yes, how many?	N/A
19. Audio/visual recording	Did the research use audio or visual recording to collect the data?	Methods
20. Field notes	Were field notes made during and/or after the inter view or focus group?	Methods
21. Duration	What was the duration of the inter views or focus group?	Methods
22. Data saturation	Was data saturation discussed?	Methods
23. Transcripts returned	Were transcripts returned to participants for comment and/or correction?	N/A

(continued)

No. Item	Guide questions/description	Reported on Page #
Domain 3: analysis and findings		
Data analysis		
24. Number of data coders	How many data coders coded the data?	Methods
25. Description of the coding tree	Did authors provide a description of the coding tree?	N/A
26. Derivation of themes	Were themes identified in advance or derived from the data?	Methods
27. Software	What software, if applicable, was used to manage the data?	NVivo
28. Participant checking	Did participants provide feedback on the findings?	Strengths and limitations
Reporting		
29. Quotations presented	Were participant quotations presented to illustrate the themes/findings? Was each quotation identified? e.g. participant number	Results
30. Data and findings consistent	Was there consistency between the data presented and the findings?	Relationship to existing knowledge
31. Clarity of major themes	Were major themes clearly presented in the findings?	Results
32. Clarity of minor themes	Is there a description of diverse cases or discussion of minor themes?	Discussion

Once you have completed this checklist, please save a copy and upload it as part of your submission. When requested to do so as part of the upload process, please select the file type: *Checklist*. You will NOT be able to proceed with submission unless the checklist has been uploaded. Please DO NOT include this checklist as part of the main manuscript document. It must be uploaded as a separate file.

CHAPTER 22

SQUIRE (Standards for Quality Improvement Reporting Excellence)

Samuel J. Huber[1], Greg Ogrinc[2] and Frank Davidoff[3]

[1] *University of Rochester School of Medicine and Dentistry, Rochester, NY, USA*
[2] *Dartmouth Medical School, Hanover, NH, USA*
[3] *Annals of Internal Medicine, Philadelphia, PA, USA*

Timetable

2005	Draft guidelines developed: initial step in consensus process
2008	SQUIRE guidelines and E&E document published in a supplement to the journal *Quality and Safety in Health Care*
2013	Formal revision of the 2008 version of SQUIRE was initiated, with revised version (SQUIRE 2.0) expected in 2015

Name of guideline

The Standards for Quality Improvement Reporting Excellence (SQUIRE) guidelines provide recommendations for authors reporting on healthcare quality improvement (QI) activities and improvement research [1].

Improvements in healthcare come from many sources – basic and clinical research, changes in health policy, better financing – but the SQUIRE guidelines apply specifically to improving patient outcomes by data-driven changes in the delivery of care at the level of systems and organizations. Many of the principles and methods of system-level improvement now being applied in healthcare were developed in industry.

Improving the performance of the healthcare delivery system – that is, increasing the appropriateness, accuracy, and consistency of clinical care – requires changing human behavior. Like all social change programs, interventions that change human behavior differ importantly from the usual clinical interventions that affect human biology and the course of disease. Thus, improvement programs are strongly and inescapably context dependent (with implications for generalizability); the interventions

Guidelines for Reporting Health Research: A User's Manual, First Edition. Edited by David Moher, Douglas G. Altman, Kenneth F. Schulz, Iveta Simera and Elizabeth Wager.
© 2014 John Wiley & Sons, Ltd. Published 2014 by John Wiley & Sons, Ltd.

are usually complex and consist of multiple components; and their implementation is reflexive (i.e., they are designed to evolve continuously in response to feedback).

As a consequence, evaluating improvement interventions is a hybrid discipline that draws on both hypothesis-testing experimental methods of natural science and observational methods of social science [2]. These conceptual and pragmatic complexities increase the challenge of writing about improvement work, and explain why the focus of the SQUIRE guidelines is on the unique content of improvement programs rather than on particular study designs.

The goals of the guidelines are to increase the breadth and frequency of published reports of QI by encouraging and guiding authors; to improve the utility of QI reports by enhancing their transparency, comprehensiveness, and rigor; and to encourage reflection on the epistemology of QI work.

History/development

Development of the SQUIRE guidelines began around 2004 in response to concern that the results of QI projects were inadequately reported in the biomedical literature; important elements of methods, context, and the interventions themselves were often incompletely described or missing altogether [3]. Moreover, the number of published reports of system-level improvement appeared to be small relative to the explosion of clinical improvement activity since the early 1990s. The developers of SQUIRE proposed that consensus-based publication guidelines might be useful not only to authors in this rapidly developing but inadequately understood area, but also to editors, peer reviewers, and funding agencies.

In 2005, building on the Quality Improvement Report guidelines published earlier [4], the SQUIRE developers began a consensus development process by publishing an initial draft set of guidelines [5]. Authors, journal reviewers, and publication guideline experts were invited to comment on this draft, and authors and editors were recruited to "road test" the guidelines by applying them as they wrote up their work. In addition, several stakeholders in healthcare improvement were asked to provide formal commentaries on the draft, which were published in subsequent issues of *Quality and Safety in Health Care*.

With grant support from the Robert Wood Johnson Foundation, the draft guidelines were then revised in April 2007 during a two-day meeting attended by 30 stakeholders, including clinicians, improvement experts, editors, and statisticians. The resulting version was revised further in three cycles of a Delphi process involving an international group of over 50 consultants. Finally, a diverse group of authors created an explanation and elaboration (E&E) document that expanded on each item in the guidelines and provided published examples of each guideline item. The guidelines themselves and a description of the development process were then published in a supplement to *Quality and Safety in Health Care* in 2008 [1], along with the E&E document [6], and several commentaries [7, 8]. The article containing the guidelines was also published concurrently in several other journals [9–12].

When to use this guideline (what types of studies it covers)

The SQUIRE guidelines can be helpful in describing the evaluation of system-level improvement projects of any size or scope. They are of particular use in reporting formal, planned, empirical studies on the development and testing of improvement interventions [1]. Authors reporting their experiences with less formal, local improvement interventions may find the quality improvement report (QIR) structure more appropriate [4, 8], although the more detailed and systematic consensus-developed SQUIRE guidelines can provide useful additional background in describing less formal studies.

Previous versions

In its early years, the editorial team of the journal *Quality in Health Care* (subsequently *Quality and Safety in Health Care*, now *BMJ Quality and Safety*), which was launched in 1992, was struck by the gap between the volume of excellent applied QI work and the dearth of published QI projects. A key issue appeared to be the lack of structured guidance for authors, as well as concern that the standard IMRaD structure was unsuited to such reports. In 1999, the editors therefore published a guided structure for QIRs (Table 22.1) [4], which was subsequently adopted and promoted by the *BMJ* [13].

Table 22.1 Structure for quality improvement reports (QIR). From Ref 4.

- Brief description of context: relevant details of staff and function of department, team, unit, patient group
- Outline of problem: what were you trying to accomplish?
- Key measures for improvement: what would constitute improvement in view of patients?
- Process of gathering information: methods used to assess problems
- Analysis and interpretation: how did this information help your understanding of the problem?
- Strategy for change: what actual changes were made, how were they implemented, and who was involved in the change process?
- Effects of change: did this lead to improvement for patients – how did you know?
- Next steps: what you have learnt/achieved and how will you take this forward?

Current version

The SQUIRE guidelines consist of 19 items that authors should consider including in reports of healthcare improvement interventions (Table 22.2) [1]. The items and their descriptions are presented in table form in the published articles, and are available in checklist form on the SQUIRE website (http://squire-statement.org). A shorter, slightly simplified version

Table 22.2 SQUIRE guidelines.

- These guidelines provide a framework for reporting formal, planned studies designed to assess the nature and effectiveness of interventions to improve the quality and safety of care.
- It may not always be appropriate or even possible to include information about every numbered guideline item in reports of original studies, but authors should at least consider every item in writing their reports.
- Although each major section (i.e., Introduction, Methods, Results, and Discussion) of a published original study generally contains some information about the numbered items within that section, information about items from one section (e.g., the Introduction) is also often needed in other sections (e.g., the Discussion).

Text section; item number and name	Section or item description
Title and abstract	*Did you provide clear and accurate information for finding, indexing, and scanning your paper?*
1. Title	(a) Indicates that the article concerns the improvement of quality (broadly defined to include the safety, effectiveness, patient-centeredness, timeliness, efficiency, and equity of care) (b) States the specific aim of the intervention (c) Specifies the study method used (e.g., "A qualitative study," or "A randomized cluster trial")
2. Abstract	Summarizes precisely all key information from various sections of the text using the abstract format of the intended publication
Introduction	*Why did you start?*
3. Background Knowledge	Provides a brief, nonselective summary of current knowledge of the care problem being addressed, and characteristics of organizations in which it occurs
4. Local problem	Describes the nature and severity of the specific local problem or system dysfunction that was addressed
5. Intended improvement	(a) Describes the specific aim (changes/improvements in care processes and patient outcomes) of the proposed intervention (b) Specifies who (champions, supporters) and what (events, observations) triggered the decision to make changes, and why now (timing)

Table 22.2 (*Continued*)

Text section; item number and name	Section or item description
6. Study question	States precisely the primary improvement-related question and any secondary questions that the study of the intervention was designed to answer
Methods	*What did you do?*
7. Ethical issues	Describes ethical aspects of implementing and studying the improvement, such as privacy concerns, protection of participants' physical well-being, and potential author conflicts of interest, and how ethical concerns were addressed
8. Setting	Specifies how elements of the local care environment considered most likely to influence change/improvement in the involved site or sites were identified and characterized
9. Planning the intervention	(a) Describes the intervention and its component parts in sufficient detail that others could reproduce it
	(b) Indicates main factors that contributed to choice of the specific intervention (e.g., analysis of causes of dysfunction; matching relevant improvement experience of others with the local situation)
	(c) Outlines initial plans for how the intervention was to be implemented: e.g., *what* was to be done (initial steps; functions to be accomplished by those steps; how tests of change would be used to modify intervention), and *by whom* (intended roles, qualifications, and training of staff)
10. Planning the study of the intervention	(a) Outlines plans for assessing how well the intervention was implemented (dose or intensity of exposure)
	(b) Describes mechanisms by which intervention components were expected to cause changes, and plans for testing whether those mechanisms were effective
	(c) Identifies the study design (e.g., observational, quasi-experimental, experimental) chosen for measuring impact of the intervention on primary and secondary outcomes, if applicable
	(d) Explains plans for implementing essential aspects of the chosen study design, as described in publication guidelines for specific designs, if applicable (see, e.g., www.equator-network.org)
	(e) Describes aspects of the study design that specifically concerned internal validity (integrity of the data) and external validity (generalizability)
11. Methods of evaluation	(a) Describes instruments and procedures (qualitative, quantitative, or mixed) used to assess (a) the effectiveness of implementation, (b) the contributions of intervention components and context factors to the effectiveness of the intervention, and (c) primary and secondary outcomes
	(b) Reports efforts to validate and test reliability of assessment instruments
	(c) Explains methods used to assure data quality and adequacy (e.g., blinding; repeating measurements and data extraction; training in data collection; collection of sufficient baseline measurements)

(Continued)

Table 22.2 (*Continued*)

Text section; item number and name	Section or item description
12. Analysis	(a) Provides details of qualitative and quantitative (statistical) methods used to draw inferences from the data (b) Aligns unit of analysis with level at which the intervention was implemented, if applicable (c) Specifies degree of variability expected in implementation, change expected in primary outcome (effect size), and ability of study design (including size) to detect such effects (d) Describes analytic methods used to demonstrate effects of time as a variable (e.g., statistical process control)

Results
13. Outcomes
	What did you find?
	
	(a) Nature of setting and improvement intervention
	
	  i. Characterizes relevant elements of setting or settings (e.g., geography, physical resources, organizational culture, history of change efforts) and structures and patterns of care (e.g., staffing, leadership) that provided context for the intervention
	  ii. Explains the actual course of the intervention (e.g., sequence of steps, events or phases; type and number of participants at key points), preferably using a timeline diagram or flow chart
	  iii. Documents degree of success in implementing intervention components
	  iv. Describes how and why the initial plan evolved, and the most important lessons learned from that evolution, particularly the effects of internal feedback from tests of change (reflexiveness)
	
	(b) Changes in processes of care and patient outcomes associated with the intervention
	
	  i. Presents data on changes observed in the care delivery process
	  ii. Presents data on changes observed in measures of patient outcome (e.g., morbidity, mortality, function, patient/staff satisfaction, service utilization, cost, care disparities)
	  iii. Considers benefits, harms, unexpected results, problems, failures
	  iv. Presents evidence regarding the strength of association between observed changes/improvements and intervention components/context factors
	  v. Includes summary of missing data for intervention and outcomes

Discussion 14. Summary	*What do the findings mean?* (a) Summarizes the most important successes and difficulties in implementing intervention components, and main changes observed in care delivery and clinical outcomes (b) Highlights the study's particular strengths

Table 22.2 (*Continued*)

Text section; item number and name	Section or item description
15. Relation to other evidence	Compares and contrasts study results with relevant findings of others, drawing on broad review of the literature; use of a summary table may be helpful in building on existing evidence
16. Limitations	(a) Considers possible sources of confounding, bias, or imprecision in design, measurement, and analysis that might have affected study outcomes (internal validity) (b) Explores factors that could affect generalizability (external validity), for example: representativeness of participants; effectiveness of implementation; dose–response effects; features of local care setting (c) Addresses likelihood that observed gains may weaken over time, and describes plans, if any, for monitoring and maintaining improvement; explicitly states if such planning was not done (d) Reviews efforts made to minimize and adjust for study limitations (e) Assesses the effect of study limitations on interpretation and application of results
17. Interpretation	(a) Explores possible reasons for differences between observed and expected outcomes (b) Draws inferences consistent with the strength of the data about causal mechanisms and size of observed changes, paying particular attention to components of the intervention and context factors that helped determine the intervention's effectiveness (or lack thereof), and types of settings in which this intervention is most likely to be effective (c) Suggests steps that might be modified to improve future performance (d) Reviews issues of opportunity cost and actual financial cost of the intervention
18. Conclusions	(a) Considers overall practical usefulness of the intervention (b) Suggests implications of this report for further studies of improvement interventions
Other information	*Were there other factors relevant to the conduct and interpretation of the study?*
19. Funding	Describes funding sources, if any, and role of funding organization in design, implementation, interpretation, and publication of study

of SQUIRE is also available on the SQUIRE website at http://squire-statement.org/assets/pdfs/SQUIRE_guidelines_short.pdf accompanied by a glossary of terms at http://squire-statement.org/assets/pdfs/SQUIRE_glossary.pdf.

The guidelines are organized in the traditional IMRaD format (Introduction, Methods, Results, and Discussion). This format is appropriate for reporting original research studies since it addresses the four key questions the authors of all such studies need to answer: Why did you do what you did? How did you do it? What did you find? and What does it all mean?

Extensions and/or implementations

Extensions of the SQUIRE guidelines being considered include a narrower version for use in writing abstracts of improvement work and a broader version (or a linked set of shortened versions), perhaps merged with the Quality Improvement Report guidelines [4, 8], that could assist in reporting projects across the entire spectrum of improvement work, from case reports to highly structured experimental studies.

Recognizing that the efficacy of improvement projects can and should be evaluated using a variety of study designs, the SQUIRE guidelines make it clear that authors may need to apply both SQUIRE and another guideline that addresses their project's particular study design, for example, the CONSORT guidelines for a randomized controlled trial, or the STROBE guidelines for an observational study [14].

Translations of SQUIRE into Japanese, Norwegian, and Spanish are now available on the SQUIRE website.

Related activities

Evaluating the impact of SQUIRE

The value of publication guidelines will ultimately be determined by assessment of their impact on the completeness, accuracy, and transparency of published reports. The SQUIRE development group has therefore begun a qualitative investigation of the strengths, limitations, and usefulness of SQUIRE, now that enough time has elapsed for the guidelines to have had a meaningful impact.

Learning how SQUIRE is actually used in practice

Little is known about how users actually apply publication guidelines during the writing, editing, review, and publication of reports of bio-medical studies [15]. The SQUIRE developers are therefore interested in supporting studies of this important question, and the SQUIRE website actively encourages authors and others to post blogs about their experiences of using SQUIRE.

Although SQUIRE was created mainly to assist authors in writing reports of improvement work, a number of improvement leaders, including the Academy for Large Scale Change in the UK's National Health Service, currently use SQUIRE in planning improvement projects. The SQUIRE developers therefore believe the guidelines may have important potential in upgrading the planning and execution of improvement work.

To encourage and support these uses, the developers have posted on the SQUIRE website a number of user responses to the following questions:

- What have you found most interesting about SQUIRE?
- How has SQUIRE helped in writing about your improvement work?
- Has SQUIRE influenced how you plan for future work?

Using SQUIRE as an educational tool

The SQUIRE development group and others have used SQUIRE as an educational framework in over 25 local, national, and international seminars, both to encourage publication and introduce participants to system-level improvement work. SQUIRE has also been used to support the teaching of writing skills, most notably in the writers' collaboration with the Dartmouth-Hitchcock Leadership and Preventive Medicine Residency.

How best to use the guideline

Authors

The SQUIRE guidelines and accompanying E&E document can be used by authors of all experience levels in writing about improvement projects. Informal and formal feedback suggest that experienced authors will find the SQUIRE guidelines more useful than those who are newer to the process of writing; this feedback also suggests that many authors will find SQUIRE most useful in revising the initial draft of a report, rather than in creating the initial draft of the report itself. Authors who have used the SQUIRE guidelines to construct a manuscript "shell" early in the course of an improvement project may find it easier to prepare the paper when the project has matured. Experienced authors can benefit from reminders in SQUIRE about aspects of improvement they know are important but that are sometimes overlooked.

Peer reviewers

Because the SQUIRE guidelines represent consensus opinion on the elements required for effective descriptions of QI interventions, they may be useful to reviewers in assessing the nature and quality of improvement projects, judging the completeness and coherence of manuscripts reporting on those projects, and making informed, targeted suggestions for revisions.

Editors

Early experience demonstrated that overly literal application of publication guidelines can result in the production of awkward, almost unreadable text [16]. The published instructions for use of SQUIRE, therefore, stress the important editorial point that "although each major section (that is, Introduction, Methods, Results, and Discussion) of a published original study generally contains some information about the numbered items within that section [of SQUIRE], information about items from one section (for example, the Introduction) is also often needed in other sections (for example, the Discussion)" [1]. Providing detailed information on all 19 items may result in manuscripts that are longer than can be accommodated in print; in that case editors might consider publishing some information as appendices in electronic form only.

Institutional review boards/ethics reviewers

Distinguishing between clinical research and improvement activities can be a vexing problem for researchers, improvers, journal editors, and institutional review boards (IRBs) alike. Because clinical research serves interests other than those of the participants, all research studies involving human participants are required to undergo ethics review by an IRB or other such body. Improvement activities, in contrast, are intended solely or primarily to provide direct benefit to those who participate in them; in that sense, system-level improvement is an extension of clinical care rather than a research undertaking [17]. Nonetheless, improvement, like all clinical care, has its own inherent ethical concerns, primarily the need to protect privacy, provide respect for persons, avoid clinical harms, and disclose possible conflicts of interest. QI activity therefore needs to be open to appropriate ethical scrutiny, just as the ethics of clinical care is governed by its own set of review mechanisms. Individual improvement projects can, of course, also be primarily intended to answer specific research questions about the efficacy and mechanisms of improvement interventions, in which case the plans or protocols for implementing and studying those interventions need to be referred for ethics review by an IRB or equivalent mechanism. A SQUIRE-based instrument for making the distinction between clinical research and quality improvement has recently been described [18].

Funding agencies

Foundations and government agencies increasingly fund the implementation and evaluation of healthcare improvement programs. The SQUIRE guidelines provide a consensus framework of the elements of improvement programs that are most likely to be associated with meaningful change. They can therefore provide funders with criteria for evaluating the potential strength of proposals that request funding support.

Development process

See the information in the section on History/Development.

Evidence of effectiveness of guideline

Although no formal study of the effectiveness of the SQUIRE guidelines has been published, as of this writing the initial 2005 draft guidelines have been cited over 114 times. Moreover, in the 4 years following publication of the 2008 version of SQUIRE, 83 published papers on healthcare improvement indicated they had used them in formulating their reports (see e.g., 19–22); the E&E document had been cited 22 times.

Total hits on the SQUIRE website have continued at about 2000 per month (between 1300 and 1600 unique hits per month) since September 2012; the maximum number of hits was 2440 in May 2013. Hits in recent months have come from between 60 and 80 different countries, with a maximum of 81 countries in January 2014. Users spent an average of 2–3 minutes on the site, with the longest time being over 23 minutes. Comments submitted to the website have described both the usefulness of SQUIRE and its limitations.

Endorsement and adherence

The SQUIRE guidelines were developed with financial support from the Robert Wood Johnson Foundation and with administrative support from The Dartmouth Institute for Health Policy and Clinical Practice, the Institute for Healthcare Improvement, and the journal *Quality and Safety in Health Care*. The published 2008 SQUIRE guidelines were personally endorsed by 52 individual stakeholders [1]; as of June 2010, they had been adopted as editorial policy by nine peer-reviewed clinical journals. They have been formally considered at meetings of the International Committee of Medical Journal Editors, and have been adopted by the Healthcare Information and Management of Systems Society (HIMSS) for use in their 2009 call for studies on information technology in promoting patient safety. The SQUIRE website (http://squire-statement.org) continues to receive active financial and administrative support from the Dartmouth Institute. Journal editors wishing to include the SQUIRE guidelines in their instructions for authors can register on the website.

Cautions and limitations (including scope)

The SQUIRE guidelines assume that those who do improvement work understand the many generic elements of planning, implementing, evaluating, and reporting on improvement interventions, such as choice of intervention, planning of study design, methods of data collection and analysis, distinguishing between improvement and research, or undertaking ethics review. These and many other important elements of carrying out and studying improvement work are therefore not included in SQUIRE.

Improvement science is a young discipline, and its epistemology continues to emerge. The SQUIRE guidelines are a direct outgrowth of that epistemology; they are still, therefore, a work in progress and are currently undergoing a major formal revision, with support from the Health Foundation (UK) and the Robert Wood Johnson Foundation (US); the next version (SQUIRE 2.0) is expected to be available in 2015.

Mistakes and misconceptions

The SQUIRE guidelines are not intended to apply to literature reviews, explorations of theoretical frameworks, or improvement "stories," although an understanding of the essential elements of empirical improvement work that SQUIRE provides can inform such publications.

SQUIRE, like all such reporting guidelines and checklists generally, should be used as a quick and simple tool "aimed to buttress the memory and skills of expert professionals" [18], rather than as a "straitjacket."

Creators' preferred bits

The most important aspects of SQUIRE are those that reflect the nature of data-driven, system-level improvement, which is a unique hybrid of clinical and social sciences. These include the following:

1 The central role of context:

   Item 8, Setting: "Specifies how elements of the local care environment considered most likely to influence change/improvement in the involved site or sites were identified and characterized;"

Item 11.b, Methods of evaluation: "Describes instruments and procedures (qualitative, quantitative, or mixed) used to assess ... b) the contributions of intervention components and context factors to effectiveness of the intervention;" and,

Item 13.ii, Outcomes: "Characterizes relevant elements of setting or settings (for example, geography, physical resources, organizational culture, history of change efforts), and structures and patterns of care (for example, staffing, leadership) that provided context for the intervention."

2 The complex, multicomponent nature of most improvement interventions:

Item 9.a, Planning the intervention: "Describes the intervention and its component parts in sufficient detail that others could reproduce it."

3 The evolution of improvement interventions in response to feedback:

Item 13.a.v, Nature of setting and improvement intervention: "Describes how and why the initial plan evolved, and the most important lessons learned from that evolution, particularly the effects of internal feedback from tests of change (reflexiveness)."

Future plans

See under Related Activities.

Acknowledgments

Richard Thomson kindly provided information on the development of the Quality Improvement Report guidelines.

References

1 Davidoff, F., Batalden, P., Stevens, D. *et al.* (2008) Publication guidelines for quality improvement in health care: evolution of the SQUIRE project. *Quality and Safety in Health Care*, **17** (Suppl. 1), i3–9.V.

2 Vandenbroucke, J.P. (2008) Observational research, randomized trials, and two views of medical science. *PLoS Medicine*, **5**, e67.

3 Shojania, K.G., Ranji, S.R., McDonald, K.M. *et al.* (2006) Effects of quality improvement strategies for type 2 diabetes on glycemic control: a meta-regression analysis. *JAMA*, **296** (4), 427–440.

4 Moss, F. & Thomson, R. (1999) A new structure for quality improvement reports. *Quality and Safety in Health Care*, **8**, 76.

5 Davidoff, F. & Batalden, P. (2005) Toward stronger evidence on quality improvement. Draft publication guidelines: the beginning of a consensus project. *Quality and Safety in Health Care*, **14**, 319–325.

6 Ogrinc, G., Mooney, S.E., Estrada, C. *et al*. (2008) The SQUIRE (Standards for QUality Improvement Reporting Excellence) guidelines for quality improvement reporting: explanation and elaboration. *Quality and Safety in Health Care*, **17** (Suppl. 1), i13–i32.

7 Stevens, D.P. & Thomson, R. (2008) SQUIRE arrives – with a plan for its own improvement. *Quality and Safety in Health Care*, **17** (Suppl. 1), i1–i2.

8 Thomson, R.G. & Moss, F.M. (2008) QIR and SQUIRE: continuum of reporting guidelines for scholarly reports in healthcare improvement. *Quality and Safety in Health Care*, **17** (Suppl. 1), i10–i12.

9 Davidoff, F., Batalden, P., Stevens, D. *et al*. (2008) Publication guidelines for improvement studies in health care: evolution of the SQUIRE Project. *Annals of Internal Medicine*, **149** (9), 670–676.

10 Davidoff, F., Batalden, P., Stevens, D. *et al*. (2008) Publication guidelines for quality improvement studies in health care: evolution of the SQUIRE project. *Journal of General Internal Medicine*, **23** (12), 2125–2130.

11 Davidoff, F., Batalden, P., Stevens, D. *et al*. (2009) Publication guidelines for quality improvement studies in health care: evolution of the SQUIRE project. *BMJ*, **338**, a3152.

12 Davidoff, F., Batalden, P.B., Stevens, D.P. *et al*. (2008) Development of the SQUIRE Publication Guidelines: evolution of the SQUIRE project. *Joint Commission Journal on Quality and Patient Safety*, **34** (11), 681–687.

13 Smith, R. (2000) Quality improvement reports: a new kind of article. *BMJ*, **321**, 1428.

14 EQUATOR Network. Enhancing the QUality And Transparency Of health Research. Available from http://www.equator-network.org/. [accessed on 28 May 2010].

15 Vandenbroucke, J.P. (2009) STREGA, STROBE, STARD, SQUIRE, MOOSE, PRISMA, GNOSIS, TREND, ORION, COREQ, QUOROM, REMARK … and CONSORT: for whom does the guideline toll? *Journal of Clinical Epidemiology*, **62**, 594–596.

16 Rennie, D. (1995) Reporting randomized controlled trials. An experiment and a call for responses from readers. *JAMA*, **273** (13), 1054–1055.

17 Lynn, J., Baily, M.A., Bottrell, M. *et al*. (2007) The ethics of using quality improvement methods in health care. *Annals of Internal Medicine*, **146** (9), 666–673.

18 Ogrinc, G., Nelson, W.A., Adams, S.P., & O'Hara, A.E. (2013) An instrument to differentiate between clinical research and quality improvement. *IRB*, **35** (5), 1–8.

19 Kievit, J., Krukerink, M. & Marang-van de Mheen P.J. (2010) Surgical adverse outcome reporting as part of routine clinical care. *Quality and Safety in Health Care*, **19** (6), e20.

20 Lynch, J.R., Frankovich, E., Tetrick, C.A. & Howard, A.D. (2010) Improving influenza vaccination in dialysis facilities. *American Journal of Medical Quality*, **25** (6), 416–428.

21 Needham, D.M., Korupolu, R., Zanni, J.M. *et al*. (2010) Early physical medicine and rehabilitation for patients with acute respiratory failure: a quality improvement project. *Archives of Physical Medicine and Rehabilitation*, **91** (4), 536–542.

22 Schechter, M.S. & Gutierrez, H.H. (2010) Improving the quality of care for patients with cystic fibrosis. *Current Opinion in Pediatrics*, **22** (3), 296–301.

CHAPTER 23

REMARK (REporting Recommendations for Tumor MARKer Prognostic Studies)

Douglas G. Altman[1], Lisa M. McShane[2], Willi Sauerbrei[3], Sheila E. Taube[4] and Margaret M. Cavenagh[5]

[1] *Centre for Statistics in Medicine, University of Oxford, Oxford, UK*
[2] *Biometric Research Branch, National Cancer Institute, Bethesda, MD, USA*
[3] *Department of Medical Biometry and Medical Informatics, University Medical Center, Freiburg, Germany*
[4] *ST Consulting, Bethesda, MD, USA*
[5] *Cancer Diagnosis Program, Division of Cancer Treatment and Diagnosis, National Cancer Institute, Bethesda, MD, USA*

Name of guideline

REporting recommendations for tumor MARKer prognostic studies (REMARK).

History/development

The development of guidelines for the reporting of tumor marker studies was a major recommendation from the first International Meeting on Cancer Diagnostics (from Discovery to Clinical Practice: Diagnostic Innovation, Implementation, and Evaluation) sponsored by the US National Cancer Institute and the European Organisation for Research and Treatment of Cancer (NCI-EORTC). The purpose of the meeting in Nyborg, Denmark, in July 2000 was to discuss issues, accomplishments, and barriers in the field of cancer diagnostics. Poor study design and analysis, assay variability, and inadequate reporting of studies were identified as some of the major barriers to progress in this field. Several working groups were set up after the Nyborg meeting and were charged with identifying achievable goals in particular areas where progress could be made in the short term. One group addressed statistical issues of poor design and analysis, and reporting of tumor marker prognostic studies. The group identified the development of reporting guidelines for prognostic studies of tumor markers as its priority, and the REMARK recommendations were the end result [1–5].

Guidelines for Reporting Health Research: A User's Manual, First Edition. Edited by David Moher, Douglas G. Altman, Kenneth F. Schulz, Iveta Simera and Elizabeth Wager.
© 2014 John Wiley & Sons, Ltd. Published 2014 by John Wiley & Sons, Ltd.

Table 23.1 REMARK checklist. [1–5].

INTRODUCTION

1   State the marker examined, the study objectives, and any pre-specified hypotheses.

MATERIALS AND METHODS

Patients

2   Describe the characteristics (e.g., disease stage or comorbidities) of the study patients, including their source and inclusion and exclusion criteria.
3   Describe treatments received and how chosen (e.g., randomized or rule-based).

Specimen characteristics

4   Describe type of biological material used (including control samples), and methods of preservation and storage.

Assay methods

5   Specify the assay method used and provide (or reference) a detailed protocol, including specific reagents or kits used, quality control procedures, reproducibility assessments, quantitation methods, and scoring and reporting protocols. Specify whether and how assays were performed blinded to the study endpoint.

Study design

6   State the method of case selection, including whether prospective or retrospective and whether stratification or matching (e.g., by stage of disease or age) was used. Specify the time period from which cases were taken, the end of the follow-up period, and the median follow-up time.
7   Precisely define all clinical endpoints examined.
8   List all candidate variables initially examined or considered for inclusion in models.
9   Give rationale for sample size; if the study was designed to detect a specified effect size, give the target power and effect size.

Statistical analysis methods

10   Specify all statistical methods, including details of any variable selection procedures and other model-building issues, how model assumptions were verified, and how missing data were handled.
11   Clarify how marker values were handled in the analyses; if relevant, describe methods used for cutpoint determination.

RESULTS

Data

12   Describe the flow of patients through the study, including the number of patients included in each stage of the analysis (a diagram may be helpful) and reasons for dropout. Specifically, both overall and for each subgroup extensively examined, report the number of patients and the number of events.
13   Report distributions of basic demographic characteristics (at least age and sex), standard (disease-specific) prognostic variables, and tumor marker, including the numbers of missing values.

Table 23.1 *(Continued)*

Analysis and presentation

14   Show the relation of the marker to standard prognostic variables.
15   Present univariable analyses showing the relation between the marker and outcome, with the estimated effect (e.g., hazard ratio and survival probability). Preferably provide similar analyses for all other variables being analyzed. For the effect of a tumor marker on a time-to-event outcome, a Kaplan–Meier plot is recommended.
16   For key multivariable analyses, report estimated effects (e.g., hazard ratio) with confidence intervals for the marker and, at least for the final model, all other variables in the model
17   Among reported results, provide estimated effects with confidence intervals from an analysis in which the marker and standard prognostic variables are included, regardless of their statistical significance.
18   If done, report results of further investigations, such as checking assumptions, sensitivity analyses, and internal validation.

DISCUSSION

19   Interpret the results in the context of the pre-specified hypotheses and other relevant studies; include a discussion of limitations of the study.
20   Discuss implications for future research and clinical value.

The REMARK checklist (Table 23.1) was finalized in about 2002 but publication was delayed as we hoped to have simultaneous publication of a short paper introducing REMARK and a long "Explanation and Elaboration" (E&E) paper. As it became clear that writing an E&E paper would be extremely time consuming, a decision was made to publish the short paper introducing the checklist in 2005 while the writing process for the E&E paper continued. That decision proved wise, as the E&E paper was not published until 2012 [6, 7].

As an additional way to improve the reporting of key information, we developed a two-part REMARK *profile* that was first presented in a paper on the reporting of prognostic studies [8] and further elaborated in the E&E paper. As illustrated in Table 23.2, the first part gives details about how the marker of interest was handled in the analysis, which further variables were available for analysis, and a concise summary of the study participant characteristics. The participant summary provides key information about the patient population, inclusion and exclusion criteria, and the number of eligible patients and numbers of events for each outcome in the full data set.

Exploratory analyses play an important role in prognostic marker studies. In general, several analyses are conducted, of which only some are fully reported, with the results of others mentioned only briefly in the text (and easily overlooked) or not reported at all. This selective practice gives rise to biased results and biased interpretation and should be avoided. To help the reader to understand the multiplicity of analyses and better assess

Table 23.2 Example of the REMARK profile illustrated using data from a study of ploidy in patients with advanced ovarian cancer.

a) Patients, treatment and variables

Study and marker	Remarks
Marker (If non-binary: how was marker analyzed? continuous or categorical. If categorical, how were cutpoints determined?)	M = ploidy (diploid, aneuploid)
Further variables (variables collected, variables available for analysis, baseline variables, patient and tumor variables)	v1 = age, v2 = histologic type, v3 = grade, v4 = residual tumor, v5 = stage, v6 = ascites[a], v7 = estrogen[a], v8 = progesterone[a], v9 = CA-125[a]

Patients	n	Remarks
Assessed for eligibility	257	*Disease*: Advanced ovarian cancer, stage III and IV *Patient source*: Surgery 1982 to 1990, University Hospital Freiburg *Sample source*: Archived specimens available
Excluded	73	General exclusion criteria[b], non-standard therapy[b], coefficient of variation > 7%[b]
Included	184	Previously untreated. *Treatment*: all had platinum based chemotherapy after surgery
With outcome events	139	Overall survival: death from any cause

b) Statistical analyses of survival outcomes

Analysis	Patients	Events	Variables considered	Results/remarks
A1: Univariable	184	139	M, v1 to v5	Table 2, Figure 1
A2: Multivariable	174	133	M, v1, v3 to v5	Table 3 [v2 omitted because many missing data; Backward selection, see text]
A3: Effect for ploidy adjusted for v4	184	139	M, v4	Figure 2 [Based on result of A2]
A4: Interaction ploidy and stage	175	133	M, v1, v2, v4, v5	See text
A5: Ploidy in stage subgroups				
v5 = III	128	88	M	Figure 3
v5 = IV	56	51	M	Figure 4

[a] Not considered for survival outcome as these factors are not considered as 'standard' factors and/or number of missing values was relatively large; [b]values not given in the paper.
Source: Altman *et al.* 2012 [8].

and interpret the results, the second part of the REMARK profile gives an overview of all analyses performed and the data used in them.

The REMARK E&E paper [6, 7] provides a detailed explanation of each of the checklist items including examples of good reporting.

When to use this guideline (what types of studies it covers)

REMARK primarily focuses on studies of single prognostic markers, but most of the recommendations apply equally to other types of prognostic studies, including studies of multiple markers, studies to develop prognostic models, and studies to predict response to treatment. As predictive markers are best investigated in randomized controlled trials, the CONSORT statement is also relevant for such studies (see Chapter 9). The REMARK recommendations should also be useful in specialties other than cancer as little of the content is cancer specific.

Current version

Checklist and introductory article: 2005 [1–5].
Explanation and elaboration (E&E): 2012 [6, 7].

Previous versions

None.

Extensions and/or implementations to be aware of

No extensions have been published. However, as we note in the E&E paper, the recommendations largely apply also to studies of other types of tumor markers, such as predictive markers. Furthermore, REMARK can be used for prognostic studies outside oncology and some examples of such are noted in the E&E paper.

Related activities

Mallett *et al.* [8] conducted an evaluation of adherence to certain key elements of REMARK in the pre-REMARK era. They showed that reporting of key information, such as the number of outcome events in all patients and in subgroups, was poor. Sigounas *et al.* [9] used a 47-item checklist including 43 items based on REMARK to evaluate reporting in 184 studies of prognostic markers for outcome of acute pancreatitis. They found that 12 of the 47 items were reported in less than 10% of studies.

How best to use the guideline

Researchers preparing to publish results of prognostic marker studies will benefit from reviewing the REMARK recommendations to ensure that they have adequately reported all aspects of their work. Review of the REMARK checklist and the E&E paper can also be beneficial in the planning and analysis stages of a study to serve as a reminder of issues that are important to consider, and the information that is necessary to collect in order to maximize the usefulness and interpretability of the study results. In addition, the E&E paper contains discussions of some basic study design and analysis issues that provide a helpful review and motivate the recommended reporting items. The didactic material is presented in boxes and through elaborations of certain items. For example, item 10 has eight subheadings, from "Preliminary data preparation" to "Model validation," which guide the reader through the multitude of steps often involved in the analysis of a tumor marker study. The extensive list of references provides an additional resource for researchers.

Development process

The NCI-EORTC Statistics Subcommittee, co-chaired by Lisa McShane and Doug Altman, had nine members, split approximately evenly between the United States and Europe and between statisticians and nonstatisticians (clinicians, pathologists, laboratory researchers). The work of the Subcommittee was carried out through teleconferences and email. After one early conference call including all members, the development of the guideline was mainly done by email with occasional face-to-face discussions among those most actively involved in drafting the guidelines. The name REMARK was adopted late in the process, after a long struggle to find an acronym that fully captured the idea of guidelines for the reporting of tumor marker studies.

We always intended to accompany the initial REMARK paper by a longer explanatory paper. Preparing that paper took many years but the long E&E paper was finally published in 2012 [6, 7]. It includes detailed explanations of the background and evidence relevant to the 20 items on the REMARK checklist, and is written in the same style as E&E papers that accompanied other consensus guidelines: CONSORT, STROBE, STARD, and PRISMA (see Chapters 9, 17, 19, and 24). The E&E paper is the product of extensive deliberations, with many face-to-face meetings and numerous interactions among the four authors over several years. We benefited from comments from several experts on a near-final version in 2010 that helped us finalize the text.

The 2012 E&E paper is based on the 2005 checklist. The authors resisted the temptation to update the checklist when preparing the E&E, apart from two trivial wording changes for greater internal consistency. The E&E paper does, however, incorporate a new recommendation to present key aspects of the study in the form of a tabular "REMARK profile."

Evidence of effectiveness of guideline

We are not aware of any direct comparisons on reporting of studies before and after REMARK was published, nor between journals that do or do not recommend (endorse) REMARK to contributors. Mallett *et al.* [8] conducted a review of the reporting of items from the REMARK guidelines in prognostic studies of tumor markers published in higher impact journals from January 2006 to April 2007, shortly after publication of REMARK in August 2005. None of the papers referenced REMARK. Therefore, this study summarizes the reporting of prognostic marker studies in the pre-REMARK era.

A comparison to more recent publications is planned (see future plans).

Endorsement and adherence

A growing number of oncology journals are including a requirement or recommendation for authors to adhere to the REMARK reporting guidelines in their instructions to authors and reviewers. As a sign of its broader recognition, the Uniform Requirements for Manuscripts Submitted to Biomedical Journals, published by the International Committee of Medical Journal Editors (ICMJE), recommends that authors consult appropriate reporting guidelines, including REMARK. The REMARK guidelines are among the reporting resources listed by the EQUATOR Network (http://equator-network.org/) and the US National Library of Medicine (http://www.nlm.nih.gov/services/research_report_guide.html). The Program for the Assessment of Clinical Cancer Tests (PACCT) Strategy Group of the US National Cancer Institute has strongly endorsed REMARK. In contrast, the observation that as of 2012 only three of the original five journals that published REMARK specifically address it in their instructions to authors demonstrates the need to continue efforts to encourage greater endorsement and adherence.

Cautions and limitations (including scope)

Like other reporting guidelines, REMARK represents a minimum standard for reporting.

Creators' preferred bits

Item 17: "Among reported results, provide estimated effects with confidence intervals from an analysis in which the marker and standard prognostic variables are included, regardless of their statistical significance."

Adherence to this item will help ensure that all published studies provide results that are adjusted for similar factors. Such results would considerably improve the ability of systematic reviews to assemble comparable results from multiple studies.

REMARK profile: Structured reporting of study methods helps readers judge a study. Wide uptake of the REMARK profile would ensure that key information about a marker study is easily accessible, and would enable readers to place the reported results in the context of all analyses performed.

Future plans

We will monitor the literature and periodically consider whether an update is needed. We may consider extensions.

We hope to repeat the Mallett study [8] with more recent publications to evaluate any improvement in reporting over time.

References

1 McShane, L.M., Altman, D.G., Sauerbrei, W. *et al.* (2005) REporting recommendations for tumour MARKer prognostic studies (REMARK). *British Journal of Cancer*, **93**, 387–391.

2 McShane, L.M., Altman, D.G., Sauerbrei, W. *et al.* (2005) Reporting recommendations for tumor marker prognostic studies (REMARK). *Journal of the National Cancer Institute*, **97**, 1180–1184.

3 McShane, L.M., Altman, D.G., Sauerbrei, W. *et al.* (2005) REporting recommendations for tumour MARKer prognostic studies (REMARK). *European Journal of Cancer*, **41**, 1690–1696.

4 McShane, L.M., Altman, D.G., Sauerbrei, W. *et al.* (2005) Reporting recommendations for tumor marker prognostic studies. *Journal of Clinical Oncology*, **23**, 9067–9072.

5 McShane, L.M., Altman, D.G., Sauerbrei, W. *et al.* (2005) REporting recommendations for tumor MARKer prognostic studies (REMARK). *Nature Clinical Practice Oncology*, **2**, 416–422.

6 Altman, D.G., McShane, L.M., Sauerbrei, W. & Taube, S.E. (2012) Reporting recommendations for tumor marker prognostic studies (REMARK): explanation and elaboration. *BMC Medicine*, **10**, 51.

7 Altman, D.G., McShane, L.M., Sauerbrei, W. & Taube, S.E. (2012) Reporting recommendations for tumor marker prognostic studies (REMARK): explanation and elaboration. *PLoS Medicine*, **9**, e1001216.

8 Mallett, S., Timmer, A., Sauerbrei, W. & Altman, D.G. (2010) Reporting of prognostic studies of tumour markers: a review of published articles in relation to REMARK guidelines. *British Journal of Cancer*, **102**, 173–180.

9 Sigounas, D.E., Tatsioni, A., Christodoulou, D.K. *et al.* (2011) New prognostic markers for outcome of acute pancreatitis: overview of reporting in 184 studies. *Pancreas*, **40**, 522–532.

CHAPTER 24

PRISMA (Preferred Reporting Items for Systematic Reviews and Meta-Analyses)

David Moher[1], Douglas G. Altman[2] and Jennifer Tetzlaff[3]

[1] *Clinical Epidemiology Program, Ottawa Hospital Research Institute, Ottawa, ON, Canada*
[2] *Centre for Statistics in Medicine, University of Oxford, Oxford, UK*
[3] *Ottawa Methods Centre, Clinical Epidemiology Program, Ottawa Hospital Research Institute, Ottawa, ON, Canada*

Timetable

Name of reporting guideline initiative	Notes	Consensus meeting date	Reporting guideline publication
QUOROM		October 1996	1999
PRISMA	Expanded the remit of QUOROM	June 2005	2010: 1. Statement 2. Explanation and elaboration paper

Name of guideline

The Preferred Reporting Items for Systematic reviews and Meta-Analyses (PRISMA) statement is a guidance for authors reporting a systematic review and/or meta-analysis of randomized trials and other types of research designs evaluating a healthcare intervention, such as a drug, device, operative procedure, or psychological counseling [1]. PRISMA can be used by peer reviewers and editors reviewing a submission of a systematic review and/or meta-analysis. PRISMA can also be used by readers wanting to gauge the validity of the results of systematic reviews and meta-analyses.

Guidelines for Reporting Health Research: A User's Manual, First Edition. Edited by David Moher, Douglas G. Altman, Kenneth F. Schulz, Iveta Simera and Elizabeth Wager.
© 2014 John Wiley & Sons, Ltd. Published 2014 by John Wiley & Sons, Ltd.

History/development

The PRISMA statement represents an extensive update and expansion of the QUality Of Reporting Of Meta-analyses (QUOROM) statement, a guideline primarily for reporting meta-analyses of randomized trials [2]. The PRISMA checklist differs in several respects from the QUOROM checklist. There are new items: (1) asking authors to report on the existence of a protocol and, if so, how it can be accessed (item 5), (2) asking authors to describe any assessments of risk of bias in the review, such as selective outcome reporting within the included studies (item 12), and (3), asking authors to provide information on any sources of funding (item 27). Generally, the PRISMA checklist "decouples" several items present in the QUOROM checklist and, where applicable, several checklist items are linked to improve consistency across the systematic review report.

The flow diagram has also been modified. Before including studies and providing reasons for excluding others, the review team must first search the literature. This search results in records. Once these records have been screened and eligibility criteria applied, a smaller number of articles will remain. The number of included articles might be smaller (or larger) than the number of studies, because articles may report on multiple studies and results from a particular study may be published in several articles. To capture this information, the PRISMA flow diagram now requests information on these phases of the review process.

When to use this guideline (what types of studies it covers)

The PRISMA statement can be used to report systematic reviews and meta-analyses involving healthcare interventions as described above (see Name of Guideline section). We have used the Cochrane Collaboration definition for both, namely, a systematic review being a review of a clearly formulated question that uses systematic and explicit methods to identify, select, and critically appraise relevant research, and to collect and analyze data from the studies that are included in the review. Statistical methods (meta-analysis) may or may not be used to analyze and summarize the results of the included studies. A meta-analysis refers to the use of statistical techniques in a systematic review to integrate the results of included studies.

Previous version

Several articles published in the late 1980s found that the quality of reporting of meta-analyses was inadequate [3–5]. To help remedy this situation, an international group developed a guidance called the QUOROM statement, which focused on the reporting of meta-analyses of randomized trials. The QUOROM statement, including an 18-item checklist and flow diagram, was published in 1999 in the *Lancet* [2].

Current version

The PRISMA statement consists of some brief text explaining the development of the reporting guideline, a 27-item checklist, and a four-phase flow diagram. The checklist guides authors on how best to report the title, abstract, methods, results, discussion, and funding of a systematic review and/or meta-analysis. The checklist is a minimum list of items (and not meant to be overly comprehensive as to the issues) that can be included in a report of a systematic review and meta-analysis. While the flow diagram provides guidance on how to report the flow of records and articles through the identification, screening, eligibility, and included studies section of a systematic review and/or meta-analysis.

Along with the statement, the PRISMA group also published a PRISMA explanation and elaboration paper [6]. The process of completing this 21,000 word document included developing a large database of exemplars to highlight how best to report each checklist item, and identifying a comprehensive evidence base to support the inclusion of each checklist item, whenever possible. The explanation and elaboration document was completed after several face-to-face meetings and numerous iterations among several meeting participants, after which it was shared with the whole group for additional revisions and final approval.

The PRISMA statement is currently published in eight journals [7–14], one of which is open access [7]. The remaining journals provide free access to the statement. The PRISMA explanation and elaboration paper is published in one open-access journal [6] and the *Annals of Internal Medicine*, *BMJ*, and *Journal of Clinical Epidemiology*.

Extensions and/or implementations

Two extensions of PRISMA have been published to date. PRISMA for abstracts [15] was recently published and focuses on providing guidance on writing abstracts for systematic reviews and includes a 12-item checklist. PRISMA for equity (PRISMA-E) provides authors with guidance for reporting equity-focused systematic reviews (e.g., interventions targeted at a disadvantaged population) and includes a 13-item checklist [16]. Other extensions are in various stages of development including PRISMA for protocols, individual patient data meta-analysis, and network meta-analysis. Any further extensions will be announced and registered on the EQUATOR website as guidelines under development (www.equator-network.org).

Other types of systematic reviews and meta-analyses exist, such as diagnostic accuracy and prognostic reviews, and genetic association reviews. We do not think PRISMA is ideally suited for reporting these reviews even though some elements of the review process will be similar to reporting reviews of randomized trials and other types of research designs evaluating a healthcare intervention. Similarly, PRISMA is likely not ideal for reporting some of the variants of qualitative systematic reviews, such as realist reviews and meta-narrative reviews.

Related activities

An essential part of completing any systematic review and meta-analysis is searching the literature to identify relevant studies to include. Inadequately reported searches prohibit interested readers from repeating what the authors did. Likewise, without accurate and transparent reporting of the search strategies it is difficult, and at times impossible, to update the original systematic review searches. Andrew Booth has developed the STARLITE [17] mnemonic for reporting literature searches (sampling strategy, type of study, approaches, range of years, limits, inclusion and exclusions, terms used, electronic sources). We encourage authors and others to consult STARLITE when reporting and peer reviewing this part of a systematic review and/or meta-analysis report.

How best to use the guideline

Authors

The process of conducting a systematic review can be a complex one and authors may not always remember the various steps they took to complete it. Use of the PRISMA checklist and flow diagram can be a helpful reminder for authors to report whether or not the steps were completed and, if so, how. The order and format of the checklist items are not essential to follow when reporting a systematic review and/or meta-analysis. Similarly, all of the checklist items do not necessarily have to be completed affirmatively. It is possible that authors elected not to complete certain parts of the review process as outlined in PRISMA. The PRISMA statement was not developed so as to pass judgment on what authors did or did not do. PRISMA has been developed to help authors accurately and transparently report the process of completing their systematic review and meta-analysis.

Peer reviewers

Peer reviewers like others are busy people and will likely only have a limited time to review any systematic review and meta-analysis. Likewise, it is human nature to sometimes forget aspects of the systematic review process, and using the checklist can facilitate a thorough peer review of all the steps the authors took completing their systematic review and/or meta-analysis.

Editors

Editors can use the checklist in many ways; two may be useful for manuscript decision making. By asking authors to complete and include a populated checklist as part of the submission process, editors can gauge the level of detail provided by the authors. This will facilitate editors helping readers being able to judge the validity of the results for their own decision making. When editors include the PRISMA checklist as part of the guidance for completing a peer review, they are helping ensure a thorough review process. From the perspective of authors, peer reviewers, and editors, using the same checklist is likely to facilitate communication about the clarity, accuracy, and transparency of the systematic review report.

Development process

A three-day meeting was held in Ottawa, Canada, in June 2005 with 29 participants, including review authors, methodologists, clinicians, medical editors, and a consumer. Prior to the meeting, the executive team completed a number of activities: (1) a systematic review of studies examining the quality of reporting of systematic reviews, (2) a comprehensive literature search to identify methodological and other articles that might inform the meeting, especially in relation to modifying checklist items, and (3) an international survey of review authors, consumers, and groups commissioning or using systematic reviews and meta-analyses to ascertain views of QUOROM, including the merits of the existing checklist items.

During the meeting, the results of the three activities mentioned above were presented. After these discussions, each QUOROM checklist item was discussed as to whether it should be retained or deleted based partly on the evidence base collected prior to the meeting. Additional checklist items for consideration were also discussed. Only items deemed essential were retained or added to the checklist. A strategy for producing the PRISMA statement and PRISMA explanation and elaboration paper were also discussed. Finally, a knowledge translation strategy was discussed.

Shortly after the meeting, a draft of the PRISMA checklist was circulated to the group, including those invited to the meeting but unable to attend.

After several iterations, the checklist was approved by the PRISMA group. The checklist was subsequently pilot tested. Simultaneously, the PRISMA statement was drafted by the executive team and after several iterations was approved by the group. After the statement was drafted, a small group of PRISMA group members drafted the PRISMA explanation and elaboration paper. As with the summary paper, the explanation and elaboration paper was iterated by the larger group and ultimately approved by them.

Evidence of effectiveness of guideline

We are unaware of any evaluations as to whether the use of the PRISMA checklist and/or flow diagram is associated with an improved quality of reporting of systematic reviews and meta-analyses. We plan completing such an assessment and encourage others to do likewise.

Endorsement and adherence

Thus far PRISMA is endorsed by about 200 journals, the Cochrane Collaboration, and the Council of Science Editors. We are actively seeking endorsement by other journals and editorial groups. We are unaware of any data on journal adherence to the PRISMA statement.

Journals and editorial groups wanting to endorse PRISMA can do so by registering on the PRISMA website. We recommend citing one of the original versions of PRISMA, the PRISMA explanation and elaboration paper, and the PRISMA website in their "Instructions to Authors."

Cautions and limitations (including scope)

The PRISMA checklist is not intended as an instrument to evaluate the quality of a systematic review or meta-analysis. Nor is it appropriate to use the checklist to construct a quality score.

The PRISMA statement was developed to report a broad spectrum of systematic reviews and meta-analyses. That said, it is of limited use in other types of systematic reviews, such as diagnostic test ones (see Extensions and/or implementations). For example, assessing the risk of bias is a key concept in conducting a systematic review, but the items used to assess this in a diagnostic review are likely to focus on issues such as the spectrum of patients and the verification of disease status, which differ from reviews of interventions. The flow diagram will also need adjustments when reporting meta-analysis of individual patient data.

Creators' preferred bits

Search

The search strategy is an essential part of the (conduct and) report of any systematic review. Searches may be complicated and iterative particularly when reviewers search unfamiliar databases or their review is addressing a broad or new topic. Reviewing a search strategy allows interested readers to assess the comprehensiveness and completeness of the search and to repeat it. Making searches available also facilitates updating a review. Some editors will argue that publishing a complete search strategy for one of the main electronic databases will take up too much space, particularly given the expense of journal page "real estate." Although publishing search strategies will require page space, most journals have an Internet presence where search strategies can be posted.

Protocols of systematic reviews

A protocol is important because it pre-specifies the objectives and methods of the systematic review. For instance, a protocol specifies outcomes of primary interest, how reviewers will extract information about those outcomes, and methods that reviewers might use to quantitatively summarize the outcome data. Having a protocol, and registering a set of minimum information about a systematic review, can help restrict the likelihood of biased post hoc decisions in review methods, such as selective outcome reporting biases [10], address excessive duplication of systematic reviews, and improve transparency.

On February 22, 2011, the Centre for Reviews and Dissemination, University of York, launched PROSPERO, an international prospective register of systematic review protocols (http://www.metaxis.com/PROSPERO/). Authors can register their prospective protocols free of charge. PROSPERO consists of 22 mandatory items and 18 optional items. Several journals and groups now endorse systematic review protocol registration. At the time of writing, more than 2200 protocols from more than 65 countries have been registered on PROSPERO.

Flow diagram

As it is said a picture – in this case a flow diagram – is worth a thousand words. The flow diagram is a great way for authors to report the flow of records and papers throughout the systematic review process. Some authors have been innovative in using a flow diagram to explain the flow of information through complex reviews. A flow diagram also enables readers to understand which papers made it into the systematic review and various meta-analyses, if completed.

Future plans

We plan on evaluating whether the use of the PRISMA statement is associated with improvements in the quality of reporting of systematic reviews and meta-analyses. A 2004 assessment of the quality of reporting of systematic reviews [18] is likely a useful baseline (prior to the introduction of PRISMA) measure. Here, the sample frame was a complete month of PubMed, enhancing generalizability of the results. Many evaluations limit their sampling frame, and their generalizability, to either a few journals of high-impact factors in a particular content area or the top five general and internal medicine journals.

References

1 Moher, D., Liberati, A., Tetzlaff, J. *et al.* (2009). Preferred Reporting Items for Systematic Reviews and Meta-Analyses: the PRISMA Statement. *PLoS Medicine*, **6** (7), e1000097. doi:10.1371/journal.pmed.1000097.

2 Moher, D., Cook, D.J., Eastwood, S. *et al.* (1994) Improving the quality of reporting of meta-analysis of randomized controlled trials: the QUOROM statement. *Lancet*, **354**, 1896–1900.

3 Mulrow, C.D. (1987) The medical review article: state of the science. *Annals of Internal Medicine*, **106**, 485–488.

4 Sacks, H.S., Berrier, J., Reitman, D. *et al.* (1987) Metaanalysis of randomized controlled trials. *New England Journal of Medicine*, **316**, 450–455.

5 Sacks, H.S., Reitman, D., Pagano, D. & Kupelnick, B. (1996) Meta-analysis: an update. *Mount Sinai Journal of Medicine*, **63**, 216–224.

6 Liberati, A., Altman, D.G., Tetzlaff, J., *et al.* (2009) The PRISMA statement for reporting systematic reviews and meta-analyses of studies that evaluate health care interventions: explanation and elaboration. *PLoS Medicine*, **6**, e1000100. doi:10.1371/journal.pmed.1000100.

7 Moher, D., Liberati, A., Tetzlaff, J. *et al.* (2010) Preferred reporting items for systematic reviews and meta-analyses: the PRISMA Statement. *International Journal of Surgery*, **8** (5), 336–341.

8 Moher, D., Liberati, A., Tetzlaff, J. *et al.* (2009) Preferred reporting items for systematic reviews and meta-analyses: the PRISMA Statement. *Journal of Clinical Epidemiology*, **62** (10), 1006–1012.

9 Moher, D., Liberati, A., Tetzlaff, J. *et al.* (2009) Preferred reporting items for systematic reviews and meta-analyses: the PRISMA Statement. *Zhong Xi Yi Jie He Xue Bao*, **7** (9), 889–896. [Chinese].

10 Moher, D., Liberati, A., Tetzlaff, J. *et al.* (2009) Preferred reporting items for systematic reviews and meta-analyses: the PRISMA Statement. *Physical Therapy*, **89** (9), 873–880.

11 Moher, D., Liberati, A., Tetzlaff, J. *et al.* (2009) Preferred reporting items for systematic reviews and meta-analyses: the PRISMA Statement. *Open Medicine*, **3** (2), 123–130.

12 Moher, D., Liberati, A., Tetzlaff, J. *et al.* (2009) Preferred reporting items for systematic reviews and meta-analyses: the PRISMA Statement. *Annals of Internal Medicine*, **151** (4), 264–269, W64.

13 Moher, D., Liberati, A., Tetzlaff, J. *et al.* (2009) Preferred reporting items for systematic reviews and meta-analyses: the PRISMA Statement. *PLoS Medicine*, **6** (7), e1000097.

14 Moher, D., Liberati, A., Tetzlaff, J. *et al.* (2009) Preferred reporting items for systematic reviews and meta-analyses: the PRISMA Statement. *BMJ*, **339**, b2535.

15 Beller, E.M., Glasziou, P.P., Altman, D.G. *et al.* (2013) PRISMA for abstracts: reporting systematic reviews in journal and conference abstracts. *PLoS Medicine*, **10** (4), e1001419. doi:10.1371/journal.pmed.1001419.

16 Welch, V., Petticrew, M., Tugwell, P. *et al.* (2012) PRISMA Equity 2012 Extension: Reporting Guidelines for Systematic Reviews with a Focus on Health Equity. *PLoS Medicine*, **9** (10), e1001333. doi:10.1371/journal.pmed.1001333.

17 Booth, A. (2006) "Brimful of STARLITE": toward standards for reporting literature searches. *Journal of the Medical Library Association*, **94**, 421–429.

18 Moher, D., Tetzlaff, J., Tricco, A.C. *et al.* (2007) Epidemiology and reporting characteristics of systematic reviews. *PLoS Medicine*, **4** (3), e78. doi:10.1371/journal.pmed.0040078.

Section/topic	#	Checklist item	Reported on page #
TITLE			
Title	1	Identify the report as a systematic review, meta-analysis, or both.	
ABSTRACT			
Structured summary	2	Provide a structured summary including, as applicable: background; objectives; data sources; study eligibility criteria, participants, and interventions; study appraisal and synthesis methods; results; limitations; conclusions and implications of key findings; systematic review registration number.	
INTRODUCTION			
Rationale	3	Describe the rationale for the review in the context of what is already known.	
Objectives	4	Provide an explicit statement of questions being addressed with reference to participants, interventions, comparisons, outcomes, and study design (PICOS).	
METHODS			
Protocol and registration	5	Indicate if a review protocol exists, if and where it can be accessed (e.g., Web address), and, if available, provide registration information including registration number.	
Eligibility criteria	6	Specify study characteristics (e.g., PICOS, length of follow-up) and report characteristics (e.g., years considered, language, publication status) used as criteria for eligibility, giving rationale.	
Information sources	7	Describe all information sources (e.g., databases with dates of coverage, contact with study authors to identify additional studies) in the search and date last searched.	
Search	8	Present full electronic search strategy for at least one database, including any limits used, such that it could be repeated.	
Study selection	9	State the process for selecting studies (i.e., screening, eligibility, included in systematic review, and, if applicable, included in the meta-analysis).	

(continued)

Section/topic	#	Checklist item	Reported on page #
Data collectiona process	10	Describe method of data extraction from reports (e.g., piloted forms, independently, in duplicate) and any processes for obtaining and confirming data from investigators.	
Data items	11	List and define all variables for which data were sought (e.g., PICOS, funding sources) and any assumptions and simplifications made.	
Risk of bias in individual studies	12	Describe methods used for assessing risk of bias of individual studies (including specification of whether this was done at the study or outcome level), and how this information is to be used in any data synthesis.	
Summary measures	13	State the principal summary measures (e.g., risk ratio, difference in means).	
Synthesis of results	14	Describe the methods of handling data and combining results of studies, if done, including measures of consistency (e.g., I^2) for each meta-analysis.	

Section/topic	#	Checklist item	Reported on page #
Risk of bias across studies	15	Specify any assessment of risk of bias that may affect the cumulative evidence (e.g., publication bias, selective reporting within studies).	
Additional analyses	16	Describe methods of additional analyses (e.g., sensitivity or subgroup analyses, meta-regression), if done, indicating which were pre-specified.	

RESULTS

Section/topic	#	Checklist item	Reported on page #
Study selection	17	Give numbers of studies screened, assessed for eligibility, and included in the review, with reasons for exclusions at each stage, ideally with a flow diagram.	
Study characteristics	18	For each study, present characteristics for which data were extracted (e.g., study size, PICOS, follow-up period) and provide the citations.	
Risk of bias within studies	19	Present data on risk of bias of each study and, if available, any outcome level assessment (see item 12).	
Results of individual studies	20	For all outcomes considered (benefits or harms), present, for each study: (a) simple summary data for each intervention group (b) effect estimates and confidence intervals, ideally with a forest plot.	

Section/topic	#	Checklist item	Reported on page #
Synthesis of results	21	Present results of each meta-analysis done, including confidence intervals and measures of consistency.	
Risk of bias across studies	22	Present results of any assessment of risk of bias across studies (see Item 15).	
Additional analysis	23	Give results of additional analyses, if done (e.g., sensitivity or subgroup analyses, meta-regression [see Item 16]).	

DISCUSSION

Summary of evidence	24	Summarize the main findings including the strength of evidence for each main outcome; consider their relevance to key groups (e.g., healthcare providers, users, and policy makers).	
Limitations	25	Discuss limitations at study and outcome level (e.g., risk of bias), and at review-level (e.g., incomplete retrieval of identified research, reporting bias).	
Conclusions	26	Provide a general interpretation of the results in the context of other evidence, and implications for future research.	

FUNDING

Funding	27	Describe sources of funding for the systematic review and other support (e.g., supply of data); role of funders for the systematic review.	

From: Moher D, Liberati A, Tetzlaff J, Altman DG, The PRISMA Group (2009). Preferred Reporting Items for Systematic Reviews and Meta-Analyses: The PRISMA Statement. PLoS Med 6(6): e1000097. doi:10.1371/journal.pmed1000097.
For more information, visit: www.prisma-statement.org.

PART III

CHAPTER 25

Statistical Analyses and Methods in the Published Literature: The SAMPL Guidelines*

Thomas A. Lang[1] and Douglas G. Altman[2]

[1] *Tom Lang Communications and Training International, Kirkland, WA, USA*
[2] *Centre for Statistics in Medicine, University of Oxford, Oxford, UK*

> "Have they reflected that the sciences founded on observation can only be promoted by statistics? ... If medicine had not neglected this instrument, this means of progress, it would possess a greater number of positive truths, and stand less liable to the accusation of being a science of unfixed principles, vague and conjectural."
>
> Jean-Etienne Dominique Esquirol, an early French psychiatrist, quoted in The Lancet, 1838. [1]

Introduction

The first major study of the quality of statistical reporting in the biomedical literature was published in 1966 [2]. Since then, dozens of similar studies have been published, every one of which has found that a high percentage of articles contain errors in the application, analysis, interpretation, or reporting of statistics or in the design or conduct of research (see, e.g., Refs [3–19]). Furthermore, many of these errors are serious enough to call the authors' conclusions into question [8,9,12,17]. The problem is made worse by the fact that most of these studies are of the world's leading peer-reviewed general medical and specialty journals.

Although errors have been reported in complex statistical procedures [19–22], paradoxically, most errors are found in basic, not advanced,

---

*First published as: Lang T, Altman D. Basic statistical reporting for articles published in clinical medical journals: the SAMPL Guidelines. In: Smart P, Maisonneuve H, Polderman A (eds). *Science Editors' Handbook*, European Association of Science Editors, 2013. NOTE: In this chapter, the text is identical to the original publication, but the references documenting the incidence of statistical errors have been updated.

---

statistical methods [23]. Perhaps advanced methods are suggested by consulting statisticians, who perform the analyses competently, but it is also true that authors are far more likely to use, in general, only elementary statistical methods, if they use any at all [23–26]. Still, articles with major errors continue to pass editorial and peer review and to be published in leading journals.

The truth is that the problem of poor statistical reporting is longstanding, widespread, potentially serious, concerns mostly basic statistics, and yet is largely unsuspected by most readers of the biomedical literature [27].

More than 30 years ago, O'Fallon *et al.* recommended that "standards governing the content and format of statistical aspects should be developed to guide authors in the preparation of manuscripts" [28]. Despite the fact that this call has since been echoed by several others [29–32], most journals have not included in their "Instructions for Authors" more than a paragraph or two about reporting statistical methods and results [33]. However, given that most statistical errors concern basic statistics, a comprehensive – and comprehensible – set of reporting guidelines might improve the documentation of statistical analyses.

The SAMPL guidelines are designed to be included in a journal's "Instructions for Authors." These guidelines tell authors, journal editors, and reviewers how to report basic statistical methods and results. Although these guidelines are limited to the most common statistical analyses, they are nevertheless sufficient to prevent most of the reporting deficiencies routinely found in scientific articles.

Unlike most of the other guidelines in this book, these guidelines were not developed by a formal consensus-building process, but they do draw considerably from other published guidelines [27, 34–37]. In addition, a comprehensive review of the literature on statistical reporting errors reveals near universal agreement on how to report the most common methods [27].

Statistical analyses are closely related to research methodologies, which must also be properly documented. We do not provide such guidance here. Instead, we refer readers to other chapters in this book and to the EQUATOR Network website (www.equator-network.org). Guidelines for reporting methodologies include items on reporting statistics, but the guidelines presented here are more specific and complement, rather than duplicate, those in the methodology guidelines [38–40].

We welcome feedback and anticipate the need to update these guidelines in due course.

Guiding principles for reporting statistical methods and results

Our first guiding principle for statistical reporting comes from The International Committee of Medical Journal Editors, whose "Uniform

Requirements for Manuscripts Submitted to Biomedical Journals" include the following excellent statement about reporting statistical analyses:

> "**Describe statistical methods with enough detail to enable a knowledgeable reader with access to the original data to verify the reported results**. [Emphasis added.] When possible, quantify findings and present them with appropriate indicators of measurement error or uncertainty (such as confidence intervals). Avoid relying solely on statistical hypothesis testing, such as P values, which fail to convey important information about effect size. References for the design of the study and statistical methods should be to standard works when possible (with pages stated). Define statistical terms, abbreviations, and most symbols. Specify the computer software used." [33, 41]

Our second guiding principle for statistical reporting is to **provide enough detail that the results can be incorporated into other analyses**. In general, this principle requires reporting the descriptive statistics from which other statistics are derived, such as the numerators and denominators of percentages, especially in risk, odds, and hazards ratios. Likewise, P values are not sufficient for reanalysis. Needed instead are descriptive statistics for the variables being compared, including the sample size of the groups involved, the estimate (or "effect size") associated with the P value, and a measure of precision for the estimate, usually a 95% confidence interval.

General principles for reporting statistical methods

Preliminary analyses

- Identify any statistical procedures used to modify raw data before analysis. Examples include mathematically transforming continuous measurements to make distributions closer to the normal distribution, creating ratios or other derived variables, and collapsing continuous data into categorical data or combining categories.

Primary analyses

- Describe the purpose of the analysis.
- Identify the variables used in the analysis and summarize each with descriptive statistics.
- When possible, identify the smallest difference considered to be clinically important.
- Describe fully the main methods for analyzing the primary objectives of the study.
- Make clear which method was used for each analysis, rather than just listing in one place all the statistical methods used.

- Verify that the data conformed to the assumptions of the test used to analyze them. In particular, specify whether (1) skewed data were analyzed with nonparametric tests, (2) paired data were analyzed with paired tests, and (3) the underlying relationship analyzed with linear regression models was linear.
- Indicate whether and how any allowance or adjustments were made for multiple comparisons (performing multiple hypothesis tests on the same data).
- Report how any outlying data were treated in the analysis.
- Say whether tests were one- or two-tailed and justify the use of one-tailed tests.
- Report the alpha level (e.g., 0.05) that defines statistical significance.
- Name the statistical program used in the analysis.

Supplementary analyses

- Describe the methods used for any ancillary analyses, such as sensitivity analyses, imputation of missing values, or testing of assumptions underlying the methods of analysis.
- Identify post hoc analyses, including unplanned subgroup analyses, as exploratory.

General principles for reporting statistical results

Reporting numbers and descriptive statistics

- Report numbers – especially measurements – with an appropriate degree of precision. For ease of comprehension and simplicity, round as much as is reasonable. For example, mean age can often be rounded to the nearest year without compromising either the clinical or the statistical analysis. If the smallest meaningful difference on a scale is 5 points, scores can be reported as whole numbers; decimals are not necessary.
- Report the total sample and group size for each analysis.
- Report the numerators and denominators for all percentages.
- Summarize data that are approximately normally distributed with means and standard deviations (SD). Use the form mean (SD), not mean ± SD.
- Summarize data that are not normally distributed with medians and interpercentile ranges, ranges, or both. Report the upper and lower boundaries of interpercentile ranges and the minimum and maximum values of ranges, not just the size of the range.
- Do NOT use the standard error of the mean (SE) to indicate the variability of a data set. Use SDs, interpercentile ranges, or ranges instead.
- Display most if not all data in tables or figures. Tables present exact values, and figures provide an overall assessment of the data [42, 43].

Reporting risk, rates, and ratios

- Identify the type of rate (incidence rates; survival rates), ratio (odds ratios; hazards ratios), or risk (absolute risks; relative risks), being reported.
- Identify the quantities represented in the numerator and denominator (e.g., the number of men with prostate cancer divided by the number of men in whom prostate cancer can develop).
- Identify the time period over which each rate applies.
- Identify any unit of population (i.e., the unit multiplier: e.g., ×100; ×10,000) associated with the rate.
- Consider reporting a measure of precision (a confidence interval) for estimated risks, rates, and ratios.

Reporting hypothesis tests

- State the hypothesis being tested.
- Identify the variables in the analysis and summarize the data for each variable with the appropriate descriptive statistics.
- If possible, identify the minimum difference considered to be clinically important.
- For equivalence and noninferiority studies, report the largest difference between groups that will still be accepted as indicating biological equivalence (the equivalence margin).
- Identify the name of the test used in the analysis. Report whether the test was one- or two-tailed and for paired or independent samples.
- Confirm that the assumptions of the test were met by the data.
- Report the alpha level (e.g., 0.05) that defines statistical significance.
- Report a measure of precision, such as a 95% confidence interval, at least for primary outcomes, such as differences or agreement between groups, diagnostic sensitivity, and slopes of regression lines.
- Do NOT use the SE of the mean to indicate the precision of an estimate. The SE is essentially a 68% confidence coefficient: use the 95% confidence coefficient instead.
- Although not preferred for confidence intervals, if desired, P values should be reported as equalities when possible and to one or two decimal places (e.g., $P = 0.03$ or 0.22) not as inequalities (e.g., $P < 0.05$). Do NOT report "NS"; give the actual P value. The smallest P value that need be reported is $P < 0.001$, except in studies of genetic associations.
- Report whether and how adjustments, if any, were made for multiple statistical comparisons.
- Name the statistical software program used in the analysis.

Reporting association analyses

- Describe the association of interest.
- Identify the variables used and summarize each with descriptive statistics.
- Identify the test of association used.
- Indicate whether the test was one- or two-tailed. Justify the use of one-tailed tests.
- For *tests* of association (e.g., a *chi*-square test), report the *P* value of the test (because association is defined as a statistically significant result).
- For *measures* of association (i.e., the *phi* coefficient), report the value of the coefficient and a confidence interval. Do not describe the association as low, moderate, or high unless the ranges for these categories have been defined. Even then, consider the wisdom of using these categories, given their biological implications or realities.
- For primary comparisons, consider including the full contingency table for the analysis.
- Name the statistical program used in the analysis.

Reporting correlation analyses

- Describe the purpose of the analysis.
- Summarize each variable with the appropriate descriptive statistics.
- Identify the correlation coefficient used in the analysis (e.g., Pearson, Spearman).
- Confirm that the assumptions of the analysis were met.
- Report the alpha level (e.g., 0.05) that indicates whether the correlation coefficient is statistically significant.
- Report the value of the correlation coefficient. Do not describe correlation as low, moderate, or high unless the ranges for these categories have been defined. Even then, consider the wisdom of using these categories given their biological implications or realities.
- For primary comparisons, report the (95%) confidence interval for the correlation coefficient, whether or not it is statistically significant.
- For primary comparisons, consider reporting the results as a scatter plot. The sample size, correlation coefficient (with its confidence interval), and *P* value can be included in the data field.
- Name the statistical program used in the analysis.

Reporting regression analyses

- Describe the purpose of the analysis.
- Identify the variables used in the analysis and summarize each with descriptive statistics.
- Confirm that the assumptions of the analysis were met. For example, in linear regression, indicate whether an analysis of residuals confirmed the assumption of linearity.

- Report how any outlying values were treated in the analysis.
- Report how any missing data were treated in the analyses.
- For either simple or multiple (multivariable) regression analyses, report the regression equation.
- For multiple regression analyses: (1) report the alpha level used in the univariate analysis, (2) report whether the variables were assessed for (a) colinearity and (b) interaction, and (3) describe the variable selection process by which the final model was developed (e.g., forward-stepwise; best subset).
- Report the regression coefficients (beta weights) of each explanatory variable and the associated confidence intervals and P values, preferably in a table.
- Provide a measure of the model's "goodness-of-fit" to the data (the coefficient of determination, r^2, for simple regression and the coefficient of multiple determination, R^2, for multiple regression).
- Specify whether and how the model was validated.
- For primary comparisons made with simple linear regression analysis, consider reporting the results graphically, in a scatter plot, showing the regression line and its confidence bounds. Do not extend the regression line (or the interpretation of the analysis) beyond the minimum and maximum values of the data.
- Name the statistical program used in the analysis.

Reporting analyses of variance (ANOVA) or of covariance (ANCOVA)

- Describe the purpose of the analysis.
- Identify the variables used in the analysis and summarize each with descriptive statistics.
- Confirm that the assumptions of the analysis were met. For example, indicate whether an analysis of residuals confirmed the assumptions of linearity.
- Report how any outlying data were treated in the analysis.
- Report how any missing data were treated in the analyses.
- Specify whether the explanatory variables were tested for interaction, and if so, how these interactions were treated.
- If appropriate, report in a table the P value for each explanatory variable, the test statistics, and, where applicable, the degrees of freedom for the analysis.
- Provide an assessment of the goodness-of-fit of the model to the data, such as R^2.
- Specify whether and how the model was validated.
- Name the statistical program used in the analysis.

Reporting survival (time-to-event) analyses

- Describe the purpose of the analysis.

- Identify the dates or events that mark the beginning and the end of the time period analyzed.
- Specify the circumstances under which data were censored.
- Specify the statistical methods used to estimate the survival rate.
- Confirm that the assumptions of survival analysis were met.
- For each group, give the estimated survival probability at appropriate follow-up times, with confidence intervals, and the number of participants at risk for death at each time. It is often more helpful to plot the cumulative probability of not surviving, especially when events are not common.
- Report median survival times, with confidence intervals, which is often useful to allow results to be compared with those of other studies.
- Consider presenting the complete results in a graph (e.g., a Kaplan–Meier plot) or a table.
- Specify the statistical methods used to compare two or more survival curves.
- When comparing two or more survival curves with hypothesis tests, report the *P* value of the comparison.
- Report the regression model used to assess the associations between the explanatory variables and survival or time-to-event.
- Report a measure of risk (e.g., a hazard ratio) for each explanatory variable, with a confidence interval.

Reporting Bayesian analyses

- Specify the pretrial probabilities ("priors").
- Explain how the priors were selected.
- Describe the statistical model used.
- Describe the techniques used in the analysis.
- Identify the statistical software program used in the analysis.
- Summarize the posterior distribution with a measure of central tendency and a credibility interval.
- Assess the sensitivity of the analysis to different priors.

References

1 Esquirol, J.E.D. Cited in: Pearl, R. (1941) *Introduction to Medical Biometry and Statistics,* WB Saunders, Philadelphia.
2 Schor, S. & Karten, I. (1966) Statistical evaluation of medical journal manuscripts. *JAMA,* **195**, 1123–1128.
3 Prescott, R.J. & Civil, I. (2013) Lies, damn lies and statistics: errors and omission in papers submitted to Injury 2010-2012. *Injury,* **44**, 6–11.
4 Fernandes-Taylor, S., Hyun, J.K., Reeder, R.N. & Harris, A.H. (2011) Common statistical and research design problems in manuscripts submitted to high-impact medical journals. *BMC Research Notes,* **4**, 304.
5 Bosker, T., Mudge, J.F. & Munkittrick, K.R. (2013) Statistical reporting deficiencies in environmental toxicology. *Environmental Toxicology and Chemistry,* **32** (8), 1737–1739.

6 Vesterinen, H.M., Egan, K., Deister, A., *et al.* (2011) Systematic survey of the design, statistical analysis, and reporting of studies published in the 2008 volume of the Journal of Cerebral Blood Flow and Metabolism. *Journal of Cerebral Blood Flow and Metabolism*, **31**, 1064–1072. [Erratum in: *Journal of Cerebral Blood Flow and Metabolism* 2011, 31, 1171].

7 Kim, J.S., Kim, D.K., Hong, S.J. (2011) Assessment of errors and misused statistics in dental research. *International Dental Journal*, **61**, 163–167.

8 Lee, H.J. & Jung, S.K. (2011) The use of statistical methodology in articles in medical journals and suggestions for the quality improvement of the Pediatric Allergy and Respiratory Disease. *Pediatric Allergy and Respiratory Disease*, **21**, 144–155.

9 Yim, K.H., Nahm, F.S., Han, K.A. & Park, S.Y. (2010) Analysis of statistical methods and errors in the articles published in the Korean Journal of Pain. *Korean Journal of Pain*, **23**, 35–41.

10 Al-Benna, S., Al-Ajam, Y., Way, B. & Steinstraesser, L. (2010) Descriptive and inferential statistical methods used in burns research. *Burns*, **36** (3), 343–346.

11 Robinson, P.M., Menakuru, S., Reed, M.W. & Balasubramanian, S.P. (2009) Description and reporting of surgical data – scope for improvement? *Surgeon*, **7** (1), 6–9.

12 Afshar, K., Jafari, S., Seth, A., *et al.* (2009) Publications by the American Academy of Pediatrics Section on Urology: the quality of research design and statistical methodology. *Journal of Urology*, **182** (Suppl. 4), 1906–1910.

13 Barbosa, F.T. & de Souza, D.A. (2010) Frequency of the adequate use of statistical tests of hypothesis in original articles published in the Revista Brasileira de Anestesiologia between January 2008 and December 2009. *Revista Brasileira de Anestesiologia*, **60,** 528–536.

14 Neville, J.A., Lang, W. & Fleischer, A.B. Jr, (2006) Errors in the Archives of Dermatology and the Journal of the American Academy of Dermatology from January through December 2003. *Archives of Dermatology*, **142**, 737–740.

15 Kurichi, J.E. & Sonnad, S.S. (2006) Statistical methods in the surgical literature. *Journal of the American College of Surgery*, **202**, 476–484.

16 Scales, C.D. Jr,, Norris, R.D., Preminger, G.M., *et al.* (2008) Evaluating the evidence: statistical methods in randomized controlled trials in the urological literature. *Journal of Urolology*, **180**, 1463–1467.

17 Gaskin, C.J. & Happell, B. (2014) Power, effects, confidence, and significance: An investigation of statistical practices in nursing research. *International Journal of Nursing Studies*, **51**, 795–806.

18 Jaykaran, Y.P. (2011) Quality of reporting statistics in two Indian pharmacology journals. *Journal of Pharmacology and Pharmacotherapy*, **2** (2), 85–89.

19 Mikolajczyk, R.T., DiSilvestro, A. & Zhang, J. (2008) Evaluation of logistic regression reporting in current obstetrics and gynecology literature. *Obstetrics and Gynecology*, **111** (2 Pt. 1), 413–419.

20 Burton, A. & Altman, D.G. (2004) Missing covariate data within cancer prognostic studies: a review of current reporting and proposed guidelines. *British Journal of Cancer*, **91**, 4–8.

21 Mackinnon, A. (2010) The use and reporting of multiple imputation in medical research – a review. *Journal of Internal Medicine*, **268**, 586–593.

22 Abraira, V., Muriel, A., Emparanza, J.I. *et al.* (2013) Reporting quality of survival analyses in medical journals still needs improvement. *A minimal requirements proposal. Journal of Clinical Epidemiology*, **66**, 1340–1346.

23 Kim, M. (2006) Statistical methods in Arthritis & Rheumatism – current trends. *Arthritis & Rheumatism*, **54**, 3741–3749.

24 Reed, J.F. 3rd,, Salen, P. & Bagher, P. (2003) Methodological and statistical techniques: what do residents really need to know about statistics? *Journal of Medical Systems*, **27** (3), 233–238.

25 Aljoudi, A.S. (2013) Study designs and statistical methods in the Journal of Family and Community Medicine: 1994-2010. *Journal of Family and Community Medicine*, **20** (1), 8–11.

26 Lee, C.M., Soin, H.K. & Einarson, T.R. (2004) Statistics in the pharmacy literature. *Annals of Pharmacotherapy*, **38** (9), 1412–1418.

27 Lang, T. & Secic, M. (2006) *How to Report Statistics in Medicine: Annotated Guidelines for Authors, Editors, and Reviewers*, 2nd edn. American College of Physicians, Philadelphia.

28 O'Fallon, J.R., Duby, S.D., Salsburg, D.S. *et al.* (1978) Should there be statistical guidelines for medical research papers? *Biometrics*, **34**, 687–695.

29 Shott, S. (1985) Statistics in veterinary research. *Journal of the American Veterinary Medical Association*, **187**, 138–141.

30 Hayden, G.F. (1983) Biostatistical trends in Pediatrics: implications for the future. *Pediatrics*, **72**, 84–87.

31 Altman, D.G. & Bland, J.M. (1991) Improving doctors' understanding of statistics. *Journal of the Royal Statistical Society: Series A*, **154**, 223–267.

32 Altman, D.G., Gore, S.M., Gardner, M.J. & Pocock, S.J. (1983) Statistical guidelines for contributors to medical journals. *British Medical Journal*, **286**, 1489–1493.

33 Bailar, J.C. 3rd, & Mosteller, F. (1988) Guidelines for statistical reporting in articles for medical journals. Amplifications and explanations. *Annals of Internal Medicine*, **108** (2), 266–273.

34 Bond, G.R., Mintz, J. & McHugo, G.J. (1995) Statistical guidelines for the Archives of PM&R. *Archives of Physical Medicine and Rehabilitation*, **76**, 784–787.

35 Wilkinson, L., Task Force on Statistical Inference (1999) Statistical methods in psychology journals. Guidelines and explanations. *American Psychologist*, **54**, 594–604.

36 Curran-Everett, D., Benos, D.J., American Physiological Society (2004) Guidelines for reporting statistics in journals published by the American Physiological Society. *American Journal of Physiology, Endocrinology and Metabolism*, **287**, E189–E191. [Plus other journals].

37 Curran-Everett, D. & Benos, D.J. (2007) Guidelines for reporting statistics in journals published by the American Physiological Society: the sequel. *Advances in Physiology Education*, **31**, 295–298.

38 Moher, D., Schulz, K., Altman, D.G., for the CONSORT Group (2001) CONSORT statement: revised recommendations for improving the quality of reports of parallel-group randomized trials. *Annals of Internal Medicine*, **134**, 657–662.

39 Des Jarlais, D.C., Lyles, C., Crepaz, N., Trend Group. (2004) Improving the reporting quality of nonrandomized evaluations of behavioral and public health interventions: the TREND statement. *American Journal of Public Health*, **94** (3), 361–366.

40 von Elm, E., Altman, D.G., Egger, M., Pocock, S.J., Gotzsche, P.C. & Vandenbroucke, J.P. (2007) The Strengthening the Reporting of Observational Studies in Epidemiology (STROBE) Statement: guidelines for reporting observational studies. *Annals of Internal Medicine*, **147** (8), 573–577.

41 International Committee of Medical Journal Editors. Uniform requirements for manuscripts submitted to biomedical journals: writing and editing for biomedical publication, 2011. www.icmje.org [accessed on 12 December 2012].

42 Schriger, D.L., Arora, S. & Altman, D.G. (2006) The content of medical journal instructions for authors. *Annals of Emergency Medicine*, **48**, 743–749, 749.e1-4.

43 Lang, T. (2010) *How to Write, Publish, and Present in the Health Sciences: A Guide for Clinicians and Laboratory Researchers*. American College of Physicians, Philadelphia.

CHAPTER 26

Guidelines for Presenting Tables and Figures in Scientific Manuscripts

David L. Schriger
UCLA Emergency Medicine Center, Los Angeles, CA, USA

Introduction

Most reporting guidelines say far more about the reporting of methods than about the reporting of results. The imbalance is not accidental; guideline-makers, confident of their wisdom regarding the presentation of methods, are far less certain about how to optimize the reporting of results.

There is controversy regarding how much data should be presented. While tomes have been written on the tabular and graphical representation of data [1–9], the paucity of empirical evidence and the omnipresence of competing principles make it extremely challenging to distill advice into succinct guidelines. Consequently, this chapter, unlike others in this book, does not attempt to provide comprehensive guidelines for reporting tables and figures. Instead, it summarizes the principles to be considered when determining what data to present and how best to present it and offers practical tips regarding graphs commonly used in specific research designs.

What to present?

- *Make your paper consensible*. Ziman argued that scientific communications must be consensible, that is, "each message should not be so obscure or ambiguous that the recipient is unable either to give it whole-hearted assent or to offer well-founded objections" [10]. Hence, provide all the data that a colleague would want to see before rendering an opinion about the merits of your work and the reasonableness of your conclusions. Except for the simplest categorical data, figures and tables will be needed to do this efficiently.

Guidelines for Reporting Health Research: A User's Manual, First Edition. Edited by David Moher, Douglas G. Altman, Kenneth F. Schulz, Iveta Simera and Elizabeth Wager.
© 2014 John Wiley & Sons, Ltd. Published 2014 by John Wiley & Sons, Ltd.

- *Let your research protocol guide your data presentation.* If a variable was important enough to be considered in your research protocol, it is important enough to be presented in your results. If two variables are suggested to be interrelated in the theoretical model of your research [11], show that relationship in your Results section.
- *Share important findings outside your research protocol.* Serendipity plays an important role in research. Share unanticipated findings and relationships, but make it clear to readers that these are post-hoc discoveries.
- *Recognize that presentation graphics and archival graphics have different purposes and formats.* Use web-only appendices for archival tables and figures. Tables and figures in the paper should help readers understand the results, guiding them through important information and key comparisons. The tables and figures in a paper make it comprehensible; the archival tables and figures make the results comprehensive.

What format to use: figure, table, or text?

- *Figures are generally preferred for data presentation*: Except for the simplest categorical data, figures provide more information than tables and foster comparisons [12].
- *Consider hybrid formats*: One does not need to choose between a table *or* a figure. Tables with embedded figures (such as small histograms that show the distribution of a variable being presented in a table) can be highly effective [13].
- *Consider whether the structure of the data demands special treatment*: Situations that may require specialized plots include survival (survival curves), meta-analysis (forest plots, funnel plots), diagnostic test performance (Receiver Operating Characteristic (ROC) curves), and comparisons of a measurement (Bland–Altman plots).
- *Choose the most detailed format that emphasizes important comparisons*: Use the most detailed format [e.g., scatter plots of various kinds, survival curves, parallel line plots (and other methods for depicting paired data)] that shows readers the key comparison(s). Reserve lower density plots (box plots, bar graphs) and tables for the rare circumstance when it is impractical to emphasize key comparisons in a more detailed graphic.
- *Avoid formats with low data density*: The numerator for the data density calculation for a bar graph with 4 bars and nothing more is 8 (4 bar heights and 4 bar identifiers). If this graph runs two columns wide in a typical medical journal, it will have a density of roughly $8/66 \text{ cm}^2 = 0.12$ data elements/cm^2. A sentence listing the 8 bits of information would have data density $8/15 \text{ cm}^2 = 0.53$. Since medical journal readers have the cognitive capacity to picture the bar graph while reading the text, the higher density text is preferred.

General principles for tables and figures

- *Tell your story*: Use tables and figures to highlight for readers your insights into the key findings of the study. Use formats that emphasize the comparisons you want them to see. Ensure that the hierarchy of information portrayed in the graphic matches your beliefs about the relative importance of the information.
- *Don't deprive readers the chance to tell other stories*: While it is wholly appropriate to create graphics that stress your interpretation of the data, your graphics should not deprive readers of the opportunity to create alternative explanations. A table or a bar graph showing only group means deprives the reader a view of the underlying distributions. Such distributions might make clear that a difference in means is an incomplete description of the difference among groups. Similarly, additional dimensions can be included in most graphs using different symbol shapes, shades, and color. This can be done in a manner that does not compete with the main comparison but allows the reader to make important secondary comparisons.
- *Make figures and tables self-explanatory*. Readers who have a little more than a general familiarity with your topic should be able to look at any table or figure in isolation and understand what is being presented. This can be done through proper titles, clear labeling, and appropriate captions. Test your creations on colleagues to determine whether they meet this goal and refine as needed.
- *Make the readers' task easier*:
  - Abbreviate only when absolutely necessary
  - Make sure to specify the units (e.g., mg/dL) for all quantities
  - Use annotation (arrows, shading, font) to highlight key comparisons
  - Avoid repetition – place information in the highest appropriate category in the following hierarchy (title, subtitle, axis titles, axis labels, legends, captions, individual data points). For example, for a survival curve covering one month, the x-axis labels should be selected day numbers (e.g., 1, 7, 14, 21, 28) and the x-axis title should be "Time (days)" rather than having labels (Day 1 ... Day 7 ... Day 28) and axis title "Time." Similarly, if every data element in a table is in the same unit, then define the units in the title or subtitle. If columns or rows have different units but all the entries in a column or row have the same unit, then define units in the column or row header. Put units in each cell only if there is no noncontradictory higher level to place them in.

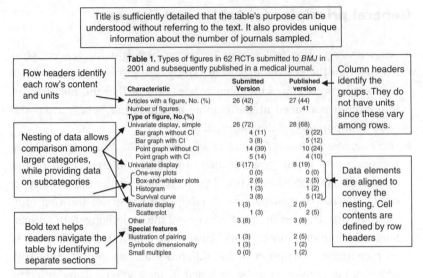

Title is sufficiently detailed that the table's purpose can be understood without referring to the text. It also provides unique information about the number of journals sampled.

Row headers identify each row's content and units

Nesting of data allows comparison among larger categories, while providing data on subcategories

Bold text helps readers navigate the table by identifying separate sections

Column headers identify the groups. They do not have units since these vary among rows.

Data elements are aligned to convey the nesting. Cell contents are defined by row headers

Table 1. Types of figures in 62 RCTs submitted to *BMJ* in 2001 and subsequently published in a medical journal.

Characteristic	Submitted Version	Published version
Articles with a figure, No. (%)	26 (42)	27 (44)
Number of figures	36	41
Type of figure, No.(%)		
Univariate display, simple	26 (72)	28 (68)
Bar graph without CI	4 (11)	9 (22)
Bar graph with CI	3 (8)	5 (12)
Point graph without CI	14 (39)	10 (24)
Point graph with CI	5 (14)	4 (10)
Univariate display	6 (17)	8 (19)
One-way plots	0 (0)	0 (0)
Box-and-whisker plots	2 (6)	2 (5)
Histogram	1 (3)	1 (2)
Survival curve	3 (8)	5 (12)
Bivariate display	1 (3)	2 (5)
Scatterplot	1 (3)	2 (5)
Other	3 (8)	3 (8)
Special features		
Illustration of pairing	1 (3)	2 (5)
Symbolic dimensionality	1 (3)	1 (2)
Small multiples	0 (0)	1 (2)

Figure 26.1 Characterisitics of high quality tables.

Source: The underlying table, taken from a paper on the quality of figures and tables in *BMJ* articles [24], is used with permission of the American College of Emergency Physicians and Elsevier.

General principles for tables

- *Don't use a table when a figure would be better*: Tables are most useful when data are counts, proportions, or percentages because there is no distribution to depict.
- *Don't use a table when text would be better*: One does not need a table to show that the binary outcome (in a cohort study) was achieved in 20% of controls and 40% of cases. The previous sentence did that perfectly, and in less space.
- *Know the purpose of your table*: Decide whether you are making a presentation table or an archival table.
- *Use the title to identify the content of the cells*: Prepare your reader for what to expect in the table. See Figure 26.1 and subsequent items for more details.
- *Ensure that the content of every cell is explained in unambiguous terms*: Make sure that column and row headers are complete and noncontradictory. Use footnotes or the caption to explain anything that might be unclear.
- *Use nesting to show stratified values, subtotals, and grand totals*: Tables can depict several layers of data. Take advantage of this feature to show readers stratified results.

General principles for figures

- *Do not use a figure when text would be better*: A bar graph depicting a control group at 20% and a treatment group at 40% on the *y*-axis "30-day survival (%)" conveys no more information than the sentence "20% of controls and 40% of treated cases were alive at 30 days."

- *Show as much data as possible*: If the number of subjects is small enough to permit depiction of each subject's result, then do so. Summary results can be superimposed in a darker shade on top of these data. If the N is too large to permit depiction of individual subject's values, use histograms or box plots to show the distribution. See Figures 26.2 and 26.3 for examples of this and subsequent items.
- *Stratify data when appropriate*: Use symbols, line types, and color to differentiate important strata in your data. This can usually be done in a way that does not distract from the main comparison but makes the stratified data available to interested readers.
- *Avoid legends when possible*: By directly labeling objects such as curves on graphs, you keep your readers' eyes on the data, the most important part of your figure. When you must use a legend, orient the items to match their orientation in the data.
- *Try rotating box plots and bar graphs 90°*: Although bars are traditionally oriented vertically, there is no good reason to do so. When identifiers are wider than box (bar) width, rotate the graphic by 90° so the identifiers can be placed to the left of each element where they can be easily read.

Make figures visually efficient:

- Subordinate all nondata elements so that they do not compete with data elements for the attention of the readers. For example, gridlines, if used, should be as thin as possible and very faint, noticeable if one seeks them out, but otherwise subordinated to the data.
- Do not use color, shading, or 3D perspective unless they serve a specific explanatory function in the graph.
- *Avoid pie charts*: A sentence or a table is preferred to a pie chart except when a large array of pie charts is used to foster comparisons (e.g., one pie for each of the 50 U.S. states).

Suggestions for specific situations

ROC curves [14–16]

- Make sure that the x- and y-axes are drawn to the same scale so the graphic is a square (not a rectangle) and the chance line is at 45°.
- Label the values of key cut points.
- Consider an insert that reveals a magnified view of the region of clinical interest. For example, if the only area of the curve that is clinically relevant is the region where sensitivity exceeds 90% and several curves lie closely together in that region, consider offering an expanded version of that region (assuming that the N is sufficient to warrant such comparison).

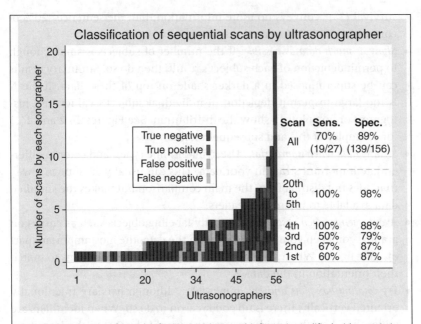

Figure 26.2 Results of a study of a Diagnostic Test. This figure is modified with permission from a paper that appeared in *Annals of Emergency Medicine* [23].

Each colored rectangle represents the ultrasound result as compared to gold standard computerized tomography for 183 scans. Studies done for a given operator are ordered from their first (at the bottom) to their most recent (at the top). Thus, the bottom row is comprised of each of the 56 operators 1st scan.

Explanation:

Many studies of diagnostic tests have two Ns, the number of tests performed and the number of persons performing the testing. It is important to be able to examine each operator's performance since there may be heterogeneity among those performing the test. To further complicate matters, each operator's skill may improve with experience (or diminish due to fatigue or boredom) and it is therefore important to examine performance over time.

Traditionally, the data from this hypothetical study might be reported as "The sensitivity was 70% (19/27) and the specificity 89% (139/156)." The figure provides far more information. It allows readers to see:

• The number of operators
• How many tests were performed by each operator
• Whether operators improved with increasing experience
• Whether performance varied among operators in general and specifically between operators who had high and low participation in the study
• Whether the two types of errors (false negatives and false positives) were more prevalent with certain operators or on initial or later scans by operators.

- Overall, this one graphic tells the story of this research project in far more detail than could be provided in text or a 2x2 table.

  Some features of the graphic worth noting:

- The x axis labels are not equally disbursed (e.g., 1,10,20...) but are chosen to make it easier for readers to calculate how many sonographers did 1 scan, 2 scans, etc. and to show that there were 56 sonographers in the study.
- The colors are carefully chosen so that the bolder shades indicate correct results, the blue squares are persons who are healthy and the red squares persons who have the condition per the gold standard test.
- The table section of this hybrid graphic provides useful information regarding how performance changes with experience.
- The caption guides readers through the figure so they can appreciate all of its nuances.

Forest plots [17, 18]

- Use the *y*-axis to aid interpretation or give information. Sort studies in a meaningful order (by year, effect size, variance, or a clinically meaningful characteristic of the study (e.g., dose used)) rather than by first author's last name. See Figure 26.3 for examples of this and subsequent items.
- When appropriate, create subgroups that include studies with similar execution, outcome measure, etc. so that readers can understand why individual study results may be heterogeneous.
- Choose an *x*-axis scale that is clinically appropriate. Consider the pros and cons of arithmetic versus multiplicative (log/odds) scales and the appropriate range for these scales. When results are tightly clustered, choose a range based on the difference that would be clinically important, not the smallest range that contains the data since the latter may make clinically unimportant differences look important.
- For studies that use counts or proportions, provide the numerators and denominators in the figure. For studies with a continuous outcome, indicate the number of subjects per group.

Survival curves [19]

- Choose a *y*-axis that is clinically appropriate. The default should be 0% to 100% as this is the natural range of such data. Smaller ranges may be used but they should not be so small (e.g., 98% – 100%) that small differences look large, unless differences of this magnitude are clinically important and the study's design supports such precision.
- When the number at risk changes during the study include relevant #s below the *x*-axis at appropriate time points.

This annotated figure illustrates some of the desirable characteristics that can be included in forest plots. Of particular importance, note that studies are not presented en masse in alphabetical order as is so often done [16]. Instead they are grouped by a meaningful stratifying variable (1° or 2° prevention) and then ordered by year of publication. This strategy makes use of the y-axis and may reveal important trends in the results that are related to the ordering variables.

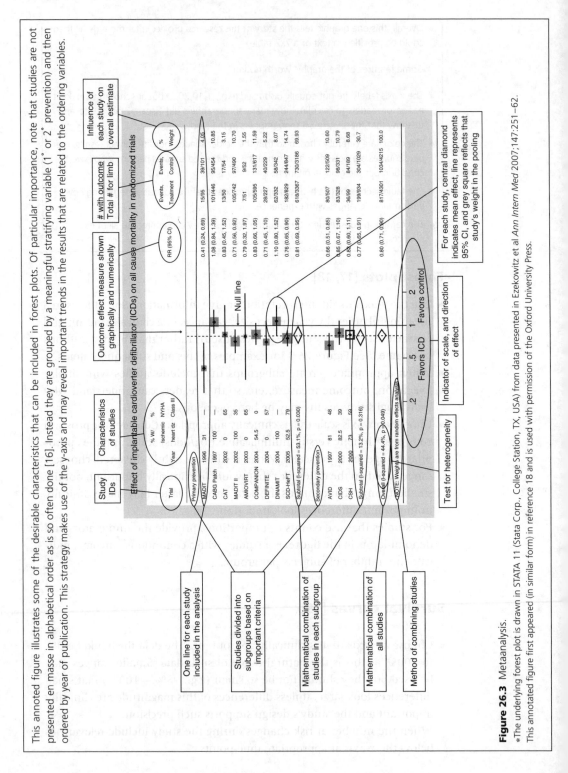

Figure 26.3 Metaanalysis.

*The underlying forest plot is drawn in STATA 11 (Stata Corp., College Station, TX, USA) from data presented in Ezekowitz et al *Ann Intern Med* 2007;147:251–62. This annotated figure first appeared (in similar form) in reference 18 and is used with permission of the Oxford University Press.

Box plots [20]

- Avoid them when the N is small enough that actual values can be shown with lines added to indicate descriptive statistics (e.g., median, mean).
- Ensure that elements of the box plot are defined. Though conventions for the representation of the median, 25th and 75th percentiles, and outlying values are standardized, there are several conventions for drawing the whiskers. Use the caption to define your format and any other nuances (e.g., if you draw the mean as well as the median).
- Depict the N each box is based on near the box identifier.
- Try to label each box directly rather than using a legend. Consider orienting the boxes horizontally so that each box's identifier is easy to read.

Bar graphs

- Always consider whether the whole bar is needed or whether a symbol identifying the height of the bar would be sufficient. When the x-axis is time, line graphs are often preferred to bar graphs.
- Are most effective when depicting data that are nested so that several comparisons are possible.
- Do not use for continuous data. A boxplot is almost always preferred.
- Do not use when there are so few bars that the information can easily be provided in a single sentence or a two-column table.
- Do not graph both sides of a binary proportion (e.g., do not graph both % male and % female, choose one).

Paired data [9, 21]

- When data are paired, use a format that shows the pairing. For small ($N < 25$) studies, a parallel coordinate line segment plot (before-and-after plot) may be effective as each subject's pre-value (on the L y-axis) and post-value (on the R y-axis) are connected by a line segment and the slopes of this family of lines provides a visual representation of how subjects changed. For larger studies, a parallel line plot is preferred. In this plot, each subject is represented by a vertical line that is drawn between pre- and post-values as measured on the y-axis. By sorting subjects from the lowest to the highest pre-value (or post-value in some cases), the patterns in the data are revealed. An alternative format is to graph each subject's pre-value on the x-axis and post-pre change on the y-axis.

Stratified data [1, 9]

- Stratification within a single plot can be achieved with shape, color, and pattern.
- Stratification can also be achieved with small multiples, repeated versions of the same graphic.

Table 1 (participant baseline characteristics) [22]

- Avoid *P*-values since no study is powered with the purpose of comparing baseline values. In randomized trials, differences are, by definition, random, so there is no point in testing to see if they are random. Furthermore, confounding can occur in the presence or absence of statistically significant differences and the presence of statistically significant differences does not imply that confounding has occurred.
- Consider hybrid formats that show minihistograms of each continuous data element [9, 13].
- When presenting binary variables (e.g., sex) present only one of the two options (there is no need to have an entry for men and an entry for women).

References

1 Tufte, E.R. (1983) *The Visual Display of Quantitative Information*, pp. 107–121, Graphics Press, Cheshire, CT.

2 Cleveland, W.S. (1985) *Elements of Graphing Data*, pp. 229–294, Wadsworth Advanced Books and Software, Monterey, CA.

3 Cleveland, W.S. (1993) *Visualizing Data*. Hobart Press, Summit, NJ.

4 Tufte, E.R. (1990) *Envisioning Information*. Graphics Press, Cheshire, CT.

5 Tufte, E.R. (1997) *Visual Explanations: Images and Quantities, Evidence and Narrative*. Graphics Press, Cheshire, CT.

6 Lang, T.A. & Secic, M. (2006) *How to Report Statistics in Medicine: Annotated Guidelines for Authors, Editors, and Reviewers*, 2nd edn. American College of Physicians, Philadephia PA, pp. 325–392.

7 Lang, T.A. (2009) *How to Write, Publish, and Present in the Health Sciences: A Guide for Physicians and Laboratory Researchers*, pp. 67–100, American College of Physicians, Philadephia PA.

8 Briscoe, M.H. (1996) *Preparing Scientific Illustrations: A Guide to Better Posters, Presentations, and Publications*, 2nd edn. Springer-Verlag, New York, NY.

9 Schriger, D.L. & Cooper, R.J. (2001) Achieving graphical excellence: suggestions and methods for creating high quality visual displays of experimental data. *Annals of Emergency Medicine*, **37** (1), 75–87.

10 Ziman, R. (1978) *Reliable Knowledge: An Exploration of the Grounds for Belief in Science*, pp. 7, Cambridge University Press, Cambridge, England.

11 Schriger, D.L. (2005) Suggestions for improving the reporting of clinical research: the role of narrative. *Annals of Emergency Medicine*, **45**, 437–443.

12 Gelman, A., Pasarica, C. & Dodhia, R. (2002) Let's practice what we preach: turning tables into graphs. *The American Statistician*, **56**, 121–130.

13 Examples include: (a) Green, S.M. *et al.* (2009) Predictors of emesis and recovery agitation with emergency department ketamine sedation: an individual-patient data meta-analysis of 8,282 children. *Annals of Emergency Medicine*, **54**, 171–180 (pages e2–4)   http://download.journals.elsevierhealth.com/pdfs/journals/0196-0644/PIIS 0196064409003722.pdf; (b) Gupta, M. *et al.* (2011) Selective use of computed tomography compared with routine whole body imaging in patients with blunt trauma. *Annals of Emergency Medicine*, doi:10.1016/j.annemergmed.2011 .06.003 (Appendix 1) http://www.annemergmed.com/article/S0196-0644%2811% 2900611-1/journalimage?loc=fx1&issn=0196-0644&src=tbl.

14 Zweig, M.H. & Campbell, G. (1993) Receiver-operating characteristic (ROC) plots: a fundamental evaluation tool in clinical medicine. *Clinical Chemistry*, **39** (4), 561–577.

15 Hanley, J.A. & McNeil, B.J. (1982) The meaning and use of the area under a receiver operating characteristic (ROC) curve. *Radiology*, **143** (1), 29–36.

16 McClish, D.K. (1989) Analyzing a portion of the ROC curve. *Medical Decision Making*, **9**, 190–195.

17 Lewis, S. & Clarke, M. (2001) Forest plots: trying to see the wood and the trees. *BMJ*, **322**, 1479–1480.

18 Schriger, D.L., Altman, D.G., Vetter, J.A., *et al.* (2010) Forest plots in reports of systematic reviews: a cross-section study reviewing current practice. *International Journal of Epidemiology*, **39**, 421–429.

19 Kaplan, E.L. & Meier, P. (1958) Non-parametric estimation from incomplete observations. *Journal of the American Statistical Association*, **53**, 457–481.

20 McGill, R., Tukey, J.W., Larsen, W.A. (1978) Variations of box plots. *The American Statistician*, **32**, 12–16. doi:10.2307/2683468.

21 McNeil, D. (1992) On graphing paired data. *The American Statistician*, **46**, 307–311.

22 Moher, D., Hopewell, S., Schulz, K.F. *et al.*, for the CONSORT Group (2010) CONSORT 2010 Explanation and Elaboration: updated guidelines for reporting parallel group randomised trial. *BMJ*, **340**, c869.

23 Kline J.A., O'Malley P.M., Tayal V.S., *et al.* Emergency clinician-performed compression ultrasonography for deep venous thrombosis of the lower extremity. *Ann Emerg Med.* 2008 Oct; **52**(4): 437–45. doi: 10.1016/j.annemergmed.2008.05.023.

24 Schriger D.L., Sinha R., Schroter S., *et al.* From Submission to Publication: A Retrospective Review of the Tables and Figures in a Cohort of Randomized Controlled Trials Submitted to the *BMJ*, *Ann Emerg Med.* 2006; **48**: 750–6 & e1–21.

CHAPTER 27

Documenting Clinical and Laboratory Images in Publications: The CLIP Principles*

Thomas A. Lang[1], Cassandra Talerico[2] and George C. M. Siontis[3]

[1] *Tom Lang Communications and Training International, Kirkland, WA, USA*
[2] *Neurological Institute Research and Development Office, Cleveland Clinic, Cleveland, OH, USA*
[3] *Clinical Trials and Evidence-Based Medicine Unit, Department of Hygiene and Epidemiology, University of Ioannina School of Medicine, Ioannina, Greece*

Introduction

Analytical images in the laboratory sciences and diagnostic images in clinical medicine differ from other figures in scientific publications because they do not simply present, organize, or summarize information, they *are* the information. For this reason alone, they should be documented well. In addition, because interpretations of these images can vary widely (sometimes notoriously so), accurate and complete documentation should be provided to support each specific interpretation. However, although the *procedures* for acquiring and interpreting many of these images are standardized and published, the information needed to document them in a scientific article remains to be specified for most. Without appropriate guidelines, documenting these images in scientific publications will almost certainly be incomplete and inconsistent, a fact confirmed by a recent study of more than 200 images from 12 major general and specialty journals [1] and in another study of 19 articles reporting the details of magnetic resonance images of 2801 breasts [2].

Most of the guidelines on documenting biomedical images in journals are self-evident. However, as imaging technologies become more complex, so too does the information needed to completely document how the images were acquired. This point is well illustrated by Warren and Graves who have identified the technical details of acquiring magnetic

---

*This chapter is reproduced with permission from *Chest* and was previously published as *Chest* 2012;141:1626–1632.

Guidelines for Reporting Health Research: A User's Manual, First Edition. Edited by David Moher, Douglas G. Altman, Kenneth F. Schulz, Iveta Simera and Elizabeth Wager.
© 2014 John Wiley & Sons, Ltd. Published 2014 by John Wiley & Sons, Ltd.

resonance images (Appendix). Thus, although we describe here the general components of documentation, specific requirements will have to be identified by the professional associations in fields that use these imaging technologies. As a result, this chapter differs from others in the book because the complete guidelines it proposes are still in the early stages of development and are awaiting contributions from the relevant associations. In the meantime, the guidelines presented here should provide both a foundation and a direction for development.

This chapter draws heavily on Chapter 10 titled "How to Document Biomedical Images for Publication" of *How to Write, Publish, and Present in the Health Sciences: A Guide for Clinicians and Laboratory Scientists* [3]. It presents some general principles for documenting images and some preliminary guidelines for documenting specific types of images. This chapter expands on those general guidelines.

Components of documentation

The guiding principle of reporting analytical and diagnostic images is to provide the information that readers need to assess the accuracy, completeness, validity, and credibility of the stated interpretation and implications of the image. The goal is to prevent missing or misleading information from reducing or distorting the accuracy of its interpretation. This guiding principle is more easily followed by always considering the six components of documentation described later. The elements in the components are intended to be prompts for consideration rather than mandatory reporting requirements.

1 What is the image of?(Report the details of the subject of the image)
- *Tell readers what, in general, they are looking at and for.* Identify the molecule, protein, cell, tissue, organ, organism, animal, body part, region, signs, or condition (in photos of patients) shown in the image.
- *State the reason for acquiring the image.* Common reasons include qualitative and quantitative analyses to establish or confirm a diagnosis, to stage a disease, or to assess the effects of treatment. If the image is used diagnostically, report the patient's presenting signs and symptoms and any differential diagnoses being considered when the image was acquired. Images of patients should not be presented unless such an image is necessary to establish or refute an important claim in the article.
- *Describe any relevant biological, historical, or physical characteristics of the sample or subject needed to understand the image.* These characteristics may include the source of specimens and how and when they were obtained for imaging. For images of patients, report any relevant demographic

(age, sex, socioeconomic status, living conditions), clinical (diagnosis, vital signs; pertinent positive and negative findings), and lifestyle (smoking status, fitness level, occupational or environmental exposures) characteristics.

2 How was the image acquired?(Report the details of the acquisition of the image)

- *Name the relevant hardware and software used to acquire the image* [2]. Identify the manufacturer's name and location and the make and model of the imaging equipment, the source of any reagents used, and the name and version of any computer programs used.
- *Describe any relevant hardware and software settings* [2], such as optical or band-pass filters, sampling algorithms, amplification, or other technical information necessary to understand how the image was acquired, which could affect the interpretation of the image.
- *Identify any procedures for preparing the sample or subject for imaging.* For analytical images, if applicable, give the details of any stains or markers used to label parts of the sample, and the nature of any positive or negative controls. For diagnostic images, if applicable, specify any contrast media used, including the dose, route, and timing of its administration relative to the acquisition of the image, and any fasting, voiding, or dietary preparations. Ideally, patients should be photographed without makeup or jewelry. Postoperative results, including scars, should never be obscured by clothing [4].
- *Note any relevant physical or environmental conditions present during image acquisition.* For clinical images, if applicable, state the conditions under which the image was taken (in the emergency department, operating room, ambulatory care center, during a stress test, etc.); identify whether the image is of a subject that is *in vivo* or *in vitro*. Postoperative photographs should always be taken after any edema from the procedure has disappeared completely [5].
- *Describe or reference the procedures or protocols used to acquire the image,* such as standard radiographic views or any evocative or suppressive techniques, used to increase the diagnostic value of the image (e.g., having patients lie still or hold their breath).
- *Describe the condition of the sample or subject during imaging.* If applicable, specify the patient's position or posture (seated; supine), state of consciousness (asleep; anesthetized), and any medications in the patient's system during imaging that might affect the image (e.g., cardiotropic drugs active during electrocardiography).

3 Why was the image selected for publication?(Report the details of the selection of the image)

- *Indicate whether the image came from a sample or subject that was part of the research population under investigation or whether it was obtained from an outside source* [1]. Images from outside sources are usually illustrative or normative of the information they convey.

- *If applicable, tell why the specific image was chosen for publication, as opposed to other related images* [1]. The representativeness or quality of the images are obvious reasons, but there may be others, such as those obtained at a particular time or under particular conditions.

- *Indicate whether the image shows a typical, extreme, or a selected case* [1]. Details of extreme and selected cases should be given [1].

- *If the image is of an extreme or a selected case, consider including an image of a typical case for comparison* [1, 4].

- *For images that are meant to be compared, such as slides with different stains or preoperative and postoperative photographs, identify any differences in the conditions under which they were acquired* [6].

4 If the image was modified, how was it changed?(Report the details of any modifications of the image)

- *Disclose any (digital) processing, modifications, or enhancements of the original image*, such as adjustments for brightness or color balance, digital manipulation with programs such as Photoshop™, or magnification, to obtain the final published image [6–8]. Such adjustments are acceptable if they are applied to the whole image and as long as they do not obscure, eliminate, or misrepresent any information present in the original image. This issue is especially relevant to laboratory images [9–11], where some basic science journals report that 25% of all accepted manuscripts have included one or more illustrations that were manipulated in ways that violated the journal's guidelines [12], but clinical images, such as digital radiographs, are also subject to intentional modification (including insurance fraud and tainting legal evidence), image reconstruction, or unintentional loss of fidelity when transmitted electronically [13, 14]. However, in clinical photographs, it is permissible to remove background elements that would distract from the subject of the image [15, 16]. Such modifications should not alter the information in the image, however.

- In basic science journals, "Do not enhance, obscure, move, remove, or introduce specific features within an image. In particular, do not: delete a band from a blot, even if it is irrelevant; add a band to a blot, even if you know for sure that such a protein or DNA fragment or RNA is present in your sample; adjust the intensity of a single band in a blot; digitally remove unwanted background elements; move a band from one part of a gel to another part, even if you do not change its size; or juxtapose pieces from different gels to compare the levels of proteins or nucleic acids. All samples should be run on the same gel." [11]

- *Make any grouping of images from different parts of the same image, gel, or from different gels, fields, or exposures, explicit in the arrangement of the figure (e.g., by using dividing lines) and in the figure legend* [11]. You may need to work with the journal to assure that image parts are placed correctly and differentiated from one another in the final publication.
- *Be ready to submit both the original and the enhanced image to the journal for comparison.* If the author cannot produce the original image when asked, some journals will reject the manuscript [17]. Many basic science journals now evaluate digital images using software designed to detect digital manipulation [8, 18].
- *Remove all patient identifiers (names, patient numbers) from the image before submission.*
- *For images of identifiable patients, obtain written permission from the patient or the patient's legal guardian.* Such permission should be sought before submitting the manuscript for publication, if not before acquiring the image. Covering the patient's eyes on the photo with a black rectangle is not sufficient to maintain anonymity and should not be used in lieu of written consent. It is not enough that the public cannot determine the patient's identity; the patient and the patient's family must likewise be unable to determine the patient's identity from the photograph [4, 16].

5 What does the image show and where does it show it?(Report the important details of the image itself)

- *Indicate what the image shows and where it shows it.* Mark the presence (or absence) of relevant details on the image with circles, arrows, inserts, outlining, or other graphic devices and include other comments in the caption or text [19]. Show scale bars, color codes, or other values if appropriate. Marks added to the image should not obscure important details.

  - *Report the resolution and any magnification of the image and describe any enhancements made to it* [4]. Remember that magnification increases the *amount of detail* that can be seen; enlargement increases only *the size of the details* that are already visible. Magnification is indicated with the appropriate multiplier: ×1000, for example.
  - *Indicate the orientation of the sample or subject in the image.* For example, identify the patient's left and right sides, the top or bottom on the subject, the angle from which the image was taken, the plane or level of any sections (e.g., a cross section at the level of the third thoracic vertebra), and whether the view is anteroposterior or posteroanterior.

6 What does the image mean?(Report the details of the *analysis* or interpretation and the implications of the image)

- *Report any quantitative or qualitative data associated with the image.* Such data may include measurements (e.g., anterior wall thickness, tumor size), or grades (e.g., New York Heart Association class IV). If color scales are used, indicate the meaning of the colors or how to interpret the color scale on the image or in the caption [1]. For laboratory images, give the criteria for identification and measurement (e.g., cell-counting or estimating procedures).
- *Describe the circumstances under which the image was analyzed or evaluated* [2]. If applicable, report the credentials of each evaluator (whether they were board certified; how many years they have worked in the field). Indicate whether certain information was provided to, or withheld from, the evaluator before the evaluation. If two or more evaluators interpreted the image, comment on their degree of agreement (e.g., "All three evaluators agreed on the following . . ."). It may also be appropriate to include a measure of intrarater or interrater agreement, such as the kappa statistic or the percentage of concordant interpretations.
- *Interpret the meaning and implications of the image in light of all the above information.* Support the interpretation with references to the features of the image (or lack thereof) and to other evidence related to the image. In all images, the possibility of confounding by artifacts should be specifically addressed [20, 21]. For clinical images, specify the criteria for the diagnosis, the treatment, or prognostic implications of a positive or a negative result, and the presence, proportion, and explanation for any equivocal diagnostic results.

Placement of information in the text

Information included in the published article to meet these guidelines may be placed in the text, under headings such as "Examination Technique," "Imaging Technique," or "Image Analysis," or in figure captions. Figure captions in clinical journals should identify the information in the image and summary information about the image's subject, acquisition, appearance, and interpretation, as space allows. Details should usually be placed in the text. Figure captions in basic science journals should also identify the information in the image but may also describe the details of sample preparation and image acquisition.

Further development

We believe that reporting guidelines should continue to be created for existing and emerging imaging technologies, and we have provided a foundation and a direction for doing so. However, we have reached the limits of our abilities to participate in the development process. As mentioned in the Introduction, specific guidelines – especially those dealing with the technical aspects of image acquisition – will have to be identified by the professionals who use these technologies and who must interpret the images they produce. Ideally, new guidelines would be approved by the appropriate professional associations and endorsed by the appropriate journals. We believe such activities are necessary because to paraphrase photographer and environmentalist, Ansel Adams, "Images are usually looked at – and seldom looked into." [22].

Acknowledgments

We thank Bart Harvey, Director of Research in Family Medicine, Director of Program Evaluation for the Physician Training program, Associate Chair of the Department of Public Health Sciences, Toronto, Canada, for his thoughtful review of early drafts of the chapter; Ruth Warren, University Department of Radiology, Cambridge, United Kingdom; Martin Graves, Consultant Clinical Scientist Cambridge University Hospitals Trust Cambridge, United Kingdom, for their substantive contributions to the guidelines on reporting magnetic resonance images.

References

1 Siontis, G.C., Patsopoulos, N.A., Vlahos, A.P. & Ioannidis, J.P. (2010) Selection and presentation of imaging figures in the medical literature. *PLoS One*, **5** (5), e10888.

2 Warren, R., Clatto, S., Macaskill, P., Black, R. & Houssami, N. (2009) Technical aspects of breast MRI – do they affect outcome? *European Radiology*, **19**, 1629–1638.

3 Lang, T. (2010) *How to Write, Publish, and Present in the Health Sciences: A Guide for Clinicians and Laboratory Scientists*. American College of Physicians, Philadelphia.

4 Aesthetic Surgery Journal. Manuscript Submission Guidelines. http://aes.sagepub .com/site/misc/ManuscriptSubmissions.xhtml [accessed on 10 August 2010].

5 Talamas, I. & Pando, L. (2001) Specific requirements for preoperative and postoperative photos used in publication. *Aesthetic Plastic Surgery*, **25** (4), 307–310.

6 Cromey, D.W. Digital Imaging: Ethics. Available from http://swehsc.pharmacy .arizona.edu/exppath/resources/pdf/Digital_Imaging_Ethics.pdf [accessed on August 10 2010].

7 (2004) Gel slicing and dicing: a recipe for disaster [Editorial]. *Nature Cell Biology*, **6**, 275. doi:10.1038/ncb0404-275.

8   Journal of Cell Science. Instructions for authors. Available from http://www
    .biologists.com/web/submissions/jcs_information.html#anchor_edit_polic [accessed
    on August 10 2010].

9   Suvarna, S.K. & Ansary, M.A. (2001) Histopathology and the 'third great lie'. When
    is an image not a scientifically authentic image? *Histopathology*, **39** (5), 441–446.

10 Tsang, A., Sweet, D. & Wood, R.E. (1999) Potential for fraudulent use of digital radio-
    graphy. *Journal of the American Dental Association*, **130** (9), 1325–1329.

11 Rossner, M. & Yamada, K.M. (2004) What's in a picture? The temptation of image
    manipulation. *Journal of Cellular Biology*, **66**, 11–15. doi:10.1083/jcb.200406019

12 Wade, N. It may look authentic; here's how to tell it isn't. New York Times, 24 January,
    2006.

13 Calberson, F.L., Hommez, G.M. & De Moor, R.J. (2008) Fraudulent use of digital
    radiography: methods to detect and protect digital radiographs. *Journal of Endodontics*,
    34 (5), 530–536. (Epub 14 March 2008).

14 Güneri, P. & Akdeniz, B.G. (2004) Fraudulent management of digital endodontic
    images. *International Endodontic Journal*, **37** (3), 214–220.

15 International Committee of Medical Journal Editors (1995) Protection of patients'
    rights to privacy. *BMJ*, **311**, 1272.

16 JAMA. Instructions for authors. http://jama.ama-assn.org/misc/ authors.dtl
    [accessed on 3 March 2008].

17 Molecular and Cellular Biology. Instructions for authors. Available from http://
    mcb.asm.org/misc/ifora.dtl [accessed on 10 August 2010].

18 Hill, E. (2008) Announcing the JCB DataViewer, a browser-based applica-
    tion for viewing original image files. *Journal of Cell Biology*, **183** (6), 969–970.
    doi:10.1083/jcb.200811132. [Editorial].

19 CHEST. Guidelines for Manuscript Preparation. http://www.chestjournal.org/misc/
    ifora.shtml [accessed on 23 March 2008].

20 Cesar, L.J., Schueler, B.A., Zink, F.E., Daly, T.R., Taubel, J.P. & Jorgenson, L.L.
    (2001) Artifacts found in computed radiography. *British Journal of Radiology*, **74** (878),
    195–202.

21 Oestmann, J.W., Prokop, M., Schaefer, C.M. & Galanski, M. (1991) Hardware and
    software artifacts in storage phosphor radiography. *Radiographics*, **11** (5), 795–805.

22 Adams, A. Great-Quotes.com, Gledhill Enterprises, 2011. http://www.great-
    quotes.com/quote/548633 [accessed on 29 April 2011].

Appendix

An excerpt from an example documenting magnetic resonance images: reporting information on the hardware and software used in image acquisition

The information provided is an excerpt from a complete example of how
to report magnetic resonance images. It illustrates the technical details
required for complete documentation and makes obvious the need for
similar documentation requirements to be developed by the professional
societies that used imaging technologies.

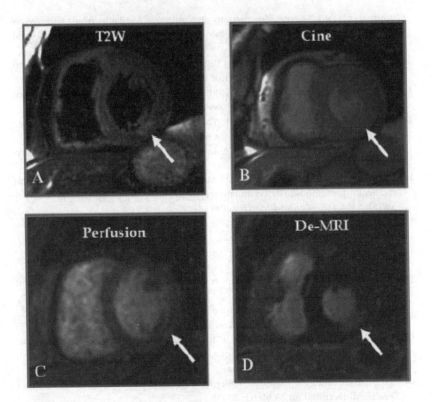

Guideline 2: Report the details of the acquisition of the image

- *Name the relevant hardware and software used to acquire the image.*

    "All patients were examined on a 1.5-Tesla magnet located in the ED (Signa HDx, GE Healthcare, Milwaukee, WI) that had an 8-element, phased-array cardiac coil."

- *Describe any relevant hardware and software settings*

    The following is the complete list of settings.

    1. *MRI scanner field strength* [T, or tesla (lower case t in tesla because it is an SI unit)] and the *scanner model* and *manufacturer* [e.g., "The images were acquired using a 3 T whole-body scanner (Signa HDx, GE Healthcare, Waukesha, WI)"].
    2. Identify the *coil* used (e.g., "The images were acquired using an 8-element cardiac array coil").
    3. *Acquisition mode*: 2D single slice, or 2D multislice, or 3D volume (for the last two modes, give the number of slices).
    4. *Acquisition plane*: State whether the plane was axial, sagittal, or coronal. For single- or double-oblique planes, identify the nearest orthogonal plane (e.g., oblique sagittal or *in vivo* orientation; parallel to the AC–PC line; cardiac short axis).

5. *Pulse sequence*: Identify the pulse sequence used (e.g., fast spin echo; spoiled gradient echo) or reference the specific sequence described in the literature. Several pulse sequences are available.

6. *Scan options*: Report any scan options relevant to image acquisition (e.g., fat suppression method; use of cardiac or respiratory gating) ("Gating" refers to coordinating image acquisition to the pulse or respiratory rate to obtain images at the same point in each cycle.) Several scan options are available.

7. *Geometry information*: Slice thickness and slice gap in millimeters (e.g., 8/2 mm). Field of view (FoV) in millimeters; the field may be different for different frequencies and phase-encoding directions (e.g., 240 × 160 mm).

8. *Acquisition matrix*: The number of frequency encoding steps times the number of phase encoding steps (e.g., 256 × 128). Specify whether the data were interpolated during reconstruction (e.g., "data were interpolated to 512 × 512 pixels").

9. *Timing information* (generally reported in microseconds): *Echo time* (TE) or *effective echo time* (TE_{eff}), if using fast spin echo sequences (e.g., $TE_{eff} = 80$ ms); *repetition time* (TR) and *inversion time* (TI), if using an inversion-recovery type sequence.

10. Other factors: *Acquisition bandwidth* (Hz/pixel); *number of signal averages* performed (e.g., 2 can be <1 for certain acquisitions, such as 0.5). For *parallel acceleration*, specify the type and the acceleration factor (e.g., SENSE factor 2).

11. *Sequence-specific factors*: For gradient echo sequences, provide the excitation flip angle, in degrees (e.g., 45°). For fast/turbo spin echo sequences, provide the echo train length (ETL).

12. For dynamic scans, report the *temporal resolution* (in milliseconds or seconds) and the number of phases acquired (e.g., "Twenty dynamic phases were acquired with a temporal resolution of 5 s").

13. If *contrast* is used, identify the agent and supplier [e.g., "(Gadovist, Bayer, Berkshire, UK)"] and report the volume administered, possibly per patient's weight (e.g., "0.2 mL/kg" or just as a total volume: "10 mL"). If the agent is administered as a bolus, state the type and manufacturer of the power injector used [e.g., "(Spectris, Medrad, PA)" and the injection rate: "5 mL/s."]. State whether any saline chaser was used, including the volume and injection rate of the saline.

14. Give the *overall scan time* for the acquisition in minutes and seconds and, if relevant to the study, mention the total examination time as well.

15. Explain any *postprocessing of the images*, including the details of any region-of-interest (ROI)-based analysis. Identify the analysis software and supplier used [e.g., "(CADstream, Merge Healthcare, Hartland, WI)"].

CHAPTER 28

Reporting Guidelines for Health Economic Evaluations: *BMJ* Guidelines for Authors and Peer Reviewers of Economic Submissions

Andrew H. Briggs[1] *and Michael F. Drummond*[2]

[1] Health Economics and Health Technology Assessment, Institute of Health & Wellbeing, University of Glasgow, Glasgow, UK
[2] University of York, York, UK

Timetable

Reporting guideline	Notes	Meeting date	Publication date
BMJ EE 1996	*BMJ* convened a working party for authors and peer reviewers of papers submitted to *BMJ* in order to improve upon the quality of published articles.	January 1995	1996 [1]

Name of guideline

The *BMJ* guideline for authors and peer reviewers of economic submissions (*BMJ* EE) was created to improve the quality of economic articles published by the *BMJ*. Although it was recognized that general guidelines for economic evaluation had been proposed by many bodies, it was observed that many economic evaluations were published in the medical literature and that few clinical journals had specific guidelines for peer reviewers to assess the quality of submitted economic evaluations. It was not the intention of the guideline to be prescriptive nor to stifle innovative methods in a rapidly evolving field, rather the emphasis was on the clarity of reporting of

Guidelines for Reporting Health Research: A User's Manual, First Edition. Edited by David Moher, Douglas G. Altman, Kenneth F. Schulz, Iveta Simera and Elizabeth Wager.
© 2014 John Wiley & Sons, Ltd. Published 2014 by John Wiley & Sons, Ltd.

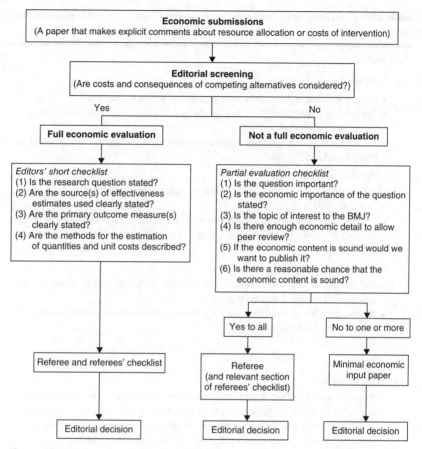

Figure 28.1 Manuscript management flow diagram and checklists for editors.

economic evaluations while avoiding duplication of those aspects that have been routinely covered in other guidelines. The guideline was published in full in the *BMJ* (formerly the *British Medical Journal*) [1]. The manuscript management flow diagram is presented in Figure 28.1 and the summary of the guideline is given in Table 28.1.

When to use the guidelines

The *BMJ* EE is focused on the *BMJ*'s submission and publication processes. Nevertheless, the guidelines are suitable for any health economic evaluations submitted to a wide range of clinical journals, and should be applicable to authors in preparing their manuscript for submission as well as providing a checklist for reviewers and editors to assess the quality of submitted manuscripts.

Table 28.1 Guidelines for authors and peer reviewers of economic submissions to the *BMJ*.

Study design

(1) Study question
- The economic importance of the research question should be outlined.
- The hypothesis being tested, or question being addressed, in the economic evaluation should be clearly stated.
- The viewpoint(s) – for example, healthcare system, society – for the analysis should be clearly stated and justified.

(2) Selection of alternatives
- The rationale for choice of the alternative programmes or interventions for comparison should be given.
- The alternative interventions should be described in sufficient detail to enable the reader to assess the relevance to his or her setting – that is, who did what, to whom, where, and how often.

(3) Form of evaluation
- The form(s) of evaluation used – for example, cost-minimization analysis, cost-effectiveness analysis – should be stated.
- A clear justification should be given for the form(s) of evaluation chosen in relation to the question(s) being addressed.

Data collection

(4) Effectiveness data
- If the economic evaluation is based on a single effectiveness study – for example, a clinical trial – details of the design and results of that study should be given – for example, selection of study population, method of allocation of subjects, whether analyzed by intention-to-treat or evaluable cohort, effect size with confidence intervals.
- If the economic evaluation is based on an overview of a number of effectiveness studies, details should be given of the method of synthesis or meta-analysis of evidence – for example, search strategy, criteria for inclusion of studies in the overview.

(5) Benefit measurement and valuation
- The primary outcome measure(s) for the economic evaluation should be clearly stated – for example, cases detected, life years, quality-adjusted life-years (QALYs), willingness to pay.
- If health benefits have been valued, details should be given of the methods used – for example, time trade-off, standard gamble, contingent valuation – and the subjects from whom valuations were obtained – for example, patients, members of the general public, healthcare professionals.
- If changes in productivity (indirect benefits) are included, they should be reported separately and their relevance to the study question should be discussed.

(6) Costing
- Quantities of resources should be reported separately from the prices (unit costs) of those resources.
- Methods for the estimation of both quantities and prices (unit costs) should be given.
- The currency and price date should be recorded and details of any adjustment for inflation, or currency conversion, should be given.

Table 28.1 (*Continued*)

(7) Modeling

- Details should be given of any modeling used in the economic study – for example, decision tree model, epidemiology model, regression model.
- Justification should be given of the choice of the model and the key parameters.

Analysis and interpretation of results

(8) Adjustments for timing of costs and benefits

- The time horizon over which costs and benefits are considered should be given.
- The discount rate(s) should be given and the choice of rate(s) justified.

If costs or benefits are not discounted, an explanation should be given.

(9) Allowance for uncertainty

- When stochastic data are reported, details should be given of the statistical tests performed and the confidence intervals around the main variables.
- When a sensitivity analysis is performed, details should be given of the approach used – for example, multivariate, univariate, threshold analysis – and justification given for the choice of variables for sensitivity analysis and the ranges over which they are varied.

(10) Presentation of results

- An incremental analysis – for example, incremental cost per life year gained – should be reported, comparing the relevant alternatives.
- Major outcomes – for example, impact on quality of life – should be presented in disaggregated and aggregated forms.
- Any comparisons with other healthcare interventions – for example, in terms of relative cost-effectiveness – should be made only when close similarity in study methods and settings can be demonstrated.
- The answer to the original study question should be given; any conclusions should follow clearly from the data reported and should be accompanied by appropriate qualifications or reservations.

Reproduced from [1] with permission from the BMJ Group Ltd.

Development process

A working party was convened by the *BMJ* in January 1995 with the object of improving the quality of health economic evaluations submitted to and published by the journal. Its task was to produce (1) guidelines for economic evaluation, together with a comprehensive supporting statement that could be easily understood by both specialist and nonspecialist readers; (2) a checklist for use by referees and authors; and (3) a checklist for use by editors.

In producing the guidelines, the working party concentrated on full economic evaluations, which are studies comparing two or more healthcare interventions and considering both costs and consequences. Many of the articles sent to the *BMJ* and other medical journals are often more broadly based "economic submissions," which comprise essentially clinical articles that report approximate cost estimates or make general statements that a given treatment was "cost effective."

The view taken by the working party was that submissions reporting partial evaluations, such as a costing study or an estimate of the value to individuals of improved health, should adhere to the relevant sections of the guidelines, as should anecdotal reports or commentaries drawing economic conclusions about alternative forms of care. In addition to a referees' (and authors') checklist, therefore, the working party produced shorter checklists to help *BMJ* editors distinguish between full economic evaluations and other types of economic submission and to help them decide which articles should be sent to referees.

Drafts of the guidelines and their supporting statement and the checklists were circulated to health economists and journal editors and were debated at the biannual meeting of the UK Health Economists' Study Group in January 1996. A survey of the members attending the meeting was used to identify those items of the full referees' checklist that should be used by editors.

Finally, in drafting the guidelines, the working party recognized that authors may not be able to address all the points in the published version of their paper. In such cases, authors may submit supplementary documents (containing, e.g., the details of any economic model used) or refer the reader to other published sources.

Current version compared to previous versions

There are no plans to update the current version of the *BMJ* EE from the original 1996 version. Nevertheless, there have been many additional guideline documents produced for economic evaluation since 1996, although few specific reporting guidelines have yet been produced. An exception would be the AMCP Format [2]. This is a set of reporting guidelines developed by the Academy of Managed Care Pharmacy in the United States, to enable pharmaceutical companies to respond to requests for economic data from health plans, within the guidelines laid down by the Food and Drug Administration. Significantly, the International Society for Pharmacoeconomics and Outcomes Research published a reporting guideline [3] as this chapter went to press. An overview of the guideline is given as part of the 'Future Plans' section below.

How best to use the guideline

The guideline is specifically designed for three groups. Firstly, for authors to understand what is required when reporting their work and submitting an article for publication in the *BMJ*. Secondly, as a checklist for reviewers to use when appraising the suitability of a submission. Finally, as a (shortened) checklist for editors to use when deciding on the manuscript's suitability for publication.

Evidence of effectiveness of guideline

A before- and after study was conducted in the editorial offices of *BMJ* and *The Lancet* to assess the effect of the *BMJ* EE on review and revision of economic submissions in two 3-month periods, during the year before and around six months after the publication of the guidelines [4]. *The Lancet* was chosen as a control journal for some parts of the study because of its similar scope and size to *BMJ* and because no concerted effort was made to promulgate the guidelines within its editorial office. "Economic submissions" were defined as those papers making explicit comments about resource allocation and/or costs of interventions. Editorial fate and changes (comparing the two time periods) in the quality of submissions (defined in terms of compliance with the guidelines) were used as the outcome variables. Editorial staff in the two journals were also surveyed about their knowledge of the guidelines, whether they had used them in their editorial assessments and whether they found them useful.

Although a number of manuscripts could not be traced to determine whether they were economic submissions, there appeared to be little difference between the two journals in numbers, quality, or editorial fate of the manuscripts. Therefore, the data were pooled. A total of 2982 manuscripts were submitted to the two journals during the "before" period, 105 (3.5%) of which were economic submissions. Of these, 27 (24.3%) were full economic evaluations and 78 (75.7%) were other economic submissions. Overall acceptance rate was 11.6% (12/105). During the "after" period, 2077 manuscripts were submitted to the two journals, 87 (4.2%) of which were economic submissions. Of these, 18 (20.7%) were full economic evaluations and 69 (79.3%) were other economic submissions. Overall acceptance rate was 6.9% (6/87). No change was found in comparing the two time periods, in the quality of submitted manuscripts, but *BMJ* editors found the guidelines and checklists useful and sent fewer economic submissions for external peer review in the "after" phase.

It was concluded that publication of the guidelines helped the *BMJ* editors improve the efficiency of the editorial process, but had no impact on the quality of papers submitted to, or published in, either journal.

Endorsement and adherence

The *BMJ* EE guidelines have not been adopted by any other journal and, as far as we are aware, no other journal has developed comparable guidelines for assessing the quality of economic submissions. Also, there is no evidence that editors in the *BMJ* have used the guidelines beyond the period shortly after their introduction. The other main set of guidelines developed by an academic group was those produced by the Public Health Services Panel on Cost-effectiveness in Health and Medicine in the United States [5]. These were widely cited and also published in *JAMA* (the *Journal of the American Medical Association*) in 1997 [6]. As far as we are aware, these guidelines were not officially adopted by any journal, although informally many economist researchers in the United States saw these as setting the standard that had to be met in making economic submissions to top journals such as the *JAMA*.

Over the past 10 years, the biggest growth has been in the development of guidelines for submission of economic data as part of the process for deciding on the reimbursement (i.e., public subsidy) of new pharmaceuticals and other technologies. About 30 jurisdictions around the world have developed such guidelines [7]. Specific examples are those developed by the Canadian Agency for Drugs and Technologies in Health in Canada [8] and the National Institute for Health and Clinical Excellence in the United Kingdom [9].

Cautions and limitations

The main criticism over the years has been that the *BMJ* guidelines can be viewed both as guidelines for methods and guidelines for reporting studies. (This confusion probably arose because of the extensive methodological discussion contained in the article that announced the guidelines.) Clearly, the guidelines are better suited to the second role. The other recurring comment has been that they have not been revised in keeping with the methodological advances in the intervening years.

Creators' preferred bits

We make our recommendations on the basis of our experience as authors and reviewers of health economic evaluations as well as editors of journals that publish health economic evaluations of the top three issues that could be used to improve reporting of health economic evaluations.
- *Disaggregation of treatment costs and cost-savings* The *BMJ* EE and many other documents emphasize the disaggregation of total costs and

quality-adjusted life-years (QALYs) when reporting results. However, it is still common for the focus of results and conclusions to be on the net total costs and QALYs. This can be particularly problematic in the economic evaluation in clinical trials where a conclusion might be that once all components of cost are taken into consideration, there is no significant cost difference between the treatment arms. This invites the potentially erroneous conclusion that the treatment arms are of equivalent cost – erroneous since this is an "absence of evidence is evidence of absence" interpretation. Particularly in the case where treatment costs under investigation are known with a high degree of certainty relative to other costs, we suggest that study treatment costs are presented separately from other costs. This is equivalent to asking two important questions: (1) Was there a difference in cost between treatments? (2) Was there any evidence of cost offsets associated with the higher cost treatment?

- *Comprehensive synthesis of the available clinical evidence* An economic evaluation is only as good as the clinical evidence on which it is based. There is a potential for bias if the economic study is based on only a subset of the available evidence. Therefore, it is important that reporting guidelines enable readers to be adequately informed about the literature searches conducted and the inclusion criteria for studies. In the case of economic evaluation, the range of relevant clinical studies often extends wider than controlled clinical trials and will include observational studies. Even when an economic evaluation is undertaken alongside a prospective clinical study, such as a randomized controlled trial, it will be important for the analyst to establish that the clinical results obtained in that study reflect the overall clinical literature [10].

  Also, it is frequently the case that there are no head-to-head clinical studies of the alternative treatments of interest. In these situations, it may be necessary for the analyst to conduct indirect or mixed treatment comparisons using Bayesian methods. This approach is often called Network Meta-analysis [11, 12]. Any new reporting framework should reflect this trend.

- *Adequate characterization of the uncertainty around estimates* Given the large number of estimates in an economic evaluation, it is inevitable that several of the parameter estimates will be subject to uncertainty. Since the publication of the *BMJ* EE, there has been considerable methodological advance in the ways that uncertainty can be characterized. In particular, many analysts favor the use of probabilistic sensitivity analysis, as this gives an overall summary assessment of the level of uncertainty in the parameter estimates, as opposed to simple sensitivity analysis, which usually assesses the impact of uncertainty in each parameter individually.[13] In addition, it has become common to present the results of economic evaluations in terms of cost-effectiveness acceptability curves or surfaces, which depict the probability of a given intervention being cost-effective at a particular threshold value, such as £30,000 per QALY [14]. Any update of reporting guidelines for economic evaluation should reflect these developments in how uncertainty is characterized and should be careful to distinguish such uncertainty from the natural heterogeneity in cost-effectiveness, which may be a function of patient characteristics, such as age, or characteristics of the condition, such as disease severity.

Future plans

There are no current plans to develop the *BMJ* EE guideline from the original 1996 version. The most recent attempt to specify reporting guidelines for economic evaluations is the CHEERS initiative from the International Society for Pharmacoeconomics and Outcomes Research (ISPOR) [3]. The acronym CHEERS refers to the Consolidated Health Economic Evaluation Reporting Standards developed by the Good Research Practices Task Force established by ISPOR. The Task Force comprised specialists in the economic evaluation of health care programmes and the editors of journals publishing cost-effectiveness studies of health care interventions. The reporting guidelines were developed through a process consistent with that of the CONSORT initiative for developing guidelines for the reporting of clinical trials [15]. The Task Force was inaugurated in 2011 and met several times over a 12-month period to draft a set of reporting guidelines, which was presented at the society's annual meeting in May 2012. Following a critical review by the membership, the Task Force Report was published by the Society's journal *Value in Health*, in 2013. Members of the *BMJ* editorial team participated in this effort.

References

1 Drummond, M.F. & Jefferson, T.O. (1996) Guidelines for the authors and peer reviewers of economic submissions to the BMJ. *BMJ*, **313**, 275.
2 Academy of Managed Care Pharmacy (2010) AMCP Format for Formulary Submissions (Version 3.0). *Journal of Managed Care Pharmacy*, **16** (1 Suppl.), S1–S29.
3 Husereau, D., Drummond, M.F., Petrou S. *et al.* (2013) Consolidated Health Economic Evaluation Reporting Standards (CHEERS): Explanation and Elaboration: A Report of the ISPOR Health Economic Evaluation Publication Guidelines Good Reporting Practices Task Force. *Value in Health*, **16**, 231–50.
4 Jefferson, T.O., Smith, R., Yi, Y. *et al.* (1998) Evaluating the BMJ guidelines on economic submissions – prospective audit of economic submissions to the BMJ and The Lancet. *JAMA*, **280** (3), 275–277.

 5 Gold, M.R., Siegel, J.E., Russell, L.B. & Weinstein, M.C. (eds) (1996) *Cost-Effectiveness in Health and Medicine*. Oxford University Press, New York.

 6 Weinstein, M.C., Siegel, J.E., Gold, M.R. *et al.* (1996) Recommendations of the panel on cost-effectiveness in health and medicine. *JAMA*, **276**, 1253–1258.

 7 International Society for Pharmacoenonomics and Outcomes Research. Pharma-coeconomic guidelines around the world. www.ispor.org/PEguidelines/index.asp [accessed on 30 July 2011].

 8 Canadian Agency for Drugs and Technologies in Health (2006) *Guidelines for the Economic Evaluation of Health Technologies*. Canada 3rd edn. CADTH, Ottawa.

 9 National Institute of Health and Clinical Excellence. (July 2008) *Guide to the Methods of Technology Appraisal*. NICE, London.

10 Sculpher, M.J., Claxton, K., Drummond, M.F. & McCabe, C. (2006) Whither trial-based economic evaluation for health care decision making? *Health Economics*, **15**, 677–687.

11 Jansen, J.P., Fleurence, R., Devine, B. *et al.* (2011 Jun) Interpreting indirect treatment comparisons and network meta-analysis for health-care decision making: report of the ISPOR Task Force on Indirect Treatment Comparisons Good Research Practices: part 1. *Value in Health*, **14** (4), 417–428.

12 Hoaglin, D.C., Hawkins, N., Jansen, J.P. *et al.* (2011) Conducting indirect-treatment-comparison and network-meta-analysis studies: report of the ISPOR Task Force on Indirect Treatment Comparisons Good Research Practices: part 2. *Value in Health*, **14** (4), 429–437.

13 Griffin, S., Claxton, K., Hawkins, N. & Sculpher, M.J. (2006) Probabilistic analysis and computationally expensive models: necessary and required? *Value in Health*, **9**, 244–252.

14 Barton, G.R., Briggs, A.H. & Fenwick, E.A.L. (2009) Optimal cost-effectiveness decisions: the role of the cost-effectiveness acceptability curve (CEAC), the cost-effectiveness acceptability frontier (CEAF), and the expected value of perfection information (EVPI). *Value in Health*, **11** (5), 886–897.

15 Moher, D., Schulz, K.F., Simera, I. & Altman, D.G. (2010) Guidance for Developers of Health Research Reporting Guidelines. *PLoS Medicine* **7** (2), e1000217.

PART IV

CHAPTER 29

Establishing a Coherent Reporting Guidelines Policy in Health Journals

Jason L. Roberts[1], Timothy T. Houle[2], Elizabeth W. Loder[3,4,5],
Donald B. Penzien[6], Dana P. Turner[2] and John F. Rothrock[7]

[1] *Headache Editorial Office, Plymouth, MA, USA*
[2] *Department of Anesthesiology, Wake Forest University School of Medicine, Winston-Salem, NC, USA*
[3] *Division of Headache and Pain, Department of Neurology, Brigham and Women's Hospital, Boston, MA, USA*
[4] *Harvard Medical School, Boston, MA, USA*
[5] *British Medical Journal, London, UK*
[6] *Department of Psychiatry, Wake Forest University School of Medicine, Winston-Salem, NC, USA*
[7] *Department of Neurology, University of Alabama at Birmingham, Birmingham, AL, USA*

Introduction

Some journals have endorsed CONSORT by simply suggesting in their Instructions for Authors that authors become familiar with the aims of that particular reporting guideline. Though this strategy is better than nothing and requires minimal effort on the part of a journal, it is more effective if journals adopt a coherent reporting standards policy.

However, journals have different needs and resources. Consequently, there is no standard application – each journal must determine what is appropriate for its circumstances and constituents. This chapter suggests the points that journals should consider in devising a reporting standards policy. It also considers the potential barriers to the successful implementation of such a policy.

The ideas presented in this chapter are drawn from our experience of launching a reporting guideline adherence policy at a mid-sized, international, medical journal: *Headache: the Journal of Head and Face Pain*.

Eight steps toward implementing a reporting standards policy

Step 1 – Identifying the needs of your journal
For a policy to be effective, it is critical that a journal first defines the scope of the problem and demonstrates how reporting guidelines can help resolve

Guidelines for Reporting Health Research: A User's Manual, First Edition. Edited by David Moher, Douglas G. Altman, Kenneth F. Schulz, Iveta Simera and Elizabeth Wager.
© 2014 John Wiley & Sons, Ltd. Published 2014 by John Wiley & Sons, Ltd.

issues of poor reporting standards. Measurable goals should also be set that can communicate the benefits of enforcing standards.

It is helpful to start by reviewing recent publications on reporting quality and adherence to guidelines such as CONSORT, PRISMA, and STROBE. The purpose of this review is to assess adherence and also to determine what reporting criteria are routinely missed. Such evidence should help the journal promote the benefits of adhering to reporting guidelines. Journals that are strict on adherence might even suggest that authors can improve their chances of publication by following the reporting guidelines.

Journals should also evaluate what other journals in their field are doing. If there has been little to no adoption of reporting guidelines, a journal will likely have to educate authors and reviewers about what the reporting guidelines are and how they should be used.

We also recommended consulting authors, reviewers, and members of the editorial board (if they are involved in decision making). Such discussion will enable a journal to shape its educational efforts better and become aware of the potential reactions to the proposed reporting standards policy.

Step 2 – Select "champions" to support and promote improving reporting standards

Working toward the launch of a reporting standards policy is generally time consuming and may be slow moving if approval from boards of directors, publishers, editorial boards, or publication committees is required. We recommend appointing a group of facilitators, or "champions," drawn from the editors, editorial office staff, and prominent thought-leaders within the field. Each group of champions would be expected to support the reporting policy and its passage through the approval process.

Editor facilitators

Editors involved with editorial decision making should be consulted at an early stage. In addition to critical input on the nature and scope of a reporting policy, the editorial board can discuss the methods for monitoring adherence to guidelines, such as incorporating a submitted reporting guideline checklist into a manuscript evaluation or using a cross-checking mechanism to ensure that a manuscript satisfies the intent of a reporting guideline.

Editorial staff

Staff can play a pivotal facilitator role. If a journal requires authors to upload a reporting guideline checklist, office staff will have to formulate a method for collecting completed checklists. This may involve online submission system reconfigurations where appropriate. Time and cost considerations, consequently, may become a factor. Editorial staff will also need to assess the effect this may have on their workload. If a mandatory policy is enforced, chasing errant authors will inevitably be required. Failure to consult with staff has the potential to lead to ill-conceived methods of enforcement that can tax workloads or lead to inconsistent application of standards as well as create scenarios that may frustrate submitting authors.

Thought leaders

Although evidence on the positive effects of reporting guidelines exists, authors likely will not be aware of this and quite possibly view the need to conform with reporting criteria (and perhaps complete a reporting checklist) as an unwelcome barrier to submission. To overcome this potentially negative perception, journals should consider involving high-profile individuals within a field to advocate the use of reporting guidelines. If thought-leaders and experienced writers recognize the need to consult reporting guidelines, then this could convince other authors of their need to do the same. Advocacy is not always "external" (i.e., educating and informing authors and reviewers) but also may be internal, convincing skeptics within a publishing house or society that positive outcomes are obtainable and that authors will not be driven away by demanding higher standards. The appointment of vocal champions, therefore, needs to take place not only after the implementation of a policy but also early in the policy development phase if an approval process needs to be completed.

Step 3 – Identifying appropriate checklists

As the goals for a reporting guideline policy are set, journals must then consider the extent of the policy. For example, will there only be a requirement for randomized controlled trials to adhere to CONSORT? Will there be additional guideline stipulations for diagnostic accuracy studies or systematic review articles? Should subject-specific adaptations of existing guidelines be considered? For example, *Headache* created an unofficial nonpharmacological, migraine-specific, adaptation of CONSORT. Editors must, therefore, select guidelines appropriate to the varieties of manuscripts submitted to their particular journal.

The EQUATOR Network website (www.equator-network.org) may be helpful in this task (see Chapter 6).

A study undertaken by the *Headache* editorial office in 2010 revealed that 63% of CONSORT-endorsing journals used more than one guideline-derived checklist. The other most commonly used guidelines were STARD (diagnostic accuracy), STROBE (observational studies in epidemiology), and MOOSE (for meta-analyses of observational studies in epidemiology). We recommend that journals take advantage of the variety of guidelines on offer and develop a policy that incorporates guidelines that fit the range of manuscript types submitted. Sometimes, this may even lead to the creation of a unique set of guidelines. At *Headache*, for example, a specific checklist for case reports was created.

Step 4 – Level of enforcement: mandatory use or recommended consultation of guidelines

With the intent and scope of a policy in place, journals must next consider the degree of enforcement. Requiring authors to complete a checklist compels them to redress omissions by forcing them to record the location of specific reporting criteria in their manuscript [1]. Checklists also enable editors and/or reviewers to quickly, and consistently, determine that at least the minimum reporting standards are met.

However, we appreciate that mandatory use of reporting guidelines is not an approach that will work for all journals. Staff time must be considered, as mandatory inclusion of a reporting guideline checklist may involve reconfiguring workflows, will require additional checking mechanisms, and potentially add delays to the peer review process if not properly thought out. Indeed, there are merits to the "recommendation approach" (i.e., "authors are strongly recommended … "). Most obviously, such an approach eliminates the possibility of author irritation. Table 29.1 includes a selection of questions to consider when determining which approach may best fit a journal.

Step 5 – Phased or complete launch of reporting policy

Journals may simply decide to construct a policy, flag its impending launch, and then implement it at a set date. However, as most journal editorial offices will attest, authors frequently demonstrate a lack of awareness of a particular publication's "author instructions." Consequently, imposition of a mandatory policy may cause disorientation for some authors. Editorial offices, therefore, need to be suitably prepared to assist.

Alternatively, journals may consider a phased approach. This potentially involves one of the following two strategies:

1 initial introduction of a single guideline, or
2 a phased launch with a simple *recommendation* to consult guidelines with the intent to move eventually toward a *mandatory* inclusion of a checklist with a submission. A phased approach allows authors to become familiar with new expectations, although this does assume that a journal regularly receives submissions from the same authors.

Step 6 – Reporting standards policy approval

Promoting good reporting may seem like a straightforward decision for a journal. Unfortunately, especially for smaller journals in a competitive publishing market, there may be perceived risks in adopting a reporting strategy. Such perceived threats are predicated on author intransigence to

Table 29.1 Issues to consider in developing a mandatory or consultative approach to using reporting guidelines.

Mandatory

Do the authors return a reporting checklist? If yes,
    Do authors upload the checklist with manuscript?
    Do authors return the completed checklist after manuscript submission?
How are checklists to be provided to authors?
    As part of the submission process (via the online submission system)
    As part of the Instructions for Authors
    As a link to sites where reporting checklists can be downloaded
    Embedded within the online Instructions for Authors
What are the administrative workflows for collecting forms?
Are reconfigurations to the online submission system required?
How is noncompliance policed (no checklist, wrong checklist, erroneously completed checklist)?
    Refuse to review the manuscript until the documentation is supplied?
    Ask for the submission of checklists with the submission of revision?
    Do nothing?
Who polices noncompliance?
    Editorial office staff
    Editor-in-chief
    Associate editors/editorial board (if applicable)
    Reviewers
How much effort will be required to chase noncompliant authors?
Are completed checklists to be made available to reviewers or just reviewed by the editorial
    team?
Strong recommendation for authors to consult guidelines
Should the submission of a checklist with the manuscript be encouraged?
Consider including notification of a policy recommending consultation of guidelines in the
    journal's Instructions for Authors
Consider including links to sites where checklists can be downloaded
Possibly include embedded versions of the checklists within the online Instructions for Authors?
Consider if the journal will assess for compliance with reporting guidelines
    If yes, how will you complete such an assessment?
    Who will assess for compliance?

---

applying extra effort or from having to take steps that may divulge previously concealed methodological flaws. Journal owners or publishers may express concern about taking steps that could repel authors toward journals with less stringent requirements.

Consequently, we recommend that journals should seek the formal support of its sponsoring society (at the Board of Directors/Governors level) or publisher before launching a reporting policy. Such official endorsement not only protects the editor from becoming a lightning rod for criticism, perhaps for "going too far," but also reinforces the policy as the official commitment of all parties to improve standards, especially in the face of complaints that efforts to accommodate improved reporting standards are burdensome.

Table 29.2 outlines some potential barriers to the launch and operation of a reporting guideline policy. These issues should be addressed or resolved before ratifying a standards policy.

Step 7 – Preparation for launch

Regardless of the type of reporting policy adopted, some simple steps can be taken ahead of launch that will boost the chances of successful implementation.

Table 29.2 Potential barriers to launching a reporting standards policy.

Barrier	Potential solution
Lack of awareness of reporting problem – unwillingness or no enthusiasm to consider a solution or take the problem seriously	Present evidence; numerous studies on the effect of reporting guidelines are available and have been highlighted by EQUATOR. Also, draw attention to the ability of reporting guidelines to provide greater transparency
Perception that applying reporting standards will be burdensome to authors – fear that authors will defect to other titles	Ensure any steps authors have to take are straightforward and meaningful; continually reinforce the benefits of reporting guidelines
Societies, publishers, and some editorial board members may fear being the first in the field to take action	Journals must consider if the potential advantages of being the first to apply standards outweigh the risks of being the first – for example, if a visible improvement in the quality of the manuscripts is evident, perhaps even measurable by an improved citation score, then the journal reacting first to the problem may then benefit by receiving better quality submissions over competing titles. Repetition of the benefits of reporting guidelines may be required
Most decision makers at the journal or society level are experienced authors who, perhaps with some justification, believe *they* suitably address reporting issues; consequently, the problem is overblown – this issue is compounded if the most vocal supporters of inertia are unfamiliar with the scale of unpublished manuscripts that still undergo peer review but are eventually rejected	Present evidence of the scale of the problem; perhaps undertake an analysis of a random sample of manuscripts
For mandatory enforcement policies that compel the use of a reporting guideline checklist, the checklist is perceived as an administrative task – some editors, society, or publisher decision makers may perceive the adoption of a checklist as excessive and advocate an approach that simply favors consultation	Outline how a reporting checklist can be utilized in the composition of a paper and subsequent evaluation by reviewers and editors. Reporting guidelines also apply consistency in reporting

The first step is to write an editorial scheduled to be published just ahead of the policy launch. Such an editorial should:

- outline the reasons for launching a reporting standards policy, detail known reporting problems, and describe the new standards expected;
- document evidence that shows the benefits of consulting reporting guideline checklists;
- explain what will be required from authors and any extra steps required at manuscript submission.

At the same time, the Instructions for Authors should be updated to reflect the new policy. Online submission and review systems may also need reconfiguring to accommodate the collection of a reporting guideline checklist. This can be done in consultation with the publisher or directly with the software system provider.

Second, the editorial office must ensure that editorial board members and reviewers are suitably trained to assess reporting checklists and/or determine if a manuscript appropriately adheres to a reporting guideline. For editorial board members, this might involve discussion at a team meeting. For reviewers, the provision of a short explanatory document, perhaps attached to the correspondence dispatched following acceptance to review a manuscript, should be considered.

Finally, we recommend that the editorial team devise short training courses to be delivered at scientific meetings, or as online courses perhaps featuring a PowerPoint presentation and the associated instruction sheets. Such courses, if resources permit, may be expanded with podcasts from the editor on why a policy is being introduced or even feature webinars around topics such as "best practices in submitting a manuscript" or "improving your chances of publication."

Step 8 – Launch

Unfortunately, unless a title is of significant size and visibility, many authors and reviewers will miss all the features mentioned in Step 7. It is critical, therefore, that a journal does not simply launch a policy and then wait passively for all parties to start adhering to new guidelines. As Table 29.3 outlines, for numerous reasons, most journals will experience a variety of challenges because of a combination of confusion, a lack of comprehension, and willful disregard, particularly if a title launches a mandatory adherence approach.

To ensure all the hard work in conceiving and preparing a policy is not undone, we recommend that journals continue with publicity efforts explaining the reporting policy. These might include writing: follow-up editorials, adding features in society newsletters, publishing positive author feedback and quotes from thought-leaders or including text in an annual "thank you" message to the recently submitting authors. Editorial

Table 29.3 Potential problems in the application of a reporting standards policy.

Barrier	Potential solution
Authors have no prior experience with reporting guidelines – uncertainty emerges leading to lots of questions or perhaps a decision by authors to submit elsewhere	Provide educational resources; ensure that editorial staff can address problems
Large number of authors with no prior record of submitting to a journal – unfamiliarity with journal guidelines leads to noncompliance; higher prevalence of authors simply "shopping around" their manuscript to any journal that will publish it	Provide clear instructions (both in the Instructions for Authors and within the online submission system); provide training resources and foster support where possible
Language barriers – authors cannot comprehend the reporting guidelines or submission instructions	Some guidelines are being translated into other languages; consider providing instructions in the languages of the most common author locations
Incomplete checklists – many forms require authors to specify on which page of the manuscript reporting criteria can be found, many leave blank when it is not appropriate to do so or answer "yes" or "no," which does not help an evaluation of reporting standards	If resources permit, journals should consider strong enforcement, especially if a new reporting standards policy is to have credibility. Otherwise, repeat authors will simply continue to perform the bare minimum or worse, just blatantly disregard the policy in future submissions
Authors complete the wrong checklist (either unintentionally or willfully) if they perceive that the checklist may mask deficiencies in their paper	Ensure consistent enforcement – request authors resupply the checklist, an approach that may best be conducted as part of a revision request, rather than at initial submission, only for the paper to quickly fail to progress through peer review
No application of reporting criteria to a manuscript, but checklist is carefully completed – experience has shown that some authors will fill out the reporting guideline checklist, but a cross-check against the manuscript finds no evidence of the presence of essential reporting criteria	Ensure consistent enforcement – request authors address the problem. Explain that the point of the reporting standards policy is not to complete a checklist, but to ensure that a manuscript suitably adopts higher standards of reporting
No application of reporting criteria to a manuscript, consultation is recommended, not mandated – if standards are not consistently or accurately evaluated; authors perceive they can make little or no effort toward applying higher standards and still get published	Continue to request reviewers and editors to be vigilant; remind authors of the benefits of reporting guidelines

Table 29.3 (*Continued*)

Barrier	Potential solution
Experienced authors believing that the rules do not apply to them	Ensure consistent enforcement no matter the seniority of the author; present evidence of inconsistent application of reporting standards; enlist the support of thought-leaders who can support a reporting standards policy
Inconsistent application of reporting standards by editors. Some manuscripts may be thoroughly vetted, others slip through peer review	Consistency is critical if reporting standards are to be taken seriously by authors. Ensure all editors are familiar with the reporting standards policy and that they agree to consistently applied standards. There should be consequences for ignoring or undermining a reporting standards policy, particularly if an editorial board or Associate Editors make recommendations regarding the suitability for publication

offices should consider reaching out to authors annually with a short training course at meetings.

Conclusion

The use of research reporting guidelines is becoming common, at least among the prestigious biomedical journals. The enforcement of standards at such journals is relatively straightforward, since authors are keen to publish under their imprimatur. However, for most other journals, challenges must be confronted. Most barriers to enforcing reporting guidelines can be mitigated with careful planning and clearly expressed intentions, supported by educational activities and continuous enforcement. To maintain the validity, or credibility, of the peer-reviewed scientific literature, it is critical that journals recognize they have the power to change the *status quo* and take the steps needed to ensure that reporting standards are followed. It is hoped that the steps described in this chapter will convince uncertain editors that the implementation of research reporting guidelines is not an insurmountable hurdle.

Reference

1 Hopewell, S., Altman, D.G., Moher, D. & Schulz, K.F. (2008) Endorsement of the CON-SORT statement by high impact factor medical journals: a survey of journal editors and journal "Instructions to Authors." *Trials*, **9**, 20.

Index

Note: "Figures are indicated by an italic f; tables are indicated by an italic t."

Guidelines for Reporting Health Research: A User's Manual, First Edition. Edited by David Moher,
Douglas G. Altman, Kenneth F. Schulz, Iveta Simera and Elizabeth Wager.
© 2014 John Wiley & Sons, Ltd. Published 2014 by John Wiley & Sons, Ltd.